"The theory underlying schema therapy offers a natural framework to understand arts and body-based therapies, and helps to apply these therapies to complex problems. This book offers a comprehensive overview of specific techniques for the different arts and body-based therapies as they can be used in the context of schema therapy. A must read for those that want to apply these techniques in a schema therapy program."

Prof. Dr Arnoud Arntz, *Faculty of Social and Behavioural Sciences, Programme Group Clinical Psychology, University of Amsterdam*

"This book presents a cogent and well-structured theoretical framework and practical guide, constituting a valuable handbook for educators and creative therapists alike. Particularly noteworthy are the unique insights it offers into engaging individuals with schema therapy through the lens of positive psychology. If you are engaged in the realm of creative arts therapies and have yet to read this book, I strongly encourage you to do so. Within its pages, you will encounter a compelling argument for exploring the advantages of utlising arts therapies, presenting powerful, playful, and poetic methods for fostering transformative and meaningful change."

Prof. Dr Dominik Havsteen-Franklin, *consultant in arts psychotherapies, professor of practice, Brunel University, London*

"Everyone will benefit from this practical guide to schema-focused working methods for arts and body-based therapies. Instructors will value the theoretical foundation grounded in expert and evidence-based information; practitioners will appreciate original intervention ideas; and students will benefit from both. Dr. Suzanne Haeyen has integrated her vast knowledge and that of other professionals into a comprehensive and accessible resource for anyone interested in a positive and growth-enhancing approach to expressive arts therapies."

Lisa D. Hinz, PhD, ATR-BC, *author,* Expressive Therapies Continuum: A Framework for Using Art in Therapy

Schema-Focused Working Methods for Arts and Body-Based Therapies

This book introduces schema-focused working methods for arts and body-based therapies, offering therapists practice-based tools to help their clients strengthen healthy patterns, self-management, and well-being on their path to recovery.

Containing 158 schema-focused working methods for different arts and body-based therapies, such as art therapy, dance therapy, drama therapy, music therapy, and body-based or psychomotor therapy, this book offers new ideas and tools for therapists to strengthen their client's adaptive schema modes: the Healthy Adult and the Happy Child. By linking arts and body-based therapies to schema-focused therapy and positive psychology, the goal is to strengthen the client's healthy patterns in emotion regulation and establish a healthier well-being.

The theoretical framework in the introduction and the scientific evidence for arts and psychomotor therapies, combined with practice-based examples, allow for a text that is broad enough for graduate creative therapy programs and specific enough to serve as a shelf reference for those in practice.

Suzanne Haeyen is professor of the research group Arts and Body-Based Therapies in Health Care at HAN University of Applied Sciences, the Netherlands. She is content coordinator for the master's program and art therapist at an expert center for personality problems. She has written several publications about arts therapies in personality disorders and has contributed to national multidisciplinary guidelines for the treatment of personality disorders.

Schema-Focused Working Methods for Arts and Body-Based Therapies

A Practical Guide

Edited by Suzanne Haeyen

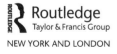
Routledge
Taylor & Francis Group

NEW YORK AND LONDON

Designed cover image: © Marieke Zwartenkot and Eugene Arts

First published 2024
by Routledge
605 Third Avenue, New York, NY 10158

and by Routledge
4 Park Square, Milton Park, Abingdon, Oxon, OX14 4RN

Routledge is an imprint of the Taylor & Francis Group, an informa business

ISBN: 9781032599588 (hbk)
ISBN: 9781032599571 (pbk)
ISBN: 9781003456988 (ebk)

DOI: 10.4324/9781003456988

Typeset in Times New Roman
by Deanta Global Publishing Services, Chennai, India

Contents

Foreword

As a clinical psychologist and schema therapist, I often find myself dealing with difficult situations in the therapeutic process. A particularly challenging experience was my introduction to group psychotherapy at a part-time treatment facility for people with a borderline personality disorder.

My colleagues and I did not manage the tension well, which resulted in participants running away, dissociating, or becoming angry. How did we eventually succeed in creating a safe environment? As psychologists and arts and body-based therapists, we began working closely together, determined to learn one another's "languages" and leverage our strengths to find new points of entry. Ultimately, we were so pleased with the results that we founded a joint institution for schema therapy.

This movement, which brings together schema therapists and arts and body-based therapists, is becoming increasingly widespread in the mental health system. On the one hand, in recent years arts and body-based therapies have—partly due to the growing body of scientific research—become an important form of therapy for people with personality disorders. On the other hand, the popularity of schema therapy is on the rise. This is an integrative form of psychotherapy inspired by diverse forms of therapy that give equal weight to thinking, feeling, and doing. Ever since its emergence, schema therapy has been applied in multidisciplinary settings in which arts and body-based therapies also play a role.

Recognizing the contribution made by arts and body-based therapists, the Dutch Register for Schema Therapy established a separate register for arts and body-based therapists: the Register for Schema-Therapeutic Practitioners. This is the only register of its kind in the world, giving arts and body-based (or psychomotor) therapists in the Netherlands a unique position within schema therapy.

Arts and body-based therapies have an important contribution to make to schema therapy. As a person-oriented therapy, schema therapy is about making contact, looking for a point of entry to connect with the client's emotional age and identify unmet basic needs, in order to restore some of what was missing in childhood. Because every therapy process is different, this calls for a great deal of creativity. One strength of arts and body-based therapies is the use of creative and body-oriented approaches to access a different, non-verbal, entry point. Another is the identification of opportunities for growth, which in turn benefits schema therapy when working with adaptive modes such as the Healthy Adult and the Happy Child.

In this book, experts in the fields of arts and body-based therapies and schema therapy describe the many ways in which you can connect with clients and meet their needs. It contains a rich collection of diverse working methods that focus on healthy behavioral patterns, self-management, and well-being. For arts and body-based therapists working with schema therapy, it offers a source of inspiration and creativity. It encourages mutual exchange between arts and body-based therapists and, by providing insight into the value of arts and body-based therapies, can foster collaboration with other mental health professionals, including psychologists and psychiatrists.

Rosi Reubsaet
Clinical psychologist, psychotherapist
Supervisor, Registered Schema Therapy, ISST, and VGCT
Co-founder and managing director, House for Schema Therapy
Co-founder, Academy of Schema Therapy

Prologue

Suzanne Haeyen, Greta Günther, and Anne-Marie Claassen

This book focuses on strengthening healthy patterns, self-management, well-being, and play through arts and body-based therapies, coupled with schema therapy and positive psychology.

Arts and body-based therapies encompass disciplines ranging from visual art, dance, drama, and music therapy to body-based or psychomotor therapy (PMT). It is an experiential form of therapy that involves recognizing one's own thought and behavioral patterns, effecting change, promoting mentalization, making healthy choices, and experiencing joy. Arts and body-based therapies are suitable for a broad target group, but particularly for those who are less verbally proficient or who cannot express their emotions well in words. In recent years, arts and body-based therapies have received increasing attention, including in scientific research. A number of evidence-based treatment protocols have been published and are in widespread use in the mental health system and private practice.

A large Dutch study on the effects of adverse childhood experiences (ACEs) on both cognition and the body recommended the use of arts and body-based therapies as entry points for treatment. As Marsman (2021, p. 148) writes, "In addition to including more body-oriented approaches, it is furthermore recommended to also include more expressive and non-verbal approaches, such as dance and movement therapy, (trauma-informed) yoga, visual art therapy, [and] drama therapy." Precisely those who experienced profound life events in childhood, she points out, often lack the verbal skills required to process trauma. Later in life, many develop personality disorders or chronic post-traumatic stress as a result of deficiencies in or traumatization of their basic childhood needs.

Arts and body-based therapies can thus make an important contribution to the observation and treatment of people with personality disorders and complex trauma. By offering experiences and eliciting or triggering emotions, thoughts, and behaviors, arts and body-based therapies can drive, perpetuate, or anchor the therapy process. Arts and body-based therapists are experts in experience-oriented work as well as direct and indirect intervention. When combined with other disciplines, arts and body-based therapies are often seen as complementary or alternative, but they can also stand alone.

Experience in mental health practice shows that arts and body-based therapies and schema therapy together form a fruitful combination (Claassen & Pol, 2015; Muste et al., 2009; Reubsaet, 2018). As suggested above, people with personality disorders or other psychological issues often do not benefit sufficiently from verbal cognitive therapy. In the event of reduced cognitive and mentalization capacities, an experiential approach may more easily pave the way for development.

Additionally, the combination of arts and body-based therapies and schema therapy may assist in identifying basic needs and values. Schema therapy offers a framework for working on stable and long-lasting personal themes involving memories, emotions, cognitions, and bodily sensations about the person himself or herself and in relation to others (Young et al., 2020). It aims to change the lens through which clients view their experiences, bringing about different perceptions and behaviors. Negative patterns, or *schemas*, are a way of assimilating negative experiences in childhood. They are created by the aforementioned deficiencies in or traumatization of a child's basic needs, such as forming secure attachments or feeling seen. In schema therapy, the term *mode* refers to a state of mind in the here and now.

Maladaptive modes prevent recovery, whereas functional modes lead to fulfillment of the basic needs required to achieve recovery and well-being. Treatment involves reducing the influence of maladaptive modes, such as the Demanding or Critical Parent, the Vulnerable or Angry Child, and strengthening the adaptive modes: the Healthy Adult and the Happy/Free Child. Schema therapy offers an experiential, playful, active, and creative approach, both direct and indirect, that has unique added value and complements arts and body-based therapies. Arts and body-based therapies, in turn, reinforce the adaptive modes. The act of doing, creating, and experiencing together in arts and body-based therapies is consistent with strengthening the Healthy Adult and Happy/Free Child modes in schema therapy.

In general, therapy tends to focus on problems, or what is not going well, rather than on clients' strengths or positive aspects. In recent years, treatment in the mental health sector has shifted from a purely symptom-oriented approach to a focus on well-being and psychological resilience. This trend can be linked to the rise of positive psychology, which assumes that optimal functioning involves not only minimizing a client's symptoms, but also identifying, appreciating, and developing opportunities, strengths, and sources of meaning (Bohlmeijer et al., 2021). Positive psychological interventions (PPIs) are increasingly applied directly and explicitly in treatments that focus on resilience and the client's capacity for recovery and well-being despite pain, discomfort, and stress. Instead of a symptom-oriented focus, they emphasize the use of adaptive strategies such as healthy patterns, self-management, reappraisal, and acceptance.

Such strategies have been found to be effective in altering feelings and reducing symptoms (Aldao et al., 2010).

In seeking to facilitate recovery or increase resilience by stimulating play, creativity, autonomy, and alternative behaviors, arts and body-based therapies fit seamlessly with the goals of positive psychology. Through its experiential nature, focus on the senses, and emphasis on doing and experiencing in the here and now, arts and body-based therapies can reinforce healthy patterns, self-management, and well-being.

Clients with personality disorders score relatively low on well-being. Given the severity of their problems, developing interventions focused on well-being targeted specifically at this group is of paramount importance. Research indicates that clients value arts and body-based therapies and view these as a suitable means of working toward this goal (Haeyen et al., 2018). The challenge for the future is to integrate therapeutic techniques in a manner that aids in the recovery of people with personality disorders. Therein lies the primary objective of this book, which aims to support and inspire arts and body-based therapists and other parties working with this target group.

Why this workbook and for whom?

In this book we link arts and body-based therapies to concepts from schema therapy and place them in the framework of positive psychology. Among arts and body-based therapists, there is a need for working methods based on arts and body-based therapies, schema therapy, and positive psychology, and clients also indicate a need for arts and body-based interventions focused on well-being (Haeyen, 2021). From this need, the idea for this book was born. First, this book is intended for arts and body-based therapists of the various disciplines, and it may also offer points of reference for adjacent disciplines.

This book describes a broad collection of *practice-based* working methods from the various arts and body-based therapies disciplines, collected from arts and body-based therapists with experience in combining arts and body-based therapies and schema therapy. These methods can be seen as *best practices* from arts and body-based therapies aimed at strengthening well-being and mental health. It provides an enriching addition to the experiential exercises described in the various books on schema therapy, but which fit more as working forms for a psychologist in the more cognitive-oriented model. Arts and body-based therapies deploy experiential techniques such as visual and play materials, instruments, and attributes combined with specific work forms, arrangements, or techniques based on creativity, fantasy, musicality, and movement within schema therapy precisely in order to work indirectly, through the material, on the treatment goals (Blokland-Vos et al., 2008; Günther et al., 2009; Haeyen, 2019).

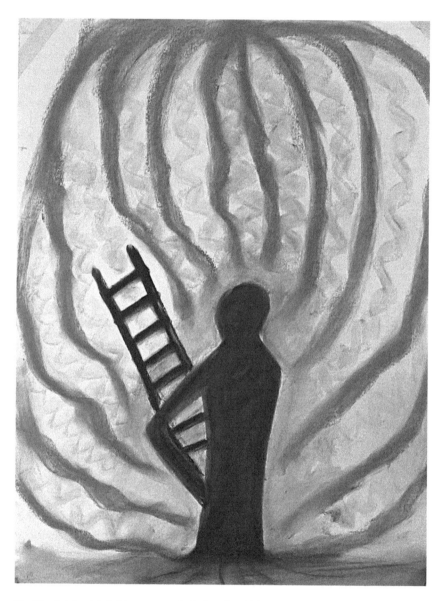

Healthy Adult with ladder as a symbol of real ambitions.

Working methods are often developed over years and therefore it is often no longer clear where exactly their origin lies, and that may not be important. After all, working methods evolve and take on new forms all the time. What is more important is that we collect, share, and thereby mix our expertise. All those who have been involved as authors of this book are listed in the Appendix with references to who provided which form of work. By recording these working methods, we stimulate professional exchange, both between the arts and body-based therapies disciplines and between arts and body-based therapies and the other disciplines. In this way, we contribute to the positive improvement and optimization of our professions for the benefit of our clients.

The working methods are experiential and directly focused on strengthening the healthy adaptive modes: the Healthy Adult and the Happy/Free Child modes. Experiential means process and experience, focusing on connecting and reconnecting with oneself and in relationship with others.

The choice to strengthen these healthy or functional modes comes from the growing realization that this is a pathway to recovery (e.g., Phagoe et al., 2022; Versluis et al., *in process*). Part of this is what one experiences in contact with the therapist. This means dwelling on experiences in the here and now and learning to better feel and express thoughts, obstacles, sadness, and anger. Feeling, doing, and thinking are central. It is about developing awareness and body consciousness. In the basic stance, the therapist must be mindful that the Healthy Adult and the Happy/Free Child receive enough attention (e.g., Yakin et al., 2020) because these modes provide the entry point to contact with the basic needs as described in schema therapy.

The experiential approach is existential and experimental. Experiential work means that it is not only about insight: change can only take place by experiencing, living through, and feeling through that which is going on, which explicitly includes the body. Existential because it is about existence itself, as one is and not as one should or could be. And experimental because exercises are used in which new behavior can be tried out.

Within schema therapy as well as within arts and body-based therapies, experiencing is used as a change mechanism. Young and colleagues (2020) add the experiential channel to the usual change channels of behavior and (conscious, verbal) cognition. These techniques are often applied to experiences we went through as children (e.g., being loved or not being loved) that contributed to a schema about ourselves. For many clients, the corrective experience of being loved is a more important contributor to change than logically exploring the tenability of the idea of being unloved (Arntz, 2016).

In the most recent book on schema therapy, the approach of *assimilative integration* of the typical schema therapy techniques such as the chair technique and imagination exercises has been chosen (Heath & Startup, 2020). In addition to the focus on therapeutic relationship, these are the earmarked experiential working methods in schema therapy. In the book edited by Heath and Startup, there is also more explicit attention paid to play and the Healthy Adult.

This book, *Schema-Focused Working Methods for Arts and Body-Based Therapies: A Practical Guide* is in line with a trend that has started when it comes to renewing the supply for schema-focused interventions. By describing interventions, we are also taking a step toward descriptions of more comprehensive practices or modules and, in time, contributing to research on these interventions and practices/modules. In general, it can be stated that there is a widely supported need for further substantiation of arts and body-based therapies, and within this, also for research aimed at methodology development, intervention description, research into mechanisms of action, and effect research, as shown in several reports and research agendas (Borgesius & Visser, 2015; Federation Arts and Body-Based Professions [FVB], 2017; MIND, 2020; P3NL, 2019).

Required basic knowledge

Within therapygenerally, certain basic rules are agreed upon together, and this is no different in arts and body-based therapies. In addition, the same specific basic rules largely apply within the various arts and body-based therapies. In arts and body-based therapies, the explicit rule with regard to safety is that one does not harm each other, oneself, or the materials. It also requires a respectful way of dealing with everyone's own way of expression. Safeguarding safety is linked to the use of appropriate expertise. Performing the working methods in this book requires this knowledge.

Arts and body-based therapists have the skills and knowledge to apply these methods responsibly and attune them to the individual possibilities, to the needs of the group and the group dynamics, and to current situations that arise. They are trained in offering accessible and inviting working methods and in being able to intervene during the process of implementation.

They can do this by using non-verbal interventions and directing the process in this way, for example, by offering materials, changing something in the working method, or by mirroring or challenging behavior during play, even when unexpected things occur. It is precisely these unexpected issues that often require adjustment or readjustment so that it is still possible to work constructively on the goals set. A basic knowledge of schema therapy and the language used is assumed.

There are many possible and necessary variations of each working method. Not all of these are described. It is up to the arts and body-based therapist to shape and apply them correctly so that they can be therapeutically correct and healing.

Depending on the client(s), it is not always necessary to discuss everything (in schema therapy language). The experience itself has an effect in itself. Verbal explication and awareness can be helpful and necessary. Reflection and evaluation can also be done in a non-verbal, experiential way.

Psychologists and other disciplines can also draw inspiration from this book. They may use the working methods as experiential techniques from a more cognitive approach (*top-down*) where arts and body-based therapists use the experiential approach more (*bottom-up*). This book offers them direct interventions to strengthen the adaptive modes.

Reading guide

Following the introduction with a description of the background framework and theory, Chapters 2 through 6 contain a wide range of working methods. Each chapter focuses on a different discipline. The aim has been an equal distribution of the number of working methods per discipline. Nevertheless, this reflects the relationship between the disciplines in the professional field and education; after all, some disciplines are more widely represented in the professional field than others.

The working methods are always based on or linked to schema therapy and zoom in on strengthening the adaptive modes, namely the Healthy Adult and the Happy/Free Child. Each working method is also indicated to which healthy ego function it connects. The overview of working methods in this book hopefully offers (arts and body-based) therapists new ideas, recognition, and the necessary tools. It may also be interesting to look at the methods used by other arts and body-based disciplines and, where possible, translate them to your own discipline.

Chapter 7 provides an up-to-date overview of the scientific rationale for arts and body-based therapies in the treatment of personality disorders.

Word of thanks

This book was created thanks to 35 co-authors who were willing to share their expert knowledge. For which, many thanks! Their names and background information can be found in the "About the editor and authors" section at the end of the book. Thanks to this fruitful collaboration, this book has grown into what it is today, and we can be proud of that! Thanks also to all the clients who gave permission to use photos of their work, to those who appear in the photos, and to the therapists/photographers who took the photos.

Everyone's contributions have made this such a rich collection! Hopefully, this book will provide inspiration for all who read and use it!

Chapter 1

Introduction

*Suzanne Haeyen, Greta Günther, and
Anne-Marie Claassen*

Summary

This chapter discusses arts and body-based therapies, why they are used in the treatment of personality disorders, and how they work. The goals of arts and body-based therapies include changing behavior patterns, learning healthy coping strategies, improving interaction with the self and others, finding healthy ways to relax, and being able to regulate emotions, stress, and impulses. These goals align well with the potential of arts and body-based therapies. In this chapter, we make the connection between the window of tolerance, well-being, positive psychology, schema therapy, and arts and body-based therapies, based on the belief that recovery for people diagnosed with personality disorders is about more than reducing symptoms. Personal and social growth, leading to improved well-being, is at least as valuable. Arts and body-based therapists use interventions aimed at enhancing well-being in addition to those designed to reduce symptoms. We describe the role of arts and body-based therapies in strengthening adaptive skills, creating healthy ego functions, and generating positive emotions.

1.1 Introduction to arts and body-based therapies

The various arts and body-based therapies work experientially through arts and body-based media, such as visual art, music, drama, play, movement, and physicality. They all have an experiential, action-oriented, and creative quality and make systematic, planned, and purposeful use, in a more or less structured way, of various working methods, materials, instruments, and props. The aim is to deploy these methods in the most scientifically rigorous way possible.

In arts and body-based therapies, feelings, thoughts, and patterns of behavior emerge through design, play, physical sensation, or movement. These offer a starting point for awareness and (self-)reflection. This occurs through observation, contact with others, impulse and emotion regulation, addressing patterns in feeling, thinking, and acting, gaining insight, experiencing, and practicing

DOI: 10.4324/9781003456988-1

different behaviors, roles, and skills (Akwa GGZ, 2019; American Art Therapy Association, 2021; British Association of Art Therapists, 2021; FVB, 2017; National Steering Committee on Multidisciplinary Guideline Development in Mental Health Care, 2008). Arts and body-based therapies work from sensing, doing, and experiencing, in the here and now. The arts and body-based therapist deploys the media methodically, in accordance with the client's personal goals.

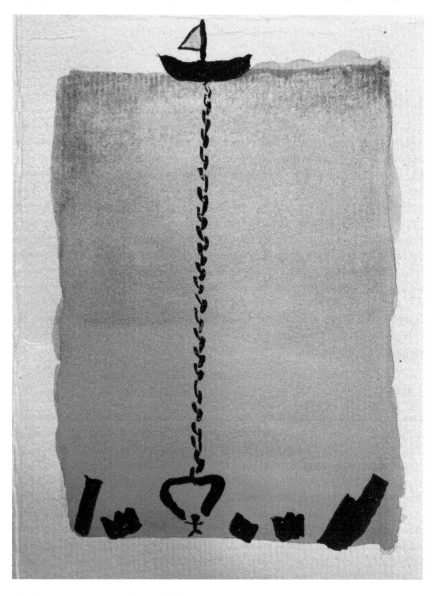

The therapy process as depicted by Wendy, age 37.

On the one hand, arts and body-based therapies are symptom based: they are aimed at eliminating, reducing, or coming to terms with problems, and preventing a relapse or new symptoms. On the other hand, the goal of arts and body-based therapies is to develop the client's well-being, adaptive skills, and personal growth (FVB, 2017; Haeyen et al., 2018). Arts and body-based therapies can aid recovery and improve resilience by encouraging play, creativity, and autonomy, and by promoting alternative behaviors.

Arts and body-based therapies are used in the treatment of personality disorders, where their experiential, action-oriented, and creative qualities offer ways of enhancing well-being. They can be part of a multidisciplinary psychotherapeutic or social psychiatric treatment strategy or used as a stand-alone treatment through private practice (Akwa GGZ, 2017; LOO VTB, 2016).

The problems faced by people diagnosed with personality disorders align well with the therapeutic mechanisms of arts and body-based therapies. The treatment goals of these clients often include:

- changing patterns of behavior;
- learning healthy coping strategies;
- improving interaction with the self and others;
- finding healthy ways to relax; and
- being able to regulate emotions, stress, and impulses.

Coping is often rigid in its persistent repetition, but is, at the same time, fluid and changeable. The more creative and intelligent clients are, the more easily they are able to let go of one coping mechanism and replace it with another. It is important to raise awareness and mirror coping; however in order to let go, clients first need a healthy alternative, preferably one that is grounded in a physical experience or memory. Arts and body-based therapies are valuable because they focus more on the nonverbal, on experiencing and doing, than treatments such as psychotherapy, which rely on verbal communication (Bruscia, 2012; Haeyen, 2018a, 2018b; Hulshof et al., 2009; Muste et al., 2009; Van Vreeswijk et al., 2008). This fits the statement of Van der Kolk (2014): "Trauma comes back as a reaction, not a memory."

1.2 Personality disorders and emotion regulation problems

Personality disorders are long-standing, rigid problems (e.g., Livesley et al., 2016) that can lead to severe personal suffering, with negative consequences for personal and professional relationships. People with personality disorders tend to have problems with self-image (identity), self-management (impulsivity, maintaining appropriate boundaries, and achieving personal goals), and/or interpersonal relationships (connectedness with others and intimacy) (American Psychiatric Association [APA], 2014; Haeyen, 2020). Personality disorders are divided into three clusters: Cluster A (the "odd, eccentric" cluster); Cluster B (the "dramatic, emotional, erratic" cluster); and Cluster C (the "anxious, fearful" cluster). They may struggle to regulate their behavior, thoughts, and feelings, and may exhibit (self-)destructive behaviors, including suicidal thoughts, negative or distorted perceptions, and affective dysregulation. Their stress levels rise regularly and intensely but decrease only slowly, and their baseline stress level is usually high (Cluster B). On the other hand, when anxiety and detachment predominate, people may not experience enough stress (Cluster C).

The *window of tolerance* (see Figure 1.1) developed by Siegel (1999) is a useful concept to this end. The window of tolerance is the optimal zone of "arousal" within which people are able to regulate their emotions, learn from new, potentially disruptive experiences, and engage in flexible thinking. As long as their arousal levels remain within this window, they can be considered to be functioning well, and personal development is possible. This is a precondition for the optimal processing of corrective emotional experiences. On the other hand, when stress levels are too high or a challenge takes too long to overcome, the autonomic nervous system takes over. The person is flung outside their window of tolerance and enters a "survival mode." This happens more commonly in children when an adult is not present to help calm them down. If an experience causes an overwhelming sense of fear, helplessness, or agony, the child may become traumatized. Severe or prolonged exposure to stress—especially at a young age—can result in lifelong disruptions to the stress response system.

People with Cluster B personality disorders often experience extreme stress, or hyperarousal. This might trigger a fight, flight, or freeze response, or cause irritation, anger, or panic. Those with a Cluster C personality disorder may have an avoidant or detached attitude, and as a result will sometimes enter a state of hypoarousal, causing them to shut down or feel unmoved, numb, listless,

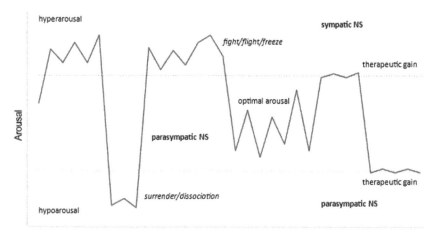

Figure 1.1 Window of tolerance (Siegel, 1999; Ogden et al., 2006) and the sympatic and parasympathic nervous system (NS).

dissociated, or absent. To benefit from therapy and be receptive to personal development, it is important that the stress level is within the window of tolerance, meaning that a person is capable of connecting with the environment and reflecting in a relatively relaxed manner.

People whose stress response system has been derailed by trauma or neglect have a narrow window of tolerance and can be triggered quickly. The therapy goal here is to broaden the window of tolerance, giving the Healthy Adult sufficient resilience to adapt to changeable and challenging circumstances.

How do coping modes relate to the window of tolerance theory? Although coping also involves fight, flight, or freeze responses, not every coping mode requires someone to be outside their optimal arousal zone. Therefore, coping is mirrored, empathic confrontations are performed, and the client is challenged to reduce the use of coping modes. Through these interventions, the therapist seeks the limits of the tolerance zone, where therapeutic gains can be made. However, a strong coping mode can conceal the boundary between the optimal zone and a state of hyper- or hypoarousal, so that the client's emotional state is not always apparent to the therapist. To aid in recognizing this, Ogden (2006) put forth the principle of the constant monitoring of body responses.

We introduce Siegel's theory here to demonstrate that sometimes people manage to stay within their window of tolerance only by sustaining their coping modes. Under such circumstances, confronting problems verbally can lead to more stress or detachment, and less exploration. Arts and body-based therapies, on the other hand, introduce alternative, helpful means of coping while working with triggers, exposure, and rescripting to ensure the necessary regulation within the working method. These tools are described in more detail below.

1.2.1 The importance of well-being

In recent years, there has been a clear trend within the mental health system for treatment to be not only symptom based, but also focused on improving well-being and strengthening mental health. Restoring people's ability to respond and adapt to life's social, psychological, and physical challenges can allow them to regain their physical and psychological/spiritual well-being and is important for living a full and meaningful life (Akwa GGZ, 2017).

This trend can be linked to progress in positive psychology, which assumes that helping people achieve their optimal functioning lies not only in minimizing their symptoms but also in discovering and nurturing their potential, strengths, and sources of fulfillment (Bohlmeijer et al., 2021). The founders of this theory (Seligman & Csíkszentmihályi, 2000) identify three pillars of study within positive psychology:

- positive experiences, such as happiness, hope, and love;
- positive traits, such as vitality, perseverance, and wisdom; and
- positive institutions, or ways in which institutions can have a positive impact on society.

Bohlmeijer (2021) describes well-being as consisting of two main components: feeling positive (life happiness and satisfaction) and being able to adapt positively to situations and life circumstances (adaptive skills and positive relationships). Both components align with various elements of the *Diagnostic and Statistical Manual of Mental Disorders, Fifth Edition* (DSM-5) levels of personality functioning (APA, 2014), and both can be linked to the Healthy Adult and the Happy/Free Child modes in schema therapy.

People with personality problems often want/need to work on identity, self-management, empathy, compassion, and intimacy. These areas are affected by a deficit in well-being, in terms of both (a lack of) positive experiences and/or positive traits. For example, well-being as it pertains to identity may consist of a certain degree of self-confidence and feeling good about oneself. As it relates to self-management, well-being may involve the ability to adapt to challenging circumstances.

Positive psychological interventions (PPIs) focus on building resilience and improving well-being using adaptive strategies, helping to develop clients' ability to deal with situations that cause pain, discomfort, and stress, and aiding recovery. Adaptive strategies include reappraisal and acceptance, which have been found to increase positive affect and reduce the clinical symptoms associated with personality disorders (Aldao et al., 2010).

According to the World Health Organization (2022), mental health involves the absence of psychological disorders and the presence of a state of well-being. Well-being is the degree to which a person feels good physically, psychologically, and socially, and consists of both feeling positive (life happiness and satisfaction) and having positive experiences (doing things that are meaningful, having positive relationships, and experiencing personal growth). Research shows that people with high levels of well-being—people who are said to be flourishing—are more creative, connected, and resilient. High levels of well-being are also associated with greater productivity, less absenteeism, lower sickness costs, and better physical health, resulting in longer life spans.

Well-being can protect against and promote recovery from psychological illness (Bohlmeijer et al., 2021). However, Keyes (2002) found that although psychological symptoms and well-being are related, they are independent. This is called the "two continua model." A person may have psychological symptoms yet score highly on well-being. Alternatively, they may have no symptoms yet score low on well-being. As artist Frida Kahlo stated: "In spite of my long illness, I feel immense joy in LIVING." To put this in schema-therapy terms: someone can function well by relying on maladaptive coping strategies but be unhappy because they do not experience the positive feelings that enable them to access the Happy/Free Child mode, or they may experience happiness and be in the Free Child mode but still have underlying psychological problems. Indeed, Wolterink and Westerhof (2018) showed that coping modes were not correlated with the presence of psychological symptoms, though increases in the strength of functional modes achieved through treatment were significantly associated with improved well-being and a reduction in symptoms.

Generally, however, people with personality disorders score significantly low on well-being (Franken et al., 2018) and commonly experience a wide range of psychological and physical problems, which severely impact their quality of life.

Psychological symptoms can be less problematic if people know how to deal with them in a way that allows them to reach their desired level of well-being. As such, it is important for a therapist to understand a client's idea of well-being. Instead of fixating on reducing a client's coping or parenting modes, schema therapists should focus explicitly on strengthening their ability to access the Healthy Adult and Happy/Free Child modes.

Even after symptom-reducing treatment, people diagnosed with personality disorders often face challenges in handling stress and dealing with the personal and professional issues of everyday life (Ng et al., 2016; Wolterink & Westerhof, 2018). Recovery for clients with personality disorders is thus about more than the mere elimination of symptoms; personal and social recovery is at least equally valuable, and they see arts and body-based therapies as a suitable means of achieving it. Research has shown that arts and body-based therapies are widely appreciated by clients (e.g., Haeyen et al., 2020; Karterud & Pedersen, 2004; Kehr, 2020; Solli et al., 2013). In practice, arts and body-based therapists highlight the importance of developing specific interventions aimed at improving well-being in addition to reducing psychological symptoms and indicate that this falls within the power of arts and body-based therapies.

1.2.2 Schema therapy and positive psychology: A development

Schema therapy, an integrative form of psychotherapy, is internationally recognized as a form of treatment for personality disorders (e.g., Bamelis et al., 2017). Derived from cognitive behavioral therapy (CBT) by Jeffrey Young, schema therapy emphasizes experiential interventions, making arts and body-based therapies a good fit. An evidence-based treatment, it is recommended as a first-line intervention in the Dutch protocol for the treatment of personality disorders (Akwa GGZ, 2017). Schema therapy is commonly used in treatment centers specializing in personality disorders, with arts and body-based therapies often forming part of the approach.

Core components of schema therapy are reducing the incidence of dysfunctional patterns (schemas and modes) and developing the Healthy Adult mode. A schema is a lens through which a person views the world, themself, and their relationships with others, based on early childhood experiences that resulted in specific patterns of thinking, feeling, and doing. Schema therapy aims to break down maladaptive schemas and strengthen adaptive schemas (the Healthy Adult and the Happy/Free Child) (Arntz & Jacob, 2012). Due to their concrete, experiential, and mentalization-based nature, arts and body-based therapies can serve as tangible tools for the operationalization of the somewhat abstract schema terminology (Claassen & Pol, 2015), and are often considered a booster, accelerator, or continuation of the psychotherapeutic process (Akwa GGZ, 2017).

Applying the principle from positive psychology that "everything you pay attention to grows" to schema therapy, the amount of attention paid to describing dysfunctional patterns may be surprising: 18 maladaptive schemas and a large number of maladaptive modes have been identified. Even "schema" and "coping mode," which were originally neutral, descriptive concepts derived from cognitive therapy, are now primarily used to refer to dysfunctional schemas and coping modes. In contrast, there are only two "functional" modes: the Healthy Adult and the Happy/Free Child.

In recent years, however, there has been a specific trend toward strengthening the functional schemas and promoting well-being. The 2015 book *Schema Therapy and the Healthy Adult: Positive Techniques from Practice* includes chapters on therapies from different disciplines (Claassen & Pol, 2015). A questionnaire that measures positive adaptive schemas has been developed (Louis et al., 2017) and validated for use with the elderly population (Videler et al., 2017). This Young Positive Schema Questionnaire (YPSQ) will also be validated for use among the adult population in the future. In addition, research on adaptive schemas focuses on positive or adaptive *reparenting* (Louis et al., 2020), or the incorporation of elements from positive psychology, such as mindfulness (Bernstein, 2020) and acceptance and commitment therapy (Roediger et al., 2018). The course Schema Therapy and the Healthy Adult, developed by Claassen & Broersen (2019), consists of ten sessions designed to aid participants in working toward the Healthy Adult.

The Healthy Adult is defined as an integrated self (Claassen & Pol, 2015) with the capacity to meet one's own needs as an independent, responsible person. Together with the Free/Happy Child—the second of the two healthy modes in schema therapy—it represents the healthy, adaptive behaviors that clients learn to access to improve their own well-being (and the well-being of others; after all, the Healthy Adult is attentive to others' needs). In schema therapy, clients learn to behave as the Healthy Adult by taking care of their own basic needs and practicing autonomy, self-management, mindfulness, and self-compassion (Claassen & Pol, 2015), in line with the healthy ego functions described later in this chapter. The Healthy Adult is thus considered an "integrated" person, not only as a mode but also as a human being (Claassen & Pol, 2014).

In short, the use of techniques focused on strengthening positive schemas can reduce symptoms associated with personality disorders (Versluis et al., 2022). Other research shows that paying specific attention to the Healthy Adult and the Vulnerable Child can also reduce symptoms (Yakin et al., 2020). All in all, there is a growing trend in schema therapy to engage with positive psychology and to employ treatment that focuses on strengthening adaptive skills and positive emotions as well as reducing the incidence of dysfunctional patterns. The approach taken in this book is that treatment should be designed based on an individual's basic needs.

1.2.3 Basic needs and the link to well-being

When we look at the origins of personality disorders, we see a clear link to deficits in universal basic needs as described in schema therapy. Basic needs are those considered essential for children to grow into healthy, mature, and functional adults and include:

- a secure attachment to others;
- autonomy, competence, and a sense of identity;
- realistic limits and self-control;
- freedom to express valid needs and feelings;
- spontaneity and play.

A working group established in 2021 with the goal of generating greater scientific support for schema therapy proposed two additional needs: the need for self-coherence and the need for fairness (Arntz et al., 2021). The basic needs align with the areas in which personality disorders most commonly arise as described in the DSM-5, namely identity, self-management, empathy, compassion, and intimacy. The degree to which a particular aspect is needed depends on a child's temperament. For example, an inhibited child will need more encouragement, while a temperamental and stimulus-oriented child may require stronger boundaries.

People with personality disorders have not learned to attend adequately to their basic needs. Due to severe neglect or trauma, they have adopted maladaptive coping modes and schemas as defense mechanisms. In schema therapy, clients regain insight into their own basic needs and those of others and learn how to start living rather than merely surviving.

1.2.4 Emotion regulation in schema therapy

One important issue for people with personality disorders is, as mentioned above, the regulation of emotions. A transdiagnostic concept, emotion regulation refers to our ability to respond to ourselves, others, and situations in a functional way (Dadomo et al., 2018). In schema therapy, problems with emotion regulation are seen as a consequence of negative early childhood experiences, such as insecure attachment, abuse, or neglect (Fassbinder et al., 2016). Unprocessed negative experiences can lead to the avoidance of, a heightened state of anxiety about, or the passive acceptance of situations in which those emotions resurface (Dadomo et al., 2018). This results in unhelpful core assumptions and, from there, early maladaptive schemas (EMS).

The different schema modes stem from different (unmet) emotional needs. A mode can be thought of as an intense emotional state involving patterns of needs, thoughts, and feelings (schemas). Each mode is associated with specific (dys)functional emotions and (dys)regulatory strategies (Dadomo et al., 2018). Modes are changeable and can be activated by both internal and external stimuli (Van Vreeswijk et al., 2012).

Child modes involve emotions such as fear, shame, sadness, or anger that went unaddressed in childhood. Dysfunctional coping modes may provide temporary stress relief but, in the long term, perpetuate dysregulated emotional states. Dysfunctional parental modes, such as the Critical or Demanding Parent, give rise to problems in emotion regulation due to incessant critical thoughts.

The Healthy Adult, on the other hand, can regulate their emotions through self-acceptance and self-restoration, and access the Happy Child mode, where they can play freely and experience positive emotions (Dadomo et al., 2018). As mentioned, the goal of schema therapy is to strengthen the Healthy Adult and Happy Child modes while reducing dysfunctional modes. Possessing healthy ego functions, as described by Arntz and Jacob (2012), means that a person is in a position to make healthy choices designed to maintain or improve their own and others' well-being. Arntz and Jacob (2012) and Young and colleagues (2003) identify several interventions through which this goal can be achieved, such as reparenting and experiential techniques.

The therapeutic context is essential here (Fassbinder et al., 2016; Heath & Startup, 2020). So too is building a good case conceptualization (see Figure 1.2). Different types of case conceptualizations are possible (Hornsveld et al., 2021); we choose a model that places the Healthy Adult at the center and identifies the tasks related to the dysfunctional modes and the child modes. This gives a powerful image of and direction to therapy. The box at the bottom also supports

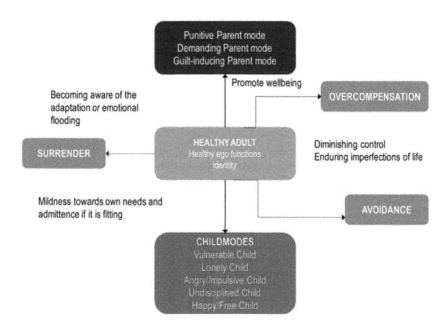

Figure 1.2 Case conceptualization: modes and coping strategies.

emotional integration when depicted as a single inner child, who can be angry, scared, hurt, or happy.

In schema therapy, the therapeutic relationship is deliberately transparent. In limited reparenting, a therapist essentially assumes the role of a parent, helping to explore needs that were frustrated in a client's childhood (Fassbinder et al., 2016). The therapist provides support, warmth, empathy, and security, in contrast to the maladaptive schemas commonly adopted by the client. The therapeutic relationship becomes a safe base from which clients can learn emotion regulation through "modeling techniques," in which clients follow their therapists' method of emotion regulation (Dadomo et al., 2018).

This process is based on creating secure attachments, which are necessary for the healthy functioning and strengthening of the Healthy Adult mode. Through empathetic confrontations, dysfunctional coping modes employed by clients are challenged. This involves identifying the cause of the maladaptive coping mode and acknowledging that, while these strategies may have served as defense mechanisms in the past, they are no longer helpful and are, in fact, hindering personal development (Fassbinder et al., 2016).

1.2.5 Adaptive modes and healthy ego functions

The Healthy Adult uses their psychological capacities to unlearn destructive patterns in order to satisfy their basic emotional needs as an independent, responsible, and well-functioning person with a positive connection to themself and their environment (Claassen & Pol, 2014). In schema therapy, clients follow the example of Healthy Adult mode set by their therapist to combat dysfunctional schemas and inspire healthy behaviors (Young et al., 2020).

The Healthy Adult is characterized by their ability to make realistic assessments of situations, conflicts, and relationships, honor commitments, perform tasks, fulfill duties, seek pleasure, and satisfy their needs in a mature manner. They are able to think about themselves and others in positive and nuanced ways and, as a result, build healthy relationships and engage in healthy activities. The Healthy Adult is disciplined, responsible, empathetic, and compassionate toward themself and others. The Healthy Adult—and consequently the Happy/ Free Child—arises by meeting the basic needs of the Vulnerable Child.

The duties of the Healthy Adult vis-à-vis the other modes serve as the guiding principles, including toward the Happy Child, because they cannot do without the Healthy Adult either. The Healthy Adult reduces the use of dysfunctional coping modes, such as the Self-Aggrandizer, the Compliant Surrenderer, or the Perfectionistic Overcontroller, and in some cases renders them redundant. The Healthy Adult teaches the Undisciplined Child discipline, thus disaffirming the Punitive or Demanding Parent modes. They offer comfort, support, acknowledgment, and hope to the Vulnerable Child, and acknowledgment and boundaries to the Angry Child. In therapeutic terms, this means establishing the basic needs required by the Vulnerable Child, and from there building on functional coping and parenting modes until the client attains the Healthy Adult mode and the therapist becomes redundant.

From a trauma perspective, it is also important to take into account that persistent parental modes occasionally serve a coping function, and there may be idealization of or identification with the perpetrator (Claassen, 2017). In this case, the parental mode is perceived as the only available friend, and the client has difficulty letting go of it. The Healthy Adult can assess this situation, choose the least harmful option, and respond in a less judgmental way to the coping strategy that was sorely needed.

> *When emotions overwhelm me and I consciously deploy a coping strategy, I actually consider that quite healthy adult behavior on my part.*

By designating maladaptive modes and schemas as survival mechanisms linked to negative experiences in childhood, clients can start to recognize the protective nature of dysfunctional behaviors. They may then be able to view themselves with greater compassion and develop the confidence to relearn how to deal with their emotions. This can be facilitated by a warm, authentic, and empathetic therapeutic relationship, which can restore clients' trust in the social world as a learning environment (epistemic trust) and erode mistrust (Fonagy & Allison, 2014; Knapen, 2017).

The Healthy Adult is able to make healthy choices in pursuit of well-being for him/herself and others. To this end, a person has six "healthy ego functions" (Haeyen, 2019):

- personality integration and formation of self-image;
- healthy emotion regulation;
- contact with one's own emotions/needs and those of others;
- healthy internal dialogue;
- testing reality and assessing situations, conflicts, and relationships; and
- seeking enjoyment and fulfillment in a mature manner.

As clients become more able to meet their basic emotional needs, they improve their emotion regulation, learn to better manage their internal dialogue, and develop self-compassion. These competencies, common to the adaptive, functional modes of the Healthy Adult and Happy/Free Child, can lead to greater well-being and resilience, which in turn improve the capacity of clients to function well and to meet their basic needs (Figure 1.3). The following section outlines the role that arts and body-based therapies can play in this regard.

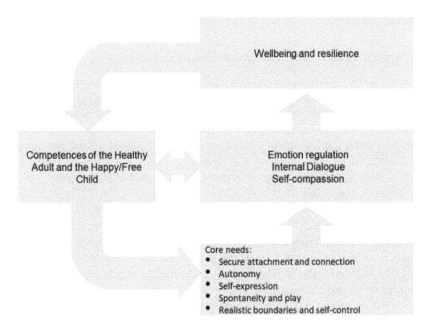

Figure 1.3 The Healthy Adult in relation to well-being and resilience, adapted from the course manual *Schema Therapy and the Healthy Adult* (Claassen & Broersen, 2019).

1.3 Arts and body-based therapies and the adaptive modes

Arts and body-based therapies typically revolve around giving expression to clients' experiences, reclaiming playfulness, letting go of perfectionism, and focusing on sensation. They liberate clients from destructive patterns, allowing them to strive in an appropriate manner to satisfy their basic emotional needs. Arts and body-based interventions have a broader focus than just the symptom or problem. Their power lies in their use of clients' existing (unconscious) competence and capacity for play, movement, and creativity.

Creativity can be understood as the Healthy Adult's capacity for flexibility and problem-solving, not only through cognitive thought but also in non-verbal ways that are more about feeling than thinking. In some cases, clients may literally establish a creative niche for their Free Child, for example by singing in a band or painting. Similarly, arts and body-based therapies stimulate strong, healthy, and mature behaviors, relating to the therapeutic principles of *empowerment* and client well-being that are central to positive psychology.

The following subsections explain how arts and body-based therapies can help strengthen the six healthy ego functions identified above.

1. Personality integration and formation of self-image

In arts and body-based therapies, inner thoughts and feelings are made visible, tangible, and concrete through experiential work, often involving arts and body-based therapeutic tools, acting, and/or movement. The relationship between the different modes, and between different sides of the self, may also be exposed. For many clients, this is the first time these sides come together, and they gain insight into the relationship between the coping and the Vulnerable Child modes. Only in this way can they come to understand the function of coping or the painful effects of a parenting mode.

Personality integration can begin as a conscious or unconscious process, with meaning always determined in consultation with the client. Clients learn to experience their emotions and bring them together in a coherent, integrated whole. Both integration and fragmentation take place at a deep level of the personality. Arts and body-based therapies, or products thereof, confirm what is apparent or reveal hidden qualities.

Self-reflection during the therapeutic process takes place in response to the development of a product. In arts and body-based therapies, this might include visual art, dance, music, dramatic play, or action/movement. Arts and body-based therapies also help to improve clients' self-image. In addition to unifying personality traits, clients work on the content of their inner self, transitioning from a negative to a positive self-image.

The arts and body-based process or product allows for distance: clients can consider themselves and their own behavioral patterns through the medium of concrete works they have created or through watching or listening to recordings of themselves. Emotions can be literally and/or figuratively released or put aside. Clients can also practice dealing differently with triggers and experience how that feels. These practices encourage clients to view themselves no longer as fragmented but rather as whole, even when intense emotions are activated—a characteristic of psychologically healthy people.

2. Healthy emotion regulation

Emotion regulation is one of the main ego functions of the Healthy Adult. Emotion or self-regulation is not only relevant for schemas with dysfunctional boundaries, such as the schema Insufficient Self-Control. Rather, all coping modes ultimately aim to regulate emotions, but dysfunctional coping modes do this in an unhelpful way.

It is assumed that the Healthy Adult can be strengthened through raised awareness. In arts and body-based therapies, different states of mind can be triggered by the various materials, techniques, and working methods employed as part of the therapeutic process. Clients become aware of their emotional reactions, recognize their basic needs, and develop alternative ways of dealing with them.

The principles of affect regulation art therapy—although developed for children ages 4–12—may be helpful in this regard:

1. The construction of self-regulation occurs in three phases: stress regulation, attention regulation, and affect regulation.
2. Interactive regulation (Rauh et al., 2021).

To promote *stress regulation*, therapists create an environment in which clients accept new experiences through interaction with another person. The goal of this phase is for clients to be able to relax in a certain space, to tolerate support and guidance, and to ask for and accept help. To promote *attention regulation*, clients undergo physical and sensory experiences that they then evaluate as pleasant or unpleasant. This simple, binary division serves as a foundation from which clients can identify basic emotions such as feeling scared, angry, happy, and sad. In the third stage, *affect regulation*, clients learn to link these emotions to affects, and to distinguish and share emotions. Clients develop awareness of the context in which they tend to experience an emotion and also become more cognizant of others' feelings, making them better equipped to participate in collaborative discussion.

Self-regulation occurs through *interactive regulation* with the caring adult. We are constantly "regulating" ourselves and others, though we are not always aware that we are doing so. Arts and body-based therapists make use of this in the context of reparenting and have a number of regulatory tools at their disposal for this purpose that can be mixed and remixed depending on the situation (Rauh et al., 2021). These "ingredients" include:

- providing structure (less–more);
- providing challenges (less–more);
- duration of the experience (shorter–longer);
- working alone or collaborating;
- task-based or process-based work;
- physical-sensory experiences (less–more);
- encouraging personal preferences (less–more);
- encouraging differentiation (less–more);
- encouraging meaning-making (less–more).

Mirroring and matching are basic elements of reparenting aimed at healthy emotion regulation and have more dimensions in the context of arts and body-based therapy than in verbal therapy. Wigram (2004) described the key role of improvisation in music therapy, with techniques ranging from warm-up to mirroring, rhythmic grounding, providing a foundation, and holding. These techniques are not only applicable in music therapy, but are also recognizable across all arts and body-based disciplines.

Bottom-up work on emotion regulation requires an open mind and the willingness to be guided. The attitude underpinning experiential work is Try it! How does it feel? An exercise can always be adjusted to make it more suitable or so that any stress it causes remains manageable. This flexibility can also help the therapist pinpoint key factors, for example: "You were startled by this big white sheet, is that right? If we fold it in half, what happens to the stress in your body? Can you translate this to challenges outside of therapy?" In this way, clients learn to integrate this flexibility into their Healthy Adult, increasing their window of tolerance.

Early experiences and their effects can emerge spontaneously from the use of materials, techniques, and working methods (Kliphuis, 1973). Herein lies the value of working with materials that provoke a certain reaction, like clay that invites kneading and squeezing or a drum kit that invites vigorous drumming. Reflecting on this leads to awareness.

A psychologically healthy person can experience several emotions or states of mind at once. Various feeling states are then integrated and are, together, adequate for the situation at hand. A person then does not become overwhelmed by negative feelings when faced with minor problems.

3. Contact with one's own emotions and needs as well as those of others

Arts and body-based therapies are strongly geared toward clients' needs and abilities. Personalized and positive challenges form the basis for further development. Through sensory experiences and movement, different topics can be explored without language. Some clients, such as those with emotionally avoidant personality disorders, find experiential work difficult or intimidating.

EXAMPLE OF BOTTOM-UP WORKING

Lisanne (age 26) is receiving individual, trauma-focused art therapy. Following her art therapist's instructions, she engages in sensorimotor work. After a brief attention and breathing exercise, standing in front of a large sheet of paper on the wall with a crayon in each hand (bilateral drawing) and her eyes closed, she begins to make movements on the paper. She is not forming any particular image, just scribbling, exploring which movement is appropriate or "feels right" in the moment. First, she scratches in small circles, not hard, not soft. "This isn't really about anything," she says.

She might change the dynamics as desired, or in response to the therapist's suggestions: "softer" or "harder," "slower" or "faster."

After a while, she moves into a harder movement in her drawing. She is asked to think about a situation in the past in which her boundaries were crossed. Her drawing becomes harder and faster.

She is now asked to indicate her limit through the movement and dynamics of scribbling, through the artwork itself, and she uses horizontal, powerful movements. After a few minutes this changes to more actively repelling vertical movements from bottom to top. The word that comes to her mind is "OUT!"

Now she wants to combine the work with paint, and she repaints the entire sheet with orange finger paint.

Ever since she was a child, Lisanne has felt dirty when experiencing this emotion, but she manages to cope with it these days, she says.

Finally, she scratches into the bottom layer of paper the word OUT!

At first it is barely noticeable. Finding this unsatisfactory, she then scratches it in more strongly, using the tip of a pair of scissors. She scratches so hard that the scissors makes holes in the paper. This way, in her opinion, it has the right emotional valence.

In the follow-up discussion, she mentions how, when faced with the traumatic situation, she was unable to do this—to signal her boundaries and push off the perpetrator. Now she wants to acknowledge her boundaries, vocalize where they lie, and she permits herself to do so.

"That felt good," she says afterwards.

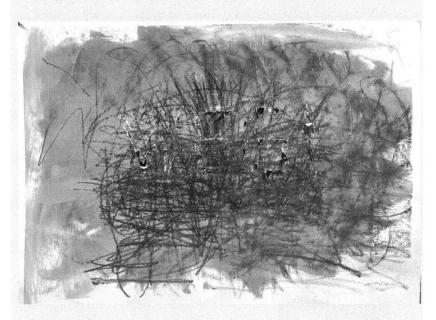

Artwork of Lisanne, bottom-up working.

Through individual or group arts and body-based therapies, clients become aware of their own feelings and needs, as well as those of others. By becoming aware of their own coping mode, they create the space to choose to respond differently. Sometimes this is a stubborn process in which the belief that their dysfunctional coping mode is necessary remains intact. They will need to get in touch with, investigate, and acknowledge their underlying basic emotions, such as fear, anger, and sadness, before they can reach Healthy Adult mode.

Arts and body-based therapies, or the resulting products, offer space for clients to get in touch with their child modes. These can be evoked by emotional reactions to materials, instruments, props, and working methods that invite play. Parenting modes may also emerge where someone strongly reproves of their own piece of work or style of play, and so fighting the Demanding and Punitive Parent can be practiced. Feelings and expressions associated with child modes can be prioritized, and clients can work on developing self-compassion (Haeyen & Heijman, 2020, 2021).

4. The healthy internal dialogue

In arts and body-based therapies, different sides of a person can be imagined, narrated, and brought into dialogue with one another. This stimulates and brings to light the internal dialogue. The follow-up discussion, in which the client reflects on the design and experience of producing the artwork, is often surprisingly perceptive. Being able to engage in an internal Socratic dialogue, aiming to identify ideas and presuppositions, is seen as evidence of the presence and growth of the Healthy Adult.

Clients report experiencing a wider range of different dynamics in arts and body-based therapies compared to other, less experiential therapies. Some perceive it as more gradual, indirect, and calm, while others find it to be more confrontational and direct. The therapist can steer this process through concrete interventions, for example, by increasing or decreasing the challenge or tactile

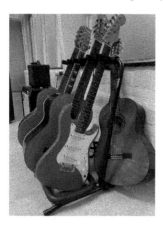

Response to instrument: desire to play or fear of failure?

input, or by intervening more or less cognitively. The manner of intervention, designed and executed by the therapist, is crucial in arts and body-based therapies. Because of this dynamic, and because other areas of the brain are also engaged, more and/or better contact can occasionally be made with deeper layers of feeling, which clients are less likely to avoid confronting. Through this, and through the search for a healthy internal dialogue, a more stable sense of self can arise, leading to healthier contact with oneself and others.

To gain control over the other modes, it is important for the Healthy Adult mode to give affirmation to the Vulnerable Child mode, to comfort and set boundaries for the Angry Child mode, and to neutralize the Punitive Parent mode.

5. Reality testing and assessing situations, conflicts, and relationships

Working with arts and body-based interventions always requires a process of actively participating on the one hand, and creating distance for reflection on the other. This encourages clients to make contact with themselves and others, and to face difficult situations or concerns, thereby fostering their development. This can be done by testing "as if" situations, where role play or game-like situations are used to mimic situations from everyday life and explore the issues that arise. This is an important strength of arts and body-based therapies (Bateman & Fonagy, 2004; Smeijsters, 2008).

In distancing, the reality check is given concrete form. The client may protest, "I can't do this, I'm not creative/musical/sporty!," but sees afterwards that they have created something that speaks to their individuality. Peer groups often reinforce this effect, because peer feedback is usually even more effective than that from the therapist. The group can also be an important witness for the child modes; for example, they can sometimes detect a client's repressed anger. Reality testing and an assessment of situations, conflicts, and relationships occur concretely through all kinds of collaborative working methods in arts and body-based therapies, which seek to identify affect and challenge and correct dysfunctional coping modes.

6. Seeking enjoyment and fulfilling needs in a mature manner

With respect to seeking enjoyment and fulfilling needs as a Healthy Adult, it is important that the client begins to see the difference between pleasure and coping. Consider the tendency to self-soothe versus seeking a healthy form of relaxation, or the tendency to overcompensate versus experiencing pleasure in human contact in a healthy way. What can replace time spent on addiction, on worrying, on keeping busy as a form of distraction? How can the client learn to set realistic boundaries? Arts and body-based therapies can help clients create literal and figurative boundaries through the structure, instruction, and setup of the working method.

In arts and body-based therapies, symptom-based and strength-based work go hand in hand, addressing symptoms while engaging in an activity with which the client feels an affinity, be it playing, making music, painting, or movement (sources of strength). Working with the client's favorite material can be satisfying in itself because it gives pleasure, which in turn leads to relaxation. This creates space to face the Vulnerable Child and possibly reveal or confront a traumatic experience. Symptom-based work means practicing what is difficult, by taking action and overcoming obstacles. It could involve, for example, working with (strength-based) concrete goals to express a shame-laden inner belief system, itself more symptom based.

A characteristic feature of arts and body-based therapies is the availability of forms of play, working methods, materials, and techniques that can replicate the experiences of everyday life. Imagination, fantasy, and play can provide a space for exploration. Therapists look for interventions with which clients have an affinity and that utilize their strengths at the same time as promoting resilience and connecting to personal therapy goals. In this way, clients can enjoy play while working indirectly on their problems. Being in therapy is then accompanied by a lightness or sense of positivity, in addition to the heaviness of facing a problem or psychological symptom.

1.3.1 Shared aspects of arts and body-based therapies

All arts and body-based therapies work indirectly and bottom-up. Through artistic, musical, dramatic, or movement-based work, different schemas, modes, and Healthy Adult traits can be triggered and explored. From there, therapists deploy both experiential and cognitive (top-down) interventions targeted toward personal therapy goals. All arts and body-based therapies are at least partially body based because motor and sensory aspects are always intertwined.

Given these common characteristics, methods may be transferrable across various arts and body-based therapies, though these methods may manifest differently in different disciplines (*form of vitality*; Stern, 2010). Aspects that are central to one form of arts and body-based therapy might also be present in another form. For example, mimicry and dramatic play might feature in music therapy, while physicality and strength may be utilized during the creative process of art therapy.

These options allow different disciplines to work together. Simultaneously enacting multiple forms of expression (e.g., body, image, sound) or translating one sensory experience into another can enhance the experience of empathy (*cross-modality*; Stern, 1985). This is theorized in the "analog process model" (Smeijsters, 2000, 2008). For example, a safe place with PMT materials can be set up in a room, followed by visual art materials; these forms of expression have a general meaning for how someone takes their place in the world. Such PMT installations or artistic images can also be called up again or embedded in imaginative exercises. This collaborative work on themes reinforces the shared, coherent framework communicated to the client.

In arts and body-based therapies, multiple theoretical principles are often linked. Schema therapy alone is often not sufficient and is thus combined with complementary principles and practices, including body-centered theories developed by Ogden et al. (2006), Pesso (Van Attekum, 2012), and Van der Kolk (2014).

Working with multiple arts and body-based therapies can give rise to challenges. For example, (arts and body-based) therapists can rush the process of achieving the Healthy Adult mode without adequately exploring difficult emotions. Clients need time and space to reflect on and process traumatic experiences. Acknowledging an experience and speaking, drawing, or singing about it are important for eventually reaching the Healthy Adult or Happy/Free Child mode.

Arts and body-based therapies can contribute to the exploration of unconscious memories through the use of indirect, physical, and non-verbal tools and working methods. They do not always require the use of a specific discourse, such as schema language. Arts and body-based therapies are experiential, supported by body language and imagery. The therapeutic relationship, the creative processes, and the products created during these processes all have an inherent therapeutic effect that can contribute to clients' personal goals.

DOUBLE SELF-PORTRAIT

Johan (age 42): "This is a dual image of myself with, in gray, the image of the Healthy Adult I am now, looking straight out into the world, and beneath it the image of me as an eight-year-old boy looking up to his brother. I gradually feel more balance between who I was then and who I am now. I notice that I have grown."

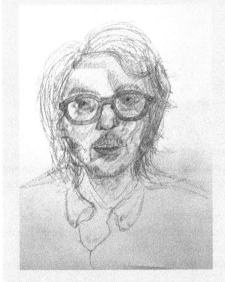

Double self-portrait.

1.3.2 Working mechanisms

Exactly how the various arts and body-based therapies work has not yet been sufficiently researched. It is hypothesized that their experiential nature is different from cognitive and verbal (psycho)therapies. Verbal therapy generally involves a top-down approach, where thinking and cognitive processes are the starting point (Van Hooren et al., 2021), while arts and body-based therapies can be seen as bottom-up, taking as their starting point concrete (emotional and sensorimotor) experiences in the body.

According to Van Hooren and colleagues (2021), the mechanisms of action of arts and body-based therapies can be ordered hierarchically, in line with the structure of the central nervous system. Starting from the lower-order processes of information processing to the higher-order processes, these are:

1. Arousal regulation.
2. Process of body perception/awareness.
3. Process of expression, creativity, and flexibility.
4. Affect and emotion regulation.
5. Regulation of higher-order cognitive processes (such as executive functions).
6. Regulation of social cognitions.

Based on a recently published systematic review ($n = 67$), De Witte and colleagues (2021) described three shared active factors for all arts and body-based therapies:

- embodiment;
- concretization;
- symbolism and metaphors.

1.3.3 Bottom-up working

Bottom-up working means starting from the body and working up to cognition. According to Levine (2012), the starting point of bottom-up working is the *somatic experience*—the ability to feel emotion at the bodily level. The concept of *felt sense* is relevant here (Gendlin, 1978). The felt sense consists solely of experiencing and feeling and is the basic element of focusing. It can be used as a compass: What do I need? What does my body need? Therapists can help clients access their felt sense by constantly monitoring their posture, facial expressions, and bodily responses.

Bottom-up work on the basis of bodily experiences helps clients to address basic emotional needs that are, in principle, also corporeal. These basic needs progress in a child's development from literal and physical to symbolic, and from concrete to abstract (Van Attekum, 1997). For example, with regard to the basic need of safety, a child is, or feels safest, in the womb, then on the lap and later when they are in their parents' thoughts and heart.

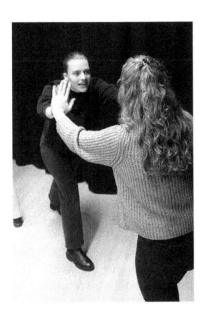

Physical depiction of a mode.

Arts and body-based therapies connect to a client's concrete bodily experiences and help to translate them, through reflection, into cognitive thought. This may be through direct or indirect work. When working *directly* in schema therapy, a therapist might ask the client to depict their coping mode in clay or portray it physically using a gesture or posture. To do this, the client must already be aware of their coping mode. An *indirect* version of this task might be to make an animal out of clay. The subsequent evaluation may then involve a discussion of how that animal defends itself in the wild, leading to whether the client recognizes these defense mechanisms in their own behavior, whether they are helpful (adaptive coping) or a hindrance (dysfunctional coping), why this coping mode was necessary, and how or by whom that need should have been fulfilled (rescripting). Assigning meaning thus follows from the *somatic experience*.

In arts and body-based therapies, the experiential techniques described in schema therapy are applied more broadly within existing exercises.

1.3.4 Multiple chair technique

The multiple chair technique involves using different chairs to represent different modes (Healthy Adult, Vulnerable Child, etc.). When a mode is identified, the client is asked to sit on the corresponding chair and respond from the perspective of that mode. This helps to clarify conflicts and emotions (Fassbinder et al., 2016) and gives rise to a dialogue between the client and these modes. In arts and body-based therapies, different modes may also be represented by symbols, materials, musical instruments, or other tools (Engelbrecht & Günther, 2019). For example, an Angry Protector might wear boxing gloves while a Vulnerable Child hides under a blanket. This directs attention to the physical aspect of the mode.

1.3.5 Imagery rescripting

Imagery rescripting (ImR) requires clients to recall an emotional situation and, with their eyes closed, visualize it clearly (Arntz & Weertman, 1999), focusing on the emotions and bodily experiences involved. Visual processing has a powerful effect on the way an experience is remembered and can thus aid in reconstructing negative images into more positive ones (Lobbestael et al., 2005; Van Vreeswijk et al., 2012). After imagining a stressful emotional situation, the client is asked to imagine a supportive figure who could make the situation better or more pleasant, perhaps by meeting the needs of the child in the imagined scene. This figure might take the form of the client themself in Healthy Adult mode or another real or imagined figure (Fassbinder et al., 2016). In this way, the situation is given a new emotional valence and clients gain insight into their own needs. It is important that both client and therapist know the schemas well and are, accordingly, able to imagine what the reconstruction should involve. Rescripting is a core intervention in schema therapy.

When arts and body-based therapists see the progress their clients are making, it can be surprising that this is not enough to break down their negative core beliefs. Corrective experiences happen in the here and now of a therapeutic situation, with support from the therapist or a group essentially playing the role of a positive parent. These experiences are important because they show clients alternative versions of events. However, past experiences are deeply ingrained, and the associated emotions are much stronger than a single positive experience in the present. ImR takes advantage of the fact that the past and present are not stored in the brain on a time line; rather, the past directly influences the present by "firing" physical warning signals. This is evident in reactions triggered by trauma. Rescripting attempts to edit the "script" (e.g., a traumatic memory) by adding an alternative response to the trauma on a new memory track.

ImR proceeds according to the following steps (Young et al., 2003):

1. Imagine a pleasant place in the present.
2. Imagine an unpleasant situation in the present.
3. Affect bridge (see below).
4. Imagine an unpleasant situation in the past.
5. "Rescript" that memory by imagining a positive end for it.
6. Return to a pleasant place in the present.

In arts and body-based therapies, this process is followed literally, as depicted in the photo on page 25. The various steps can be acted out, portrayed through sound and/or images, or imagined (Haeyen, 2007, 2018a).

1.3.5.1 Affect bridge

In ImR, the therapist monitors the client's physical and emotional reaction to an unpleasant situation in the present, before asking them to release the image of the situation but to hold onto the feeling. The therapist asks where or when else the client has felt this way. The client might recall being in a situation as a child in which they felt the same way. The therapist will ask questions such as "What do you see in front of you now? How old are you now?"

This is a technique known as the affect bridge. In arts and body-based therapies, the affect bridge can be used alongside or in response to the ImR process described above, or while working on a product. Clients can then choose a process that helps regulate their emotion, such as kneading clay.

> *When I knead clay, I feel powerful; I never have that otherwise. I can also imagine, or imagine things better, when I'm kneading at the same time.*

Clients often shift into a child mode during arts and body-based therapy; the interaction with the materials and activities is so elementary and impulse driven that it triggers their inner youth. They may suddenly feel excitable, despondent, anxious, angry, or stubborn, which in turn triggers a schema and brings out the Vulnerable Child. In this case, the therapist does not need to ask the client to

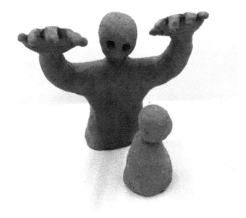

Modes of Ella, age 56, art therapy client.

imagine an unpleasant situation in the present—instead, it occurs organically (Günther, 2019).

ImR can also be used in response to a positive feeling that emerges through arts and body-based therapy by identifying the basic need that is fulfilled by the action. When a client derives satisfaction, joy, or pleasure from an action—such as working with clay, as in the previous example—the therapist draws attention to this. Often clients are unaware of positive reactions, as dysfunctional schemas have taught them to store only negative sensations. Therapist and client then discuss what basic emotional need is involved, with the therapist asking: "What does this material/action give you in this moment?" The client may reply with something along the lines of "I feel firmness and stability, so I don't have to be gentle." The therapist will then relate this to the client's past, for example by asking whether they experienced firmness and stability in their upbringing. If the client did not, the therapist can then introduce an Ideal Parent figure with the traits of the material—in this case, the firmness of the clay, which invites the client to treat it forcefully. This is followed by (imaginary) role play or dialogue, linking the concrete experience of working with the material to the deficiency in the historical scene. The client may be asked to visualize this Ideal Parent, or the experience may remain a bodily one.

This form of rescripting from something positive may seem unnecessary; after all, the client is feeling good in that moment. However, we know that clients try to fulfill the needs of their inner child according to their dysfunctional schemas. Highlighting that schemas may be at work even when they are feeling positive allows the client to distinguish between overcompensation and Healthy Adult interaction.

In arts and body-based therapies, unpleasant memories can be portrayed or narrated through material, music, or movement (Haeyen, 2019). The image can then be adapted, for example, by referring to something that has helped the client deal with this particular memory. "As your present self or as an adult today, what would you want or be able to do when you step into this situation? Is there another end to the events?"

Someone in the Healthy Adult mode can portray how they would handle the situation. The therapist might assume this role as a *rescripting figure*, but it might also be possible for the client themself or a fellow group member to reimagine the situation with a positive outcome. It often helps to call the rescripting figure the "Ideal Parent" when dealing with an interaction that a parent should have shaped (Perquin, 1986). Because clients may continue to deploy a dysfunctional coping mode (doing it alone) as they attempt to achieve the Healthy Adult mode, they may first need to see how somebody else does it and allow themselves to trust in and be supported by others. This type of ImR can also be used to address trauma-related nightmares, where the story of the nightmare is rescripted with a different, more positive outcome (Haeyen & Staal, 2021).

Every action and interaction can acquire meaning in the Quadrant Model (see Figure 1.4), be it verbal interaction, interaction between client and material, or a physical response to the self or another person. The therapist can ask the

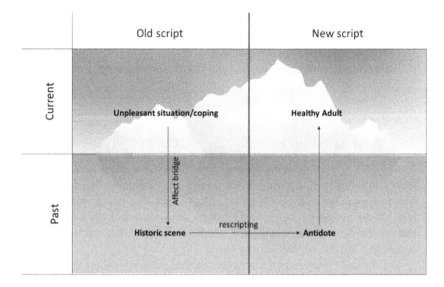

Figure 1.4 Quadrant Model (after the model of a Pesso = Structure [Perquin & Vos, 2008] applied here to schema therapy).

question, "In which quadrant can I place this observation? In the past, below the iceberg, and thus in the child reactions? Or in the present, above the iceberg, on the schema side (the old script) or the healthy functional side (new script)?" For some clients, the model is also appropriate for psychoeducation.

Through the techniques described, the client works to build their Healthy Adult while remaining within their window of tolerance, thus avoiding or at least limiting their reliance on destructive coping modes.

When a client has adequately explored past experiences in this way, following the route in the lower half of the quadrant, it may then suffice to remind them (cognitively, verbally) that they are wearing "schema-tinted" glasses, and that there are other experiences to rely on now. The client can then transition "above the iceberg"—from the old script to the new script, and from coping mode to Healthy Adult. This is a good opportunity for the client to test their newfound resilience and flexibility. The therapist should keep in mind that the client's new, healthy schema may still be fragile, and that it may be necessary to take a step back and retrace the route through the early experiences. A new, as yet unconscious memory will then likely present itself that needs rescripting. This process is repeated until the client is prepared to take the step to the Healthy Adult.

From the perspective of arts and body-based therapies, we could add another ego function to the list of healthy ego functions in Section 1.2.5. This time, it is about learning to deal with the body and using it as a kind of "compass" to identify the presence of a particular need instead of falling back into old patterns.

HEALTHY ADULT WITH BODY AS COMPASS

- "reads" the body;
- identifies which script it is following;
- can choose between healthy coping modes and new behaviors.

THE THERAPEUTIC PROCESS IN PICTURES

Denise (27) is drawing about having "killed her Vulnerable Child," in her words. In high school, she had low self-esteem and was bullied. She draws an image of a gallows with people to the right and left of it (see photo below, left). Of the people on the right, she had no expectations; of the people on the left she did (e.g., her teacher and the family doctor)—but neither group helped her. She did not feel seen or heard.

She decided that she hated her vulnerable side and that it should no longer exist. From then on, she became "the monster under her bed" (see photo below, right). In treatment, she has discovered that her vulnerable side is still in there somewhere. She continues to feel vulnerable and sad, however, and struggles to open up (see Figure 1.5).

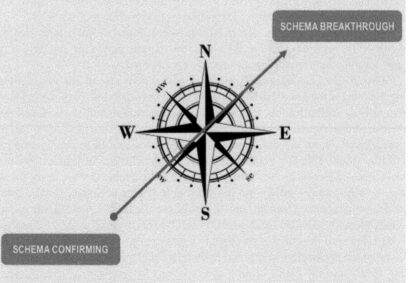

Figure 1.5 Body as compass.

(a) 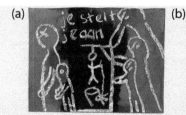   (b)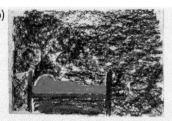

a) The end of her vulnerable side; b) The monster under her bed.

In another session, Denise speaks about how she was quite insensitive toward her mother. Her mother was often very sad and put pressure on Denise by saying things like: "if I didn't have you, I don't know what I'd do." The dangerous "sea of tears" represented the fear and anger that Denise experienced.

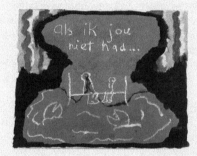

"If I didn't have you", emotional pressure from her mother.

Several sessions later, Denise makes her parents from clay. While making them, she reports that she barely wants to touch them, and after the clay dries, she wants to break the figures. She integrates the fragments into her artwork, putting them into the coffin from which she crawls as a Vulnerable Child, with flowers for herself on top.

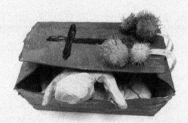

The Vulnerable Child coming back.

She refers again to how, in the past, she declared that part of herself dead. As her therapy progresses, however, she feels that it is coming back and may make her feel more like herself. She is happy about that.

This chapter has described how arts and body-based therapies, positive psychology, and schema therapy can be a fruitful combination for the treatment of personality disorders and emotion regulation problems, focusing both on reducing symptoms and improving adaptive skills and well-being.

References

American Art Therapy Association. (2021). *About art therapy?* Accessed January 15, 2021, from https://arttherapy.org/about-art-therapy/

Akwa GGZ. (2017). *Care standard personality disorder: Individualized care pathway and treatment.* GGZ Standards. Accessed September 3, 2021, from https://www.ggzstandaarden.nl/zorgstandaarden/persoonlijkheidsstoornissen-zorgstandaard-2017/individueel-zorgplan-en-behandeling/zelfmanagement

Akwa GGZ. (2019). *Generic module for arts and body-based therapies.* GGZ Standards. Accessed September 3, 2021, from https://www.ggzstandaarden.nl/generieke-modules/vaktherapie/inleiding

Aldao, A., Nolen-Hoeksema, S., & Schweizer, S. (2010). Emotion-regulation strategies across psychopathology: A meta-analytic review. *Clinical Psychology Review*, *30*(2):217–237. https://doi.org/10.1016/j.cpr.2009.11.004

American Psychiatric Association. (2014). *Handbook of classification of mental disorders: DSM-5* (M.W. Hengeveld, Supervision transl.). Boom Publishers.

Arntz, A., & Jacob, G.A. (2012). *Schema therapy in practice: An introductory guide to the schema mode approach.* Wiley-Blackwell.

Arntz, A., Rijkeboer, M., Chan, E., Fassbinder, E., Karaosmanoglu, A., Lee, C.W., & Panzeri, M. (2021). Towards a reformulated theory underlying schema therapy: Position paper of an international workgroup. *Cognitive Therapy and Research*, *45*(6):1007–1020. https://doi.org/10.1007/s10608-021-10209-5

Arntz, A., & Weertman, A. (1999). Treatment of childhood memories: Theory and practice. *Behaviour Research and Therapy*, *37*(8):715–740. https://doi.org/10.1016/S0005-7967(98)00173-9

Bamelis, L.M., Evers, S.M.A.A., Spinhoven, P., & Arntz, A (2017). Results of a multicenter randomized controlled trial of the clinical effectiveness of schema therapy for personality disorders. *American Journal of Psychiatry*, *171*(3):305–322. https://doi.org/10.1176/appi.ajp.2013.12040518

Bateman, A., & Fonagy, P. (2004). *Psychotherapy for borderline personality disorder: Mentalization-based treatment.* Oxford University Press.

Bernstein, D., Oorsouw, K. van, & Candel, I. (2020). *Creating corrective emotional experiences for youth with serious behavioral problems and their family/social networks: Integrating schema therapy and positive psychology.* INSPIRE 2020 ISST Conference Amsterdam.

Bohlmeijer, E.T., Jacobs, N., Walburg, J.A., & Westerhof, G.J. (2021). *Handbook of Positive Psychology: Theory, research, and interventions*. Boom Publishers.
British Association of Art Therapists. (2021). *What is art therapy*. Accessed January 15, 2021, from https://www.baat.org/About-Art-Therapy
Bruscia, K. (2012). *Case examples of music therapy for personality disorders*. Barcelona Publishers.
Claassen, A. (2017). The function of the punishing parent: Entry point for treatment. *PsyXpert*, 2:29–37.
Claassen, A.M.T.S., & Broersen, J. (2019). *Handbook module Schema therapy and the healthy adult*. Bohn Stafleu van Loghum.
Claassen, A.M.T.S., & Pol, S.M. (2014). The healthy adult: From mode to human. *Psychopraktijk*, 6(4):19–22. Https://doi.org/10.1007/s13170-014-0054-y
Claassen, A.M.T.S., & Pol, S.M. (2015). *Schema therapy and the Healthy Adult: Positive techniques from practice*. Bohn Stafleu van Loghum.
Dadomo, H., Panzeri, M., Caponcello, D., Carmelita, A., & Grecucci, A. (2018). Schema therapy for emotional dysregulation in personality disorders: A review. *Current Opinion in Psychiatry*, 31(1):43–49. https://doi.org/10.1097/YCO.0000000000000380
De Witte, M., Orkibi, H., Zarate, R., Karkou, V., Sajnani, N., Malhotra, B., Tin Hung Ho, R., Kaimal, G., Baker, F.A., & Koch S.C. (2021). From therapeutic factors to mechanisms of change in the creative arts therapies: A scoping review. *Frontiers in Psychology, 12*:678397. https://doi.org/10.3389/fpsyg.2021.678397
Engelbrecht, J., & Günther, G. (2019). Creating an anchor: Music therapy, psychodrama and schema therapy. In Cardinaels & Goosens (Eds.), *Making space for body and mind in therapy* (pp. 161–167). Acco.
Fassbinder, E., Schweiger, U., Martius, D., Brand-de Wilde, O., & Arntz, A. (2016). Emotion regulation in schema therapy and dialectical behavior therapy. *Frontiers in Psychology*, 7:1373. https://doi.org/10.3389/fpsyg.2016.01373
Franken, K., Lamers, S.M.A., Ten Klooster, P.M., Bohlmeijer, E.T., & Westerhof, G.J. (2018). Validation of the mental health continuum-short form and the dual continua model of well-being and psychopathology in an adult mental health setting. *Journal of Clinical Psychology*, 74(12):2187–2202. https://doi.org/10.1002/jclp.2265
Federation of Arts and Psychomotor Therapies. (2017). *Strategic Research Agenda for the Profession of Arts and body-based therapies*. Accessed October 1, 2021, from https://fvb.vaktherapie.nl/strategische-onderzoeksagenda
Fonagy, P., & Allison, E. (2014). The role of mentalizing and epistemic trust in the therapeutic relationship. *Psychotherapy*, 51(3):372–380. https://doi.org/10.1037/a0036505
Gendlin, E.T. (1978). *Focusing*. Everest House.
Günther, G. (2019). Don't let me get lost in my self-built maze - The interplay between body-centered imagery and schema therapy. In Cardinaels & Goossens (Eds.), *Making space for body a mind in therapy* (pp. 154–160). Acco.
Haeyen, S. (2007). *Not indulging but experiencing, visual therapy in personality problems*. Bohn Stafleu van Loghum.
Haeyen, S. (2018a). *Art therapy and emotion regulation problems: Theory and workbook* (C.L. Stennes, Vert). Palgrave Macmillan.
Haeyen, S. (2018b). *Effects of art therapy: The case of personality disorders clusters B/C* [dissertation]. Radboud University.

Haeyen, S. (2019). Strengthening the healthy adult self in art therapy: Using schema therapy as a positive psychological intervention for people diagnosed with personality disorders. *Frontiers in Psychology, 10*:644. https://doi.org/10.3389/fpsyg.2019.00644

Haeyen, S. (2020). *The powerful experience: Emotion and self-image regulation in personality disorders through arts and body-based therapy* [Lectureship]. HAN University of Applied Sciences.

Haeyen, S., & Heijman, J. (2020). Compassion focused art therapy for people diagnosed with a cluster B/C personality disorder: An intervention mapping study. *The Arts in Psychotherapy, 69*(20). https://doi.org/10.1016/j.aip.2020.101663

Haeyen, S., & Heijman, J. (2021). Compassion Focused Art Therapy for clients with personality disorder cluster B/C: An Intervention Mapping study. *Groups, 21*(2):22–45.

Haeyen, S., & Staal, M. (2021). Imagery rehearsal based art therapy: Treatment of posttraumatic nightmares in art therapy. *Frontiers in Psychology, 11*:628717. https://doi.org/10.3389/fpsyg.2020.628717

Haeyen, S., Hooren, S. van, Veld, W. van der, & Hutschemaekers, G. (2018). Promoting mental health versus reducing mental illness in art therapy with patients with personality disorders: A quantitative study. *The Arts in Psychotherapy, 58*(4):11–16. https://doi.org/10.1016/j.aip.2017.12.009

Heath, G., & Startup, H. (2020). *Creative methods in schema therapy: Advances and innovation in clinical practice*. Routledge.

Hornsveld, H., Bögels, H., & Grandia, H. (2021). *Schema therapy casebook: 21 real-life examples*. Bohn Stafleu van Loghum.

Hulshof, R., Pol, S., & Wentink, M. (2009). Schema-focused therapy in a clinical setting. *Groups, 4*(3):24–35.

Karterud, S., & Pedersen, G. (2004). Short-term day hospital treatment for personality disorders: Benefits of the therapeutic components. *Therapeutic Communities, 25*(1):43–54.

Kehr, T. (2020). *Report focus group 'Vaktherapie bij persoonlijkheidsstoornissen'*. HAN University of Applied Sciences. Internal Publication.

Keyes, C.L.M. (2002). The mental health continuum: From languishing to flourishing in life. *Journal of Health and Social Behavior, 43*(2):207–222. https://doi.org/10.2307/3090197

Kliphuis, M. (1973). Handling creative processes in formation and counseling. In L. Wils (Ed.), *By way of play*. Samsom.

Knapen, S. (2017). Better together: In the absence of trust, there is no capacity for change. *Journal of Psychotherapy, 43*(2):109–125. https://doi.org/10.1007/s12485-017-0177-9

Levine, H.B. (2012). The colorless canvas: Representation, therapeutic action and the creation of mind. *The International Journal of Psychoanalysis, 93*:607–629.

Livesley, W.J., Dimaggio, G., & Clarkin, J.F. (2016). Why integrated treatment? General principles of therapeutic change. In W.J. Livesley, G. Dimaggio, & J.F. Clarkin (Eds.), *Integrated treatment for personality disorder: A modular approach* (pp. 3–18). Guilford Press.

Lobbestael, J., Arntz, A., & Sieswerda, S. (2005). Schema modes and childhood abuse in borderline and antisocial personality disorders. *Journal of Behavior Therapy and Experimental Psychiatry, 36*(3):240–253. https://doi.org/10.1016/j.jbtep.2005.05.006

LOO VTB. (2016). *National domain profile bachelor programs in arts and body-based therapy professions.* LOO VTB.

Louis, J.P., Wood, A.M., & Lockwood, G. (2020). Development and validation of the positive parenting schema Inventory (PPSI) to complement the Young Parenting Inventory (YPI) for Schema Therapy (ST). *Assessment, 27*(4):766–786.

Louis, J.P., Wood, A.M., Lockwood, G., Ho, M.H.R., & Ferugson, E. (2018). Positive clinical psychology and Schema Therapy (ST): The development of the Young Positive Schema Questionnaire (YPSQ) to Complement the Young Schema Questionnaire 3 Short Form (YSQS3). *Psychological Assessment, 30*(9):1199–1213. https://doi.org/10.1037/pas0000.567

Muste, E., Weertman, A., & Claassen, A.M. (Eds.). (2009). *Handbook of clinical Schema therapy.* Bohn Stafleu van Loghum.

National Steering Committee on Multidisciplinary Guideline Development in Mental Health Care. (2008). *Multidisciplinary guideline personality disorders: Guideline for the diagnosis and treatment of adult patients with a personality disorder.* Trimbos Institute.

Ng, F.Y.Y., Bourke, M.E., & Grenyer, B.F.S. (2016). Recovery from borderline personality disorder: A systematic review of the perspectives of consumers, clinicians, family and carers. *PLoS One, 11*(8):1–21. https://doi.org/10.1371/journal.pone.0160515

Ogden, P., Minton, K., & Pain, C. (2006). *Trauma and the body: A sensorimotor approach to psychotherapy.* W.W. Norton.

Perquin, L. et al. (1986/2000). Ideal parenting exercise. *Journal of Pesso-psychotherapy.*

Perquin, L., & Vos, L., (2008). Safe deep-sea diving. *Journal of Pesso-Psychotherapy, 24*(1):8–31.

Rauh, W., Velde, I. van de, Nieuwenhuis, L., & Vlugt, S. van der (2021). First affect regulation, then self-regulation. Learning to regulate affect within the arts and body-based therapies relationship by doing and experiencing. *Journal of Arts and body-Based Therapies, 17*(3):12–19.

Roediger, E., Stevens, B.A., & Brockman, R. (2018). *Contextual schema therapy: An integrative approach to personality disorders, emotional dysregulation & interpersonal functioning.* New Harbinger Publications.

Seligman, M.E.P., & Csíkszentmihályi, M. (2000). Positive psychology: An introduction. *American Psychologist, 55*(1):5–14. https://doi.org/10.1037/0003-066X.55.1.5

Siegel, D.J. (1999). *The developing mind: How relationships and the brain interact to shape who we are.* Guilford Press.

Smeijsters, H. (2000/2008). *Handbook of creative therapy.* Coutinho.

Solli, H.P., Rolvsjord, R., & Borg, M. (2013). Toward understanding music therapy as a recovery-oriented practice within mental health care: A meta-synthesis of service users' experiences. *Journal of Music Therapy, 50*(4):244–273. https://doi.org/10.1093/jmt/50.4.244

Stern, D. (1985). *The interpersonal world of the infant.* Basic Books, Inc., Publishers,

Stern, D. (2010). *Forms of vitality: Exploring dynamic experience in psychology, the arts, psychotherapy, and development.* Oxford University Press.

Van Attekum, M. (1997/2012). *In person: Body-oriented psychotherapy according to Pesso,* 5th ed. Pearson.

Van der Kolk, B.A. (2014). *The body keeps the score: Brain, mind, and body in the healing of trauma.* Viking Penguin.

Van Hooren, S., Van Buschbach, J., Waterink, W., & Abbing, A. (2021). Mechanisms of action of arts and body-based therapies: Towards a foundation and explanation of effects - Work in progress. *Journal of Arts and body-based therapies, 17*(2):4–12.

Van Vreeswijk, M., Broersen, J., & Nadort, M. (Eds.). (2008). *Handbook of Schema therapy: Theory, practice and research.* Bohn Stafleu van Loghum.

Van Vreeswijk, M., Broersen, J., & Nadort, M. (Eds.). (2012). *The Wiley-Blackwell handbook of schema therapy: Theory, research, and practice.* John Wiley & Sons.

Versluis, Y., Bol, Y., Bouwmeester, S., & Peeters, F.P.M.L. (2022, January 24). *Strengthening the healthy adult mode: A case experimental study exploring the effects of a new schema therapy protocol in an outpatient population* (Clinical Trial NCT04466163).US Clinical Trials Registry. https://ichgcp.net/clinical-trials-registry/NCT04466163

Videler, A.C., Van Royen, R.J.J., Heijnen-Kohl, S.M.J., Rossi, G., Van Alphen, S.P.J., & Van der Feltz-Cornelis, C.M. (2017). Adapting schema therapy for personality disorders in older adults. *International Journal of Cognitive Therapy, 10*(1):62–78. https://doi.org/10.1521/ijct.2017.10.1.62

Wigram, T. (2004). *Improvisation: Methods and techniques for music therapy clinicians, educators and students.* Jessica Kingsley Publishers. 237 pages. ISBN 1-84310-048-7. $29.95 (paper), *Music Therapy Perspectives, 22*(2):128–130, https://doi.org/10.1093/mtp/22.2.128

Wolterink, T., & Westerhof, G. (2018). Verandering van schemamodi en klachten bij cliënten met complexe persoonlijkheidsproblematiek: Een naturalistische volgstudie in een klinische setting [Changing schema modes and symptoms in clients with complex personality problems: A naturalistic follow-up study in a clinical setting]. *Gedragstherapie [Behavioral Therapy], 51*(1):24–43.

World Health Organization. (2022). Fact sheet mental health. https://www.who.int/news-room/fact-sheets/detail/mental-health-strengthening-our-response

Yakın, D., Grasman, R., & Arntz, A. (2020). Schema modes as a common mechanism of change in personality pathology and functioning: Results from a randomized controlled trial. *Behaviour Research & Therapy, 126,* Article 103553. https://doi.org/10.1016/j.brat.2020.103553

Young, J.E., Klosko, J.S., & Weishaar, M.E. (2003). *Schema therapy: A practitioner's guide.* Guilford Press.

Young, J.E., Klosko, J.S., & Weishaar, M.E. (2020). *Schemagerichte therapie: Handboek voor therapeuten [Schema therapy: A practitioner's guide].* Bohn Stafleu van Loghum.

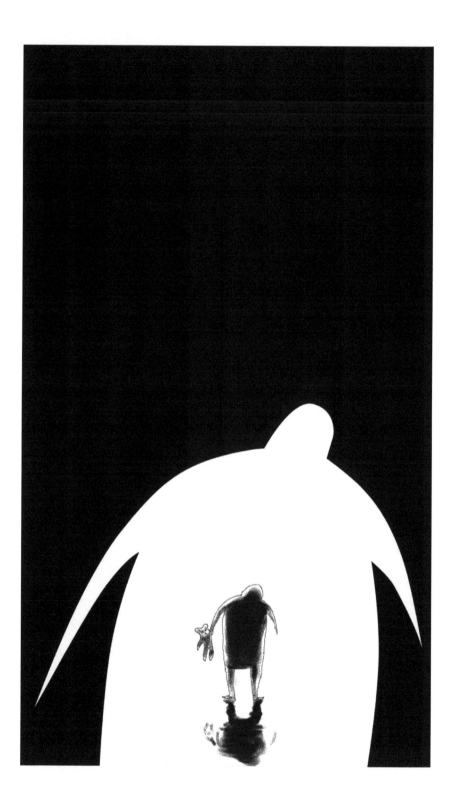

Chapter 2

Art therapy working methods

Summary

Art therapy involves methodical, focused interventions with art materials, tools, and techniques. The client gains physical, sensory, emotional, and cognitive experiences during this process. Art therapy aims at initiating processes of change, development, and/or acceptance through visual artwork (such as painting, drawing, and working with clay, wood, or stone). What makes art therapy special is that the work is tangible and concrete. The client can let it go, put it away, look back on it and experience what it is like to do things differently. Art therapy is experienced by many clients as a direct route to deeper layers of feeling. It confronts them with maladaptive and adaptive patterns in thinking, feeling, and acting within a relatively safe situation and offers them opportunities to explore and possibly change these patterns.

DOI: 10.4324/9781003456988-2

2.1 Modi setup in pictures (minimum two sessions)

Description

The therapist gives a brief introduction to the different modes and asks which one can one recognize more or less in oneself, for example, the Abandoned, Angry, or Lonely Child, the Punishing or Demanding Parent, or the Distant or Detached Protector. Also reflect on the position of the Healthy Adult. Pair this with a recent situation if necessary to make it concrete.

1. The question to the client is to choose the mode in which he (at that moment) most recognizes himself. Work out this mode with clay. Put this mode in the form of a human figure. Give this mode an appearance, pose, and size appropriate to this mode. Consider a lying, sitting, or standing figure. What expression and what effect fit it? What emotion does it convey? You have 15–20 minutes for this. You can use different colors of clay.
2. Now make a statuette of another mode that comes up after making the first one. Again, see how to shape this most appropriately. Again, you have 15–20 minutes.
3. Repeat this so that you end up with a group of different modes, at least a child mode, a parent mode, a protector mode, and a Healthy Adult mode.
4. Now dwell on what these figures do to each other, on what relationship they are to each other, and express this relationship between them by placing them in a certain way relative to each other on a surface (board or sheet of paper). Find the most appropriate arrangement. Take five minutes to do this.

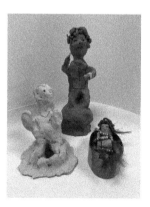

Offer the working method step by step and take two sessions for this, for example, so that the client can pay attention to each clay figure.

The debrief also requires ample time.

AIM

- Gaining insight into one's own patterns of feeling and behavior.
- Gaining insight into what position(s) one usually takes (what does the client show a lot and what does he show little? In other words, which mode does he recognize most and which mode does he avoid most).
- Examining the mutual dynamics of the modes and the different needs one has.

Connection to healthy ego functions

- Personality integration and the formation of a self-image.
- Contact with one's own feelings/needs and those of others.
- Healthy internal dialogue.

Materials

Clay: chamotte clay coarse and fine, multiple colors. Clay board and clay tools.

Group/pair/individual

- Group.
- Individually in the group.
- Individually.

Further details

- The therapist might provide additional information about the different types of schema modes:
- Vulnerable Child, Angry Child, Enraged Child, Impulsive Child, Undisciplined Child, Happy Child.
- Compliant Surrenderer, Detached Protector, Detached Self-Soother, Self-Aggrandizer, Bully and Attack Mode.
- Punitive Parent, Demanding Parent.
- Healthy Adult.

In each mode, the person has typical thoughts, beliefs, and behaviors. The same behavior can occur in different modes but has very different meanings in them. Each mode requires its own approach.

In all kinds of situations, modes can be triggered that determine thinking and behavior from past experiences. These modes get in the way of a functional response in the here and now.

This working method is consistent with a Gestalt therapeutic framework.

EVALUATION

- Describe in the order in which you made them what the different modes look like individually.
- What is important about it in terms of design?
- What mode first came to your mind and what does this tell you? And next?
- What do your different modes do to each other? In what relationship have you placed them in relation to each other? Is there a little or a lot of distance? How would you describe the contact between the modes?
- Ask for a dialogue between the various modes: "If one mode said something, who would say what? And what would this one say?" Ask the client to say this out loud from the figure of the mode. Pay attention to non-verbal signals. You can often see that there is an initial reaction that is not yet uttered (or immediately censored internally).
- Which of the other modes would answer? (Possibly have them written down so the words don't "dissipate.")
- This dialogue might be explored further.
- Which of the modes do you know best of yourself/which side do you show more often (group members may give feedback on this)? Which side less?
- Is the setup all right as it stands right now? Or would you rather change anything? Move the figures into the more desirable arrangement. How does it feel now?
- What is it like to look at this now with some distance (literally)? What insight does this give you?
- What Healthy Adult message can you get out of this? (If necessary, write it down again.)

2.2 Future view Healthy Adult

Description

Describe the future as you would like it to be. In doing so, also describe whether you have achieved your goals or are in emotional balance. Based on this, create an image or fragment that is meaningful or summarizes it. Then, write a letter from the future to your present self.

AIM

- Dialogue with yourself.
- Focused on value(s).

Connection to healthy ego functions

- Healthy internal dialogue.
- Seeking enjoyment and fulfillment in a mature way.

Materials

Pastel chalk or paint.

Group/pair/individual

- Individually in the group.
- Individually.

Further details

The final letter can be used as homework if necessary. The next time, the letter will be discussed.

EVALUATION

- Describe what your picture of the future looks like in your mind.
- How did you describe this?
- What part of it did you choose as the "core"?
- How did it feel to make this?
- Would you like to read your letter to yourself? (Do this with attention to being calm, use of voice, keeping in touch, and so on.)
- What is it like to do this? What do you feel about it?
- What are you getting out of it? (Select key sentence from letter.)

2.3 Two colors: Positive and negative

Description

Choose two colors of paint, one as a positive color and one as a negative color. The positive color represents positive emotions; you may, for example, choose a color you like. The other color represents negative emotions, which may be, for example, a color you find ugly or a color you associate with negative emotions.

You are going to make two paintings using these two colors. First, you will make one, which will take a maximum of 20 minutes. The work may be abstract or figurative. Fill the whole sheet and decide yourself how to use the colors and how much of each color. You may mix the colors if you like, but you don't have to.

Then, we look together at what strikes us about the use of color, the division of the surface, the meaning, and what else we can see. From there, you give yourself an assignment for the second piece of work in which you will use the colors in a different way. You work on this piece for a maximum of 20 minutes too.

AIM

- Gaining insight into your own patterns of emotion regulation.
- Emotion regulation.
- Taking charge of your own process.

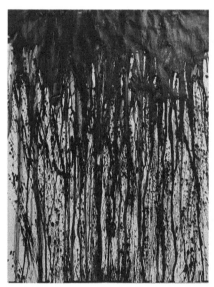 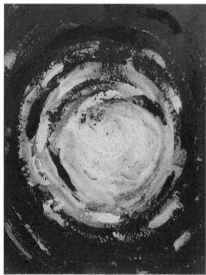

Connection to healthy ego functions

- Healthy emotion regulation.
- Contact with one's own feelings/needs and those of others.
- Healthy internal dialogue.

Materials

Acrylic paints, brushes, masking tape, two sheets of painting paper per person (50 × 65 cm).

Group/pair/individual

- Individually in the group.
- Individually.

Further details

The group can actively think along with each other when looking at the first piece of work. Explain about looking out loud, not filling in but observing and giving one's own impression and maybe checking with the creator.

There is also the possibility of creating multiple versions. Just search until you find the ideal balance.

EVALUATION

Intermediate reflection

- What tells you what is the positive color and what is the negative one?
- How are the two colors distributed?
- What is the emotional image of the work?
- What did you experience while painting? And is this reflected in the work?
- How would you actually like the division?
- What would a Healthy Adult division look like?
- What is your plan for the second piece of work?

Final evaluation

- What was it like making the second work?
- What do you think of the result?
- What emotional image does the work have now?
- Are you satisfied or would you like to try another way? (A third and fourth experiment is also possible in a subsequent session.)

2.4 Acrylic pouring: Playing from the Happy Child

Description

The assignment consists of pouring acrylic paint. Mix the acrylic paint with water in cups. The more you dilute the paint, the more the paint will run. Each thickness of paint gives a different effect. Pour the diluted paint over your canvas/sheet. You can experiment with this, for example:

- by mixing different colors;
- by mixing the colors very lightly, creating a marbled effect; or
- by mixing other materials such as glitter or beads in with the paint.

You can also use a straw or a hair dryer to spread the paint further.

Start playing and experimenting with the paint, the colors, and the effects of the paint in combination with other materials, and see if you can manage to enjoy it/be absorbed in it.

AIM

- Letting go of control.
- Experimenting and discovering and thus connecting with the Happy Child.

Connection to healthy ego functions

- Seeking enjoyment and fulfillment in a mature way.

Materials

Acrylic paint, cups, stirrers/spoons, painting canvas/wooden boards (possibly thick cardboard), glitter/beads (or other materials appropriate for experimenting with paint), straws, hair dryer, water, possibly pouring medium/varnish.

Adding hair oil may have a nice effect as well; this creates circles in the paint, and it smells nice. Adding acrylic pouring medium or varnish makes the paint even smoother.

Group/pair/individual

- Subgroups/twos or threes.
- Individually in the group.
- Individually.

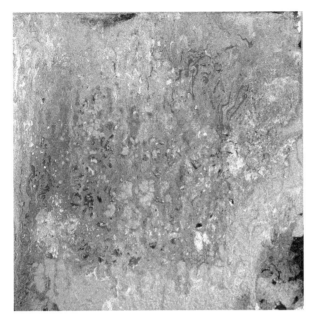

Sculptural acrylic pouring.

Further details

For clients with a high Perfectionist Over Controller, this working method may be a bit more difficult. In this case, the exercise is mainly focused on letting go of the Over Controller and the Demanding Parent; making contact with the Happy Child is often still too difficult.

For clients with schema inferiority/shame in combination with a Demanding Parent, this assignment may create a tendency to strongly compare one's own work to that of others. Here, it is important to emphasize or focus on what the client likes in his own work.

It is nice to take a picture of the work on completion and have the work looked at again after a week. As it dries, the paint often reshapes as well. Looking back at the work often gives a good Happy Child reaction.

EVALUATION

- What was it like to do this?
- What was it like to muck around and make a mess?
- What did you notice about yourself while performing the exercise?
- What modes have you encountered?

- (How) Did you manage to let go of the parent or protector mode?
- Have you felt your Happy Child and if so, at what time?
- What did you notice in contact with your group members?
- What do you like about your own piece of work and what do you like about someone else's?

2.5 Inside and outside

Description

Large sheets of paper are available (A2 size). On these are the outlines of a torso with enough white space around it. You can also have the client's torso drawn. For doing this, have the client stand with his back against a wall, with the sheet of paper behind his head and shoulders, and have someone with whom the client feels sufficiently at ease outline the silhouette with a pencil.

Clients are asked how they feel inside and how they express themselves to the outside world. Inside the outline the inner world is reflected, outside the outline one can represent how he shows himself to the outside world.

This can be done by means of shapes, colors, or words.

AIM

- Getting in touch with one's own feelings.
- Awareness of the importance of congruence between the inner/outer world; integration self-image and emotions.

Connection to healthy ego functions

- Personality integration and the formation of a self-image.
- Healthy emotion regulation.
- Healthy internal dialogue.

Materials

Various drawing and painting materials such as pastels, crayons, paints, pencils, and charcoal, paper (A2 size), possibly with an outline of a torso on it.

Group/pair/individual

- Individually in the group.

Example outline of torso.

Further details

The working method focuses on insight and can therefore be used at different stages of the therapy. For example, the assignment can be repeated after a few sessions to reveal differences between the beginning and the end of therapy. Moreover, it can help clients to see that other group members also struggle with feelings they keep inside.

The elaboration can also give an insight into the (multidisciplinary) care/ treatment team, and including the obtained "inside-outside self-images" in the team meeting may be considered. The pieces of work can represent and clarify the clients' self-image.

This working method is suitable for clients who are capable of self-reflection.

EVALUATION

After the assignment, all sheets with the torsos are hung on the wall and discussed. When doing so, also explicitly question other group members (if any):

- What stands out in the work?
- Is there a big difference to be noticed between the inner and outer world?
- Which colors did you use in your inner world and which ones in your outer world?
- At what moments in daily life is there a particular difference between your inner and outer world? What do you do in those moments?
- Do you pay much attention to your feelings inside? If not, why do you think you give this feeling no/little attention?

2.6 Happy Child assignment for someone else

Description

Devise a working method for the person sitting on your right. Do this with the Happy Child in mind. What material do you want the other person to work with and in what way? The point is that fun in playing, experimenting, and letting go are leading.

AIM

- Dare to play and experiment.
- Allowing spontaneity.

Connection to healthy ego functions

- Healthy emotion regulation.
- Getting in touch with one's own feelings and needs and those of others.
- Seeking enjoyment and fulfillment in a mature way.

Materials

Free choice, for example, ecoline, water colors, clay, spatial materials, and finger paints.

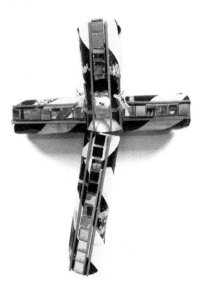

Group/pair/individual

- Group.

Further details

Suggesting something to experience spontaneity is sometimes easier for someone else than for yourself. For the other person, it is easier to go a step further in terms of challenge. Often, someone thinks of something that would be appropriate for himself as well.

When the client has performed the working method, a variation option may be offered. The client may then ask the creator for a variation option or a continuation.

EVALUATION

- What was the working method you were given?
- What was it like to do this?
- Ask the person who came up with the working method for someone else: Would you have liked to do this yourself?

2.7 Circles of power

Description

The therapist begins with the following introduction:

"How much power do you allow your past to have, a trauma, an offender?

"Does your past still influence you? This assignment is about literally stepping out of your schema and out of the influence of your past on your present. It is about taking charge of yourself, taking back control of your life. It is labor that you have to do yourself, no one can do this for you. You used to be dependent but now you can act decisively. Because you are not used to this or have not learned it, we take you by the hand with this assignment, step by step. We work in three phases.

"For the power of your past, we choose the symbol of the circle. A circle because it surrounds you from all sides and there is no way out. All sides are equally powerful. In this assignment, we are going to fill your circle of power, and you are going to gain more insight into what keeps you in your place against your will. However, we are going to break the power of these circles later. In the end you will have new choices."

Phase 1

- First, from several colored sheets of paper choose a color that appeals to you and set the sheet aside for a while. This is your "safe spot." You can also call it your comfortable spot, or the spot where you can relax, or a spot without danger.

- Then, on another sheet (A3 size or slightly smaller) draw a loose circle, it can fill the sheet completely. In the center of this circle draw a small circle, which is your core, your I, your self.
- Then, draw rings around this core that holds you captive. For each ring, choose a different color. Make a legend on the sheet explaining what each color stands for. Examples: guilt, shame, sadness, anger, distrust, abuse, neglect, abandonment, triggers, sounds, persons. Which ring feels closest, which one more on the outside?

The therapist helps the client remember to give the previously discussed details a place. """Could it be that, is it possible that I recognize ...?" The therapist points out that the position of the rings is not so important and that feelings can recur in different layers.

Dwell on the outer circle: this is the circle in which you meet other people. What does the other person get to see or feel from you?

Phase 2

- Now, out of this circle of power, you can cut yourself, your own core, the little circle in the middle with a Stanley knife (it can also be done with a scissors, but a Stanley knife gives a different, more powerful feeling motorically).
- Stick yourself on the sheet chosen previously for the safe, pleasant spot. Here, you now shape the environment (possibly from a "safe spot imagination"). The therapist allows time for you to shape the spot around the cut out bit.
- Then, continue with the circles of power: one by one, you cut apart all the rings but you leave them whole at this point.

AIM

- Addressing trauma.
- Step to the Healthy Adult: taking charge.

Connection to healthy ego functions

- Personality integration and the formation of a self-image.
- Healthy emotion regulation.

Materials

Phase 1: White and colored sheets of paper in different sizes, drawing materials.
Phase 2: Stanley knife, free material.

Group/pair/individual

- Individually in the group.
- Individually.

Further details

This is an assignment for rescripting in art therapy, which is about breaking through persistent schemas such as mistrust/abuse as well as emotional deficit, abandonment, inferiority, or submission. It can also deal with modes that have a hold on someone, for example, a Perfectionist Over Controller or a parent mode. Furthermore, it may also address themes that do not (yet) fit into a schema or mode such as "mother," "anger," "headache," and "abuse."

The prerequisite for this form of work is that the client has an understanding of modes and schemas, of how his past determines his present, that the client can mentalize and is aware of different sides in himself and is also familiar with "safe spot imagination."

Phase 1: In terms of timing, the therapist takes care that the clients do not dwell too long on each ring but fill the circle smoothly so that they are not absorbed in it too much and also to avoid flashbacks. The image of being caught in the circles themselves should not last too long. There is a danger here that powerlessness will be evoked too strongly. It is important that clients leave with the image that they have freed themselves from the circles (Phase 2).

Phase 2: Clients in this phase may have the experience that the circle of power becomes meaningless, subsides, disappears from attention. This is something they often did not think possible, which did not occur in their mindset until now; after all, everything was always related to the known circle of power.

If clients find it difficult to leave the circles whole, the therapist responds with validation, explaining that further work will be done with them, and that at a later time, tearing up or clearing is an option.

Phase 3: Coping rings sometimes do not need anything because they are a consequence of a primary schema. Once that primary schema is dealt with, coping can sometimes naturally diminish or remain "on hold" in the background. In Phase 3, clients may experience that they now have power over the rings and experience their own autonomy in making choices. By cutting the circles loose from each other, air literally comes between them, they lose their rigidity and closedness, and their grip on the client. Physically, clients experience that they are fairly thin, skinny paper rings that they can play with a bit and move around on the table in front of them. This is already part of body-centered rescripting:

moving from rigidity to movement. A fear might be: "What will be left of me?" This means that there is identification with the trauma. As an antidote, the therapist makes sure that the new pleasant spot remains near and in the clients' attention.

EVALUATION

Phase 3

"We are now going to pay attention to the different rings. Each ring needs something different, one may need to be torn up, another cleared, and in what way? Or a ring needs attention, comfort perhaps, because it deals with an important feeling. Some rings need no further action."

The therapist allows the time this takes; this is a coping process that takes some clients longer than others.

"Play around with the circles a bit and end up making two piles: disempowerment/clearing versus recognition, comfort, and care. With each circle, you have to make a choice. How can you as a Healthy Adult take care of your Vulnerable Child right now?"

Recognition, comfort and care: Is there enough comfort, recognition, and care in the new spot or do you want to further shape your spot? You can literally work with a circle on the new sheet if you want to preserve something (e.g., with a deceased person). Or you can create a new piece of work triggered by a circle.

Refuting/clearing: If you want to tear up a ring, do so! The shreds symbolize the past, what happened to you when you had no influence. Now it is your turn, and you may give this past a new shape and meaning. Therefore, you may now do whatever you want with the shreds: throw them away, knead them into clay and throw this lump of clay into the river so that they can flow away, or perhaps you want to make a symbol of strength with them. Anything goes and anything is possible. You determine the Now, in which you may literally make a countermove and step out of the circle that has held you captive for so long.

2.8 Control versus letting go

Description

Divide the group into two subgroups (max. five people per subgroup). Each group has a large sheet of paper hung on the wall.

One group is instructed to work from the theme of "control"; they must first deliberate for five minutes and agree on how they are going to make a landscape together using chalk, marker, ruler, paint, and fine brushes. The other group is instructed to work from the theme of "letting go"; they are not allowed to deliberate. They are instructed to start immediately and work together on an abstract painting using paint, water, sponges, palette knives, and coarse brushes.

Both groups work on this for 20 minutes.

Then the therapist instructs the groups to switch. The group with the theme "control" now continues on the work of the group with the theme "letting go" and vice versa. This is done for another 15–20 minutes.

AIM

- Exploring Happy Child and parent modes.
- Experiencing control and working from agreements and rules.
- Experiencing letting go and allowing play.
- Experimentation.

Connection to healthy ego functions

- Healthy emotion regulation.
- Getting in touch with one's own feelings and needs and those of others.
- Seeking enjoyment and fulfillment in a mature way.

Materials

Gouache or acrylic paint, thick pencils, markers, chalk, large sheet of paper, coarse and fine brushes, sponges, palette knives, dishwashing brush, cups of water, tape, palettes, paper/piece of cloth for the floor, and aprons.

Group/pair/individual

- Subgroups/twos or threes.

Further details

The assignment of letting go is very free. Someone may get stuck quickly because it is difficult to start without agreements or guidelines. The working method may affect everyone differently; therefore, guidance may be needed in letting go. If someone doesn't succeed, they can "join in" or examples can be given of splashing the paint/tearing the paper/mixing paint very thinly or thickly, and so on.

EVALUATION

The evaluation is all about reflecting on what the working method has evoked.

- Did you manage to experiment?
- Did your spontaneity/the Happy Child appear?
- What different things have you tried?
- What was going on in your mind when working freely and when working in a controlled/structured way?
- Was there a difference for you between the free work/letting go and the controlled/structured work?
- What fits you best?
- What would you like to develop more of?
- Are you able to let go completely in everyday life? What do you need for this?
- Would you like to do this more often?

2.9 Crisis drawing

Description

"In this session, we will reflect on an important/significant moment in your life: the moment when you or others decided it was necessary to seek professional help. Today is about the trigger for that.

"Take the sheet of paper in front of you and fold it in half once in both directions (that is, once standing format and once lying format) so that four equal areas remain.

"Number these surfaces from 1 to 4."

Meanwhile, the therapist writes down instructions on the board after the four numbers.

1. What has been the cause/run up for seeking professional help?
2. Situation outline of what has happened (the crisis/offence).
3. Consequences for others.
4. Consequences for myself.

Ask the client to render as clear an image as possible for each item, preferably with as little text as possible. Try to translate it into an image.

It is important that the therapist coordinates the extent to which it is desirable for the client to remain in contact with the therapist for support while working, or whether the client would like to be left alone for a while.

AIM

- Addressing mentalization ability.
- Review of experiences that often involve guilt or shame.
- Formulating intrinsic motivation/treatment goals.

Connection to healthy ego functions

- Healthy internal dialogue.
- Testing reality and assessing situations, conflicts, and relationships.

Materials

Drawing paper (A2 size), charcoal, and kneading eraser.

Group/pair/individual

- Individually in the group.
- Individually.

Further details

The advice is to offer this working method in the early stages of the treatment. It may be especially suitable with the forensic population. In this case, it can be called the "delict drawing," because that is slightly more guiding to establish the relationship to the crime that is central to the conviction, the so-called "index crime" and the conviction. Within the forensic framework, starting quickly with this working method immediately puts on the table where a client stands in his process and can lead to commitment to treatment/art therapy.

EVALUATION

In the evaluation, it is important to pay attention to the process and the choices made. It is also important to pay attention to what may have been left out of the picture.

It is helpful to phase the follow-up discussion by item:

1. What has been the cause/run up?

How is the run up presented? As a causal situation (often a specific short-term situation beforehand and a clear cause-and-effect)? As a reflection of self-insight (often a long-term view in which more responsibility for one's own development is taken)? Who and what have been presented? What meaning is given to this run up?

2. Situation outline of what has happened

What exactly took place? What exactly happened? Did the client present the moment (memory) or did he try to present a clear picture for the viewer? Who and what were presented? What meaning is given to this situation? With what feeling does the client look back on this?

3. Consequences for others

Who has been affected and what are the consequences? Who and what has been presented? What meaning is given to this image and what emotion is experienced with it?

4. Consequences for myself

Who and what has been presented? What does this image mean in terms of intrinsic motivation for the client and how can it best be translated into goals?

General

- What image elements stand out? Is there anything that recurs or is similar in all four drawings? How are the human images (me and the others) depicted?
- What modes have been active in the different situations?
- What modes have been active in rendering and reviewing them?
- In what way does the Healthy Adult give meaning to the situation and how does he integrate it into his own life story?
- In what way should this story be followed up?

2.10 Schema triptych past–present–future

Description

"Divide your sheet into three sections, one titled 'Past,' one titled 'Present,' and one titled 'Future.'"

"You give shape to these three sections in your own way; it can be abstract or figurative, concrete or more from a certain prevailing tone/atmosphere, with, for example, a certain schema as subject."

"The main thing is to depict something about where you came from, where you are now, and where you would like to go."

AIM

- Creating perspective regarding basic needs and the Healthy Adult (future picture).
- Creating one's own empathetic confrontation.
- Dealing with the past.

Connection to healthy ego functions

- Personality integration and the formation of a self-image.
- Contact with one's own feelings/needs and those of others.
- Healthy internal dialogue.

Materials

Drawing or painting paper (50 × 65 cm) and free choice of materials, optionally several materials mixed together; for example, acrylic paint, pastel crayons, crayons, ecoline, collage materials, markers, and/or color pencils.

Group/pair/individual

- Individually in the group.
- Individually.

Further details

If someone has difficulty getting started, it might help to ask him to start with the background, what mood, color, or degree of light and dark suits each part. A more concrete implementation can be made later.

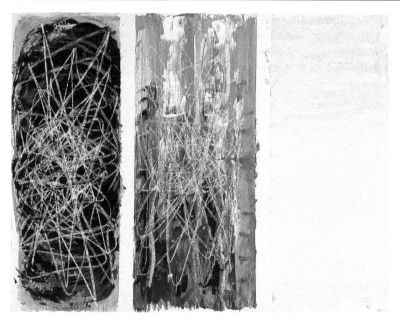

Triptych past–present–future.

EVALUATION

- What would you like to share about your piece of work and the various sections?
- What pattern/schema can be seen in your work?
- What did it take for you to get from the past to the present?
- What do you need to get from the present to the future?
- What would you like to get out of this work?

2.11 Ecoline wet and dry

Description

Make two pieces of work with ecoline. One piece by painting with ecoline on a dry sheet and the other piece by working with ecoline on a sheet that has first been made quite wet with water until there is a puddle of water on it.

You can decide what you make yourself, focus on what you feel while working, and observe your own inclinations and thoughts. A tip is not to work too fast when working with the wet sheet; slow down and watch what happens on the paper.

AIM

- Emotion regulation.
- Attention/attentiveness.
- Adaptive skills, responding from what you notice.

Connection to healthy ego functions

- Healthy emotion regulation.
- Healthy internal dialogue.
- Seeking enjoyment and fulfillment in a mature way.

Materials

Painting paper (50 × 65 cm), several colors of ecoline, water, and watercolor brushes.

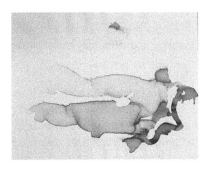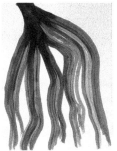

Ecoline wet and dry.

Group/pair/individual

- Individually in the group.
- Individually.

Further details

The exercise is suitable for those with high control needs. When the work is dry, the result can also be included in the experience.

Sometimes, people need one more try at doing the wet work in which they are more allowed to let things happen and do less to control them, so they learn to respond to the material and its properties.

EVALUATION

- What was it like to do this?
- What happened?
- What did you notice in yourself? What was your inclination?
- What did you do?
- What effect did this have?
- Which piece of work do you like better/did you more enjoy making?
- What was your expectation beforehand and how did it turn out?
- What worked best and how did you find out?
- What do you get out of this experience? How do you translate this to yourself and your patterns?

2.12 Edward Hopper: Writing assignment

Description

The therapist has paintings by painter Edward Hopper printed on a table (depicting one person). Discuss the mood of the paintings and what they may evoke/express.

1. The client is invited to choose a painting that most appeals to him. The therapist also chooses one work that appeals to him. The choice can be briefly explained, but that is not necessary. The assignment is to write a short story based on the chosen picture, describing a "problem." Provide the following structure: Who is this person, where is he, what is going on, why is this person alone, how does he feel? Take 10–15 minutes for this and swap sheets.
2. The therapist and the client read each other's stories.
3. The follow-up task is to finish each other's text with the goal of solving the problem for the main character. In this, offer helping questions: What does this person need? Who can help him? What needs to be done? Again, 10–15 minutes is allotted for this.

Finally, both read the stories to each other. First the therapist re-reads the client's own piece to the client, with the sequel written by the therapist. Then vice versa.

AIM

- Giving words to (sad) emotions.
- Recognizing emotional needs (in oneself and in the other person).
- Recognizing and describing fulfillment of emotional needs.

Connection to healthy ego functions

- Personality integration and the formation of a self-image.
- Contact with one's own feelings/needs and those of others.
- Healthy internal dialogue.

Materials

A series of distinctive paintings by painter Edward Hopper depicting (prefer-ably) one person in a room, paper (A4 size) (this may be line paper, but need not be), and writing utensils (pen, pencil).

Group/pair/individual

- Group.
- Subgroups/twos or threes.
- Individually.

Further details

The therapist may choose to explain in advance, or when exchanging texts, the five basic needs from schema therapy (safety and attachment, autonomy, emotion expression, spontaneity and play, and realistic boundaries) to help the client come up with what the other person's main character might need.

The therapist may choose to invite the client in advance to consciously put his own experience (or missed basic need) into the story.

The description invites the client to describe a "problem," but this can also be omitted by writing "just" a story.

This can therefore become a positive story in which there are no missed basic needs to "fix." But again, you can ask the questions: What does this person need? Who can help them with this? What needs to be done?

EVALUATION

- What was it like to do this?
- How did you give words to your main character's emotions?
- Do you recognize yourself in the main character?
- Do you recognize your own needs?
- Could you recognize the (missed) needs of the other person's main character?
- What did you find the tricky/easy part of the assignment (describing the problem or solution)? What caused this?
- Optional: What mode is the main character in?
- What would be a response to this from the Healthy Adult?

2.13 Island assignment

Description

In front of the group is a large sheet covering one or more large tables. The group assignment is to make one island together. Anything goes on the island. Here, the clients are asked to make at least one spot on the island for themselves and then to collectively see what needs there are and what can be added to the island.

Beforehand, it may be discussed what kind of island the group wants to make and what landscape elements could have a place on it. This can start with brainstorming: Is the island located in northern or southern waters? Are there rivers, lakes? Are there mountains, rocks, fields, and so on?

The instruction might be given that in designing they concentrate first on the shape of the island itself, the landscape elements in it, and the surrounding waters. This creates a base from which each can begin to make their own spot.

AIM

- Exploring one's own and common needs.
- Practicing stating one's own limits.
- Allowing play/spontaneity.

Connection to healthy ego functions

- Contact with one's own feelings/needs and those of others.
- Seeking enjoyment and fulfillment in a mature way.

Materials

Large sheet of paper, e.g., 80 × 150 cm, various drawing materials (pastel crayons may be most suitable but pencils/ markers/crayons may also be considered).
Possibly painting materials as well.

Group/pair/individual

• Group.
• Subgroups/twos or threes.

Further details

The implementation of the assignment varies with the composition of the group. Depending on the type of clients and problems, there is a difference in how the cooperation and the product is initiated.

Making the basic elements of the island together first, prevents the elaboration from remaining too superficial. One must be able to go into it, as it were, while working on it so that it comes "alive."

While working, one option is to give clients a different challenge, appropriate to their own schema dynamics. For example, consider mandatory collaboration on framed parts of their own, or instructing clients to speak out more about their needs for the shared part.

EVALUATION

• What do you notice about the island?
• What did you notice in yourself or in the other person while working?
• How do you look at your own spot? Is this a nice safe spot for you? Has it become what you had in mind?
• What modes were triggered during collaboration?
• Did you stick to your own plan or were you influenced by your group members?
• How did you challenge your own schemas in this assignment?

2.14 Nice place for the Vulnerable Child

Description

Prior to this exercise the client has already shaped a figurine of his Vulnerable Child, preferably in spatial material. If not, this could be the first part of the working method.

Create a nice place for your Vulnerable Child. Where would this child like to be? What would it need? Think of a literal environment as well as of elements that the Vulnerable Child would like or enjoy.

Make sure you use materials that the Vulnerable Child would also like. What colors, what can the material have?

Always take a moment to place the figurine of the Vulnerable Child in the created environment and take a look at how the work looks then. How does it feel and what else might the Vulnerable Child need in this nice place?

AIM

- Reflecting on one's own needs.
- Learning to care for the Vulnerable Child.
- Developing the Healthy Adult.

Connection to healthy ego functions

- Healthy emotion regulation.
- Contact with one's own feelings/needs and those of others.
- Healthy internal dialogue.

Materials

A wide range of materials can be used in this assignment, preferably materials with more soft qualities.

Examples include fabric, collage materials, pastel crayons, (water) paint, felt, cotton wool, natural materials, and feathers.

Group/pair/individual

- Individually in the group.
- Individually.

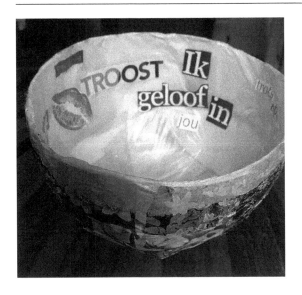

Further details

As a variation, group members can be asked to make something to add to the safe place a client has made. Here, the client can decide what he wants to add to his created place and in what way he wants to do this. The goal of the intervention is to give the client new insights into what he might need.

EVALUATION

After having placed the Vulnerable Child:

- What do you see when you look at the piece of work?
- How does the place feel now?
- Is there anything else missing? Anything else you would like to add?

At the end:

- How does it feel to see the figurine now?
- How would the Vulnerable Child feel now?
- What elements could you also apply in daily life to take good care of yourself?

2.15 Error fun

Description

The therapist introduces the term: "error fun"!

For many, fear of failure is a familiar phenomenon: the fear that "it" could go wrong, whatever "it" might be. This can manifest itself in the fear of being found out, the fear of causing something to fail, the fear of being a failure, or some other form in which something doesn't work out or you do not feel you are good or worthy enough.

Within schema therapy there are several schemas and modes that have taken root in you as part of yourself: the feeling of not doing the right thing or of not being good enough fits in with them.

How great it would be if we could stop talking about the fear of failure but could find joy in the mistakes we make.

The next assignment is about this and is an invitation to explore what happens when things are allowed to fail. What happens when everything goes horribly wrong? What happens when you may not have a plan in advance?

In this assignment, you send your Healthy Adult on vacation and get to mess around and play with paint in a carefree way. Or maybe you just want to enjoy yourself: that's okay too!

Please note: This is not an assignment in which your painting must fail, because in that case you would set yourself another task. Feel free to explore what happens when you follow your impulses and do not care about the result and everything can fail or it does not have to be anything special. Take about 10 minutes.

AIM

- Awareness of the impact of the presence of parenting modes or over-compensating modes.
- Making contact with and enjoying the Happy Child mode.

Connection to healthy ego functions

- Healthy emotion regulation.
- Contact with one's own feelings/needs and those of others.
- Seeking enjoyment and fulfillment in a mature way.

Materials

Drawing paper (A1 or A2 size, preferably on an easel or taped to a wall), paint, brushes/spatulas, painter's tape, bowls for water.

Group/pair/individual

- Subgroups/twos or threes.
- Individually in the group.
- Individually.

Further details

You can direct the instruction a little more toward making contact with the Happy Child mode (playing) or have it focus more on the Enraged/Angry or Impulsive Child mode (affect regulation), depending on the client and the underlying needs. When more contact is made with the Angry/Enraged/Impulsive Child modes, it is important to be able to *contain/guide* this well as a therapist by making sure in advance that no "damage" (paint stains) is done and to guide the client back to the Healthy Adult mode upon completion of the work.

This working method is of specific interest to clients with a strong Demanding or Punitive Parent mode.

Practice shows that clients who have had difficulty in learning to make contact with their Happy Child mode, and in whom the emotional inhibition schema is active, often finish their artwork with a large cross across their work. It is interesting to pay attention to this in the follow-up discussion. What meaning does the client himself give to this cross as it is incorporated into the image?

EVALUATION

- In the follow-up discussion, it is important to ask mainly process questions: How was the working method experienced? What was it like to do this? Were choices made? On what basis were choices made?
- Was the client able to let go of the outcome well? Were there things the client noticed about his own thoughts or feelings?
- Which mode was let go and which one was activated?
- As a Healthy Adult, what can you get out of the insights gained from this working method?
- How do you look at the final result and what title would you give it?

2.16 No rules

Description

Tape your paper to the wall and prepare a palette with different colors of paint. Stand in front of your paper and start experimenting with the paint.

You can splash, smear, and so on. There are no rules in this working method.

You get to do what you feel like doing!

Take 10 minutes to do this.

This is followed by imagining a carefree moment from your childhood: "Stand still for a moment and put down what you are doing. Stand firmly on your feet ... relax your body ... feel your shoulders drop and feel your feet firmly on the ground. If you like, you can close your eyes. Now go back in time in your thoughts and recall a moment from your childhood when you felt free and carefree. Maybe you are playing or running ... and now go all the way back to this moment and feel what it does to you. What kind of feeling does it create in your body? Try to hold on to this feeling and try to keep the moment with you now open your eyes."

After this, continue with paint splattering/painting (20 minutes). Depending on what the client wants, he may also model something of the moment from childhood.

AIM

- Addressing the Happy Child.
- Letting go of control.
- Being able to experiment.

Connection to healthy ego functions

- Contact with one's own feelings/needs and those of others.
- Seeking enjoyment and fulfillment in a mature way.

Materials

Gouache/acrylic paint, large format paper (at least 50 × 65 cm), brushes, tape, palettes, paper/piece of cloth for the floor, aprons, bowls of water.

Group/pair/individual

- Individually in the group.

Further details

The assignment is very free. Someone may get stuck quickly because it is difficult to start without guidelines. The working method may not have the same impact on everyone; therefore, personal guidance is needed in getting disengaged. If someone does not succeed, then others can "join in" or examples can be given of splashing the paint/tearing the paper/mixing paint very thinly or thickly, and so on.

It is recommended to offer this assignment later in therapy, when the client is already somewhat comfortable in the work space/therapy.

This working method is not suitable for clients in whom its free nature could lead to undesirable disruption and excessive tension.

Variations include:

- Turning on music during therapy/letting the client choose music that relaxes or disengages them.
- Have the clients take turns doing a "movement," which the others must then imitate on their sheet (e.g., moving the brush up and down quickly on the paper, applying paint with fingers). In this way, the group takes its members in tow.

EVALUATION

- Did you manage to experiment?
- Did a sense of spontaneity and play, the Happy Child, emerge?
- What different things have you tried?
- What went on in your head?
- Was there a difference between before and after imagination?
- Are you able to let go completely in everyday life? What do you need for this? And would you like to do this more often?

2.17 Group disruption assignment

Description

Each participant comes up with three disruption assignments and writes them on a note. The notes go into a jar. Examples of disruption assignments are "paint it yellow," "give your piece of work to your left neighbor," "write your life motto on it."

- Each client starts with self-selected material on his own sheet of paper for about 5 to 10 minutes.
- Each client can then take a note from the jar whenever he wants and read it aloud.
- Everyone should follow this assignment as much as possible.

The focus is on play and experimenting.

Overall assignment: Always choose how you want to do the assignment, keep doing it from within yourself, and keep looking at the whole while modeling it.

AIM

- Staying balanced when thrown off balance (Healthy Adult).
- Increasing flexibility/developing adaptive skills (Healthy Adult).
- Increasing self-expression, spontaneity, and play (Happy Child).

Connection to healthy ego functions

- Contact with one's own feelings/needs and those of others.
- Healthy internal dialogue.
- Seeking enjoyment and fulfillment in a mature way.

Materials

Drawing and painting materials, collage materials, scissors, glue, paper.

Group/pair/individual

- Group.
- Subgroups/twos or threes.
- Individually in the group.

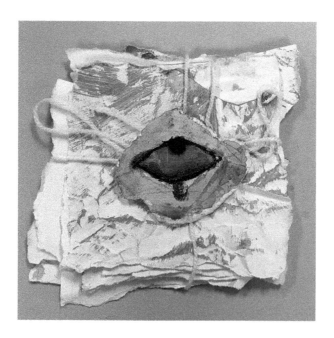

Further details

It is important to emphasize self-direction and that clients are allowed to state their boundaries. If a client doesn't want to do something, he does not have to do it. Clients are allowed to put their own twist on the assignment.

By doing it this way, fear of losing control can be curbed and clients can experience more room for experimentation, each one at their own level.

EVALUATION

- What did you experience while doing it?
- What new things did you experience?
- How did you take charge/guard boundaries yourself?
- How did your Healthy Adult side help you in this working method?
- What do you think of the result?
- What do you want to take away from this experience and how can you apply it outside of therapy?

2.18 Same piece of work

Description

We are going to do a working method with clay. In a minute, you are going to clay in silence for 10 minutes. The only assignment here is that at the end you will all have made the same piece of work. You cannot consult with each other or point at each other, but you can look at each other's work.

This assignment is about the interaction between you and the other person, about leading and following, and about basic needs and how your Healthy Adult can take care of this. (See also Haeyen, 2018c, 12.4, p. 296.)

AIM

- Getting in touch with your needs in interaction and taking care of this.
- Setting boundaries.
- Attuning to the other person.

Connection to healthy ego functions

- Contact with one's own feelings/needs and those of others.
- Healthy internal dialogue.
- Testing reality and assessing situations, conflicts, and relationships.
- Seeking enjoyment and fulfillment in a mature way.

Materials

Clay.

Group/pair/individual

- Group.

Further details

In this assignment, clients experience the dilemma of the "clash of needs." The basic needs described in schema therapy are opposites of each other. Connection and autonomy (the needs of the first and second domain) are sometimes mutually exclusive, just as realistic boundaries versus self-expression or play (third, fourth, and fifth domain) are opposites of each other.

This plays a part not only in the interaction, but also in the internal dialogue: "Do I want to connect or do I choose my own form? Will I move with the other person or do I take the risk that no one imitates me and I remain alone?"

Clients really need the basis of a Healthy Adult to benefit from this assignment, and the group must be safe.

If necessary, the therapist can do a mindfulness exercise beforehand while kneading the clay so that the clients make contact with themselves and their hands and do not get lost in the interaction.

During the exercise, the therapist frequently indicates the time remaining and, if necessary, repeats the assignment: "Make the same piece of work!" This may involve the therapist stepping into the role of an Authoritarian Boss or a Demanding Parent. It is important to explain this at the end and "step out of the role" for the clients.

The task is intensive and evocative; therefore, it is better not to have too large a group, a maximum of eight people. The Compliant Surrender mode (constantly following) and the Self-Aggrandizer mode (constantly leading) are clearly challenged in this working method. Many parent modes also come into play (I'm not doing it right).

The Angry or Detached Protector (stupid assignment/makes no difference to me anyway). Schemas such as dependence, submission, self-sacrifice, inferiority, abandonment, social isolation, and emotional deficit may be triggered.

Variations: If the assignment is judged to be very stressful, the therapist may say in advance that everyone can make their own piece of work in the second round. However, the risk is that with the stress the essence of the assignment and its power of expression will also be weakened. In that case, it is better to bring in the second assignment unannounced as a "recovery moment" afterward. Another possibility is to continue with making a piece of work that does *not* resemble the other person's work. Then clients see similarities everywhere and that too can be interesting, for example, when it comes to "submission"–counter-submission; a client with the schema submission who chooses the schema "insisting on your rights" or the Self-Aggrandizer mode as overcompensation.

EVALUATION

- Start with the open question, "This was the assignment, who would like to respond to it?"
- Then different moments during the assignment are discussed, what specifically happened in the clay (in medium language, for example, "you suddenly turned it into a ball and I didn't like that").
- What was the consequence of the interaction? What did you feel and think? What modes play a role here?

The therapist makes sure that during the follow-up discussion the dilemma of basic needs becomes palpable for the clients: you can never get this "right" in a group or in a family, there is a constant search for balance, there is ease and discomfort at the same time. The Healthy Adult can live with this continuous dynamic and even experience pleasure in it. But it does mean that sometimes we have to endure discomfort, get angry, or feel abandoned. Welcome to real life!

- How do you deal with the clash of needs and still get pleasure and fulfillment out of it?

2.19 Homage to yourself

Description

Step 1

In this working method, a self-portrait is central. Imagine that an ode to you is being made, a homage to yourself. You are being portrayed; all your (beautiful) qualities are being highlighted. The portrait may be supplemented with symbols or other additions that do justice to you.

You are going to make this piece of work with crayons: you can use color and you can make a semi-abstract representation. Use your creativity. The advantage of crayons is that you do not have to draw in great detail, and you can work more crudely. So, the trick is to highlight important features of yourself well.

Make sure you know how to portray yourself on paper in such a way that you can be proud of.

Step 2

Introduce Step 2 only after Step 1 has been carried out.

Fill the sheet (the entire background) with watercolors and combine the two to make one picture.

AIM

- Inner dialogue/self-reflection.
- Learning to validate oneself.
- More positive self-image.

Connection to healthy ego functions

- Personality integration and the formation of a self-image.
- Healthy internal dialogue.

Materials

Watercolor paper (A3 size), crayons/oil pastels, watercolors, palette, brushes, bowls for water.

Group/pair/individual

- Individually in the group.
- Individually.

Further details

This working method can emphasize a more ego-invigorating, supportive approach. With Cluster C issues this can focus on "What are you really proud of?" For Cluster B problems the focus could be more on validating any self-glorifying qualities: "What would you really like to see reflected in a homage to yourself? After all, no one knows your strong points as well as you know them and would like to see reflected."

Clients are often surprised by the effect of watercolors (sometimes activating the Happy Child). This has a positive effect on the assessment of the final result and indirectly also positively reinforces self-esteem.

EVALUATION

- How did you depict yourself? It is important to ask what needed attention and what was added to the image.
- To what extent are these qualities seen and recognized by others?
- If it was difficult to make a homage to oneself: What hinders you? What modes hinder you from being allowed to be distinctly proud?

- It is interesting to then comment on characteristics of the Happy Child: feels loved, praised, satisfied, carefree, worries little about possible judgments of others, and so on. To what extent do you succeed in making contact with the Happy Child within yourself?
- What was the effect of the layer of watercolor paint?
- What do you take away from this working method or its follow-up talk into your daily life?

2.20 Ideal Parent

Description

First focus on the Vulnerable Child. Do this through imagination or via a previously created image.

Now that you have your Vulnerable Child in view (or in mind), you can follow up with an image of an ideal, a good, a helping parent figure.

Create a picture of what your Ideal Parent would have looked like. This is a figure who does not resemble your own parents, but who may have very different characteristics. Characteristics that exactly fit the needs of this child (of you at that moment).

If possible, the therapist makes a "reversal" of the situation seen here verbally or in guided imagination. For example, in the case of a lonely child: "Then I see before me a mother who is not sitting on the couch with a headache, but who notices that her child is sad. She comes to the child and communicates that she notices her." The therapist monitors the client's reaction and may, in consultation with the client, adjust the image, if necessary, so that it becomes appropriate for the client.

The therapist asks if the client could portray this figure, brainstorms about the choice of materials or makes suggestions.

AIM

- Developing compassion for the Vulnerable Child and his needs.
- Getting in touch with Healthy Adult skills.
- Being able to accept help.

Connection to healthy ego functions

- Personality integration and the formation of a self-image.
- Contact with one's own feelings/needs and those of others.
- Testing reality and assessing situations, conflicts, and relationships.

Materials

Collage material, scissors, glue, or just free material.

Group/pair/individual

- Individually in the group.
- Individually.

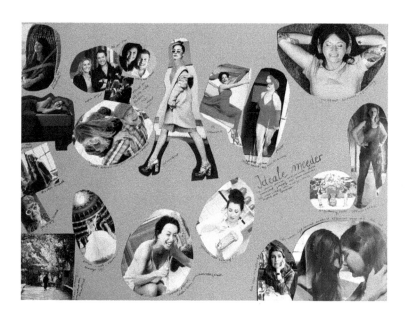

Further details

This assignment is for clients who have previously portrayed a Vulnerable Child or a traumatic situation, or have gone through rescripting.

It may also be appropriate if a client is currently in contact with a need (toward group members or therapists).

In addition to the parent modes, schema therapy often speaks of the Good, the Ideal, or the Helping Parent. This assignment is about exploring what a parent should or could have done at a particular age, in a particular situation, or throughout childhood. Age is important because behavior and needs change as the child grows.

Later in life, a need perceived as inadequate (such as wanting to sit on the therapist's lap) can be explained by this. Coming to understand this increases compassion for the Vulnerable Child.

The Ideal Parent is a precursor to the eventual Healthy Adult; it is used to explore human traits that the client ultimately wants/needs to internalize.

Another part of the Ideal Parent traits remains interactive, in that the Healthy Adult also has needs (support, touch, listening ear, etc.) that he can ask for.

An intermediate step for the client might be the realization that from the Dependent Child position he may have tried very cleverly to take care of himself, but could not actually succeed or that these attempts have led to dysfunctional coping in adulthood.

The client's own real parents who could not provide the protection, boundaries, support, or other needs remain intact as memories. This is so as not to confuse the client's perception of his past by having a real parent suddenly do that what he or she could not or did not do then.

If the client has resistance to the word "parent" from loyalty or from a schema (distrust, abandonment, emotional deficit), "figure," "person," or "animal" can also be chosen.

Clients with schemas such as self-sacrifice or distrust and the Self-Aggrandizer or Self-Soother mode often prefer to step into the role of Healthy Adult themselves and avoid accepting help. Here, it is important to nuance the extent to which this breaches or affirms schemas.

This assignment may also be seen as part of rescripting. From here, rescripting may also be employed, imaginarily or otherwise.

EVALUATION

In the follow-up discussion, the therapist and client/group look at the piece of work together. The therapist explores body reaction: Does calmness, satisfaction, happiness, relaxation occur in the body?

The therapist makes sure that no repetition of the schema has surreptitiously crept into the image. For example, when the client endures a discomfort because things are no different from how they were in the past. In this case, the therapist makes sure that the image changes so that rescripting really happens.

For example, in the case of an emotional deficit: the client makes a parent out of clay, but the Vulnerable Child figurine does not lean against the parent figure. The client explains, "Yes, there was just no other way, the clay was not stable enough, the parent would fall over."

The therapist makes the client aware that this could be a repetition of the relationship with his real mother. The client is invited to recount a situation when this was so.

Then the therapist makes the distinction between then and now very explicit by assuming the role of the Ideal Parent, speaking to the client in this way and, in agreement with the client, also depicting this in the material/piece of work. The client is asked if this is appropriate for him and if the Vulnerable Child can now entrust himself to the parent. This ultimately creates an appropriate image.

2.21 You and the causer of your schema

Description

This working method consists of three steps and can be performed after the client has become familiar with the concept of "schemas."

Step 1: Imagination

First, the client focuses on his breathing and can close his eyes. If this does not feel comfortable, he can also choose to look at a fixed point on the table or the floor.

The therapist then pays attention to proper sitting posture, abdominal breathing, body scan (feet, legs, buttocks, bottom, back, abdomen, chest, shoulders, head, jaws, frown).

The client(s) are asked to follow the story and listen carefully, to see if a picture can emerge from the words.

"You have been introduced to schemas, and we know that these deep-seated beliefs are often formed early in our lives. Often adults, and especially one or both parents, are involved in the creation of these schemas. My question to you is to go back to such a moment in which your own schema became active. You can think of a situation that had a significant impact on you, because of the message you received or perhaps never received. You don't have to think about this, just see what may come up naturally. Several images or situations may come up, this is perfectly normal and not a bad thing. Just pick one, even if you have a vague image, it is okay to pursue this.

"If you have a situation in mind, I would like to ask you to reconstruct the image as vividly as possible.

"Who are you with in this situation? Where is the situation taking place? Where are you yourself in the picture? What do you see around you? What is the temperature like? Can you perceive sounds, smells, or other sensations? What person or persons belong in the picture? What relationship do you have to each other? What does the other person do? What is your reaction? What are you thinking about in this situation? What are you feeling? How do you deal with what is happening?

"Try to reinforce the image and your sense of the situation as best you can.

"Is there any contact between you and the other person? What does that look like? Try to feel what your need is."

Step 2: Elaboration of the image

Try to fix the image you have just reconstructed as firmly as possible and develop it on the sheet in front of you, in silence. In case it feels very personal to you, you don't have to share the situation out loud later.

Step 3: Corrective messages

Pass out A4 paper and take turns responding to the image you see in front of you. Fold your own text in half and then move on to the next spot/drawing, in silence. Above all, try to look at the underlying need: What is the image you see before you asking for? What message do you want to give the creator of the image? (Link to basic needs.)

AIM

- Getting in touch with own imprinted experiences and missed needs (mentalizing abilities).
- From own Healthy Adult connecting with experiences of others (empathic ability).
- Emotionally connecting in the here and now (showing vulnerability, making contact, etc.).

Connection to healthy ego functions

- Personality integration and the formation of a self-image.
- Contact with one's own feelings/needs and those of others.
- Testing reality and assessing situations, conflicts, and relationships.

Materials

Drawing paper (A3 size), charcoal, kneading eraser, paper (A4 size), pen or marker.

Group/pair/individual

- Group.
- Individually in the group.
- Individually.

Further details

Provide a quiet (enclosed) space for this exercise and pay attention to a comfortable sitting position (especially if only stools are available for the client[s] in the art therapy room).

The advice is to do this exercise only when the client is already familiar to some degree with schema therapy, his own modes model, and can make contact with his Healthy Adult.

In a group, this exercise can only be offered when clients feel safe enough in the group.

This working method is contraindicated when there is too much risk of unwanted deregulation or when clients are influenced by medication. In the case of both mild intellectual disability and previously untreated post-traumatic stress disorder (PTSD), it is important to keep in mind that this working method needs further therapeutic pretreatment to estimate whether it can be implemented at a later stage.

It may be important to pay explicit attention to the rescripting part in the same session if it is deemed irresponsible for the individual client or the group to end the session with only the imagination (when there is a risk, for example, of drug abuse relapse, decompensation, PTSD triggers).

In the follow-up discussion, it is important to explain the importance of rescripting the situation and the different options for tackling it.

In classical rescripting, the child's own Healthy Adult or therapist steps into the image and takes care of the child's (basic) needs. Rescripting within art therapy can also mean working on the current image or creating new images or symbols. This could be an appropriate next step in the therapy process.

EVALUATION

- Share what you want to share, you don't have to share the situation itself in detail, but you can share some part of the process and any insights, for example.
- What was it like to do this?
- What child mode and which feelings belong to the situation you have put on paper?
- Think about what schema/mode of yourself belongs to this and how you can make a connection between the image on the paper and the presence of this schema in your daily life.
- What responses did you get (in Step 3)? What do you notice in them? What effect does this have on you?
- What was it like looking at other people's images and responding to them?
- Did you come across things about yourself in them that you recognize from everyday life or that relate to your own schemas/modes?

2.22 Children's photos

Description

Bring one or more photos from your childhood. At the beginning of the session, the photos will be looked at and briefly explained if necessary. Make one or more copies of them and enlarge or reduce as desired.

Stick the picture on some surface and design the space around it. You can do this on paper or spatially with wood or clay, for example. You can also work/paint over it or write words or phrases around it.

AIM

- Compassion with the Vulnerable Child mode and the needs of the child that the client has been.
- Focusing on and gaining insight into feelings regarding one's own history.

Connection to healthy ego functions

- Personality integration and the formation of a self-image.
- Healthy emotion regulation.
- Contact with one's own feelings/needs and those of others.
- Healthy internal dialogue.

Materials

For copies: Paper or plastic sheets, colored paper, kite paper, drawing and painting materials.

For elaboration: Free choice.

Group/pair/individual

- Individually in the group.
- Individually.

Further details

Copy facilities are important to be able to work with the photos. After all, many people do not like using originals. Or the opposite is the case: clients with excessive self-hatred tend to damage the photo on impulse.

When asking for preparation (picking out photos and bringing them), this may also be indicated if necessary.

For some clients, it is difficult to experience compassion and understanding with the child they once were. They call it stupid, bad, or retarded. They can pursue compassion for the child in this working method by dwelling on its needs.

Variation: Ask clients to bring one photo from the past and one photo from the present and combine them in a piece of work. Indicate in the image a relationship or connection between the two photographs (also see Haeyen, 2018, 12.10, p.306).

EVALUATION

- What did you do with the photo you brought?
- Describe your piece of work. What environment did you create for your photo?
- What material did you choose and does it fit well with it?
- What is the relationship or connection between the picture and the background? How did you visualize this?
- What is it like for you to look at this work?
- What feeling does it give you?
- What was it like being engaged with your own Vulnerable Child as a Healthy Adult?
- What other modes did you experience while working or are you experiencing now while looking?

2.23 Exploration in clay

Description

Take a handful of clay and knead it well for a while. Then roll it into a ball about the size of a mandarin. Make seven to ten balls. Take a ball in your hands and carry out one short action with it, such as squeezing, rolling, pushing, pulling, or twisting. Put the resulting shape away. Repeat this with the rest of the balls using a different action each time.

If necessary, the therapist stimulates by kneading beforehand or participating himself.

Then, look at your shapes and put them in the order of the degree to which the shape evokes something in you. Give each shape a title, naming the first thing that comes to mind. Write each title on a separate Post-it. This will give further meaning to the experience and to the shape that has emerged from the client's own strength.

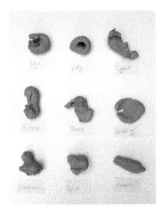

Shot actions with clay.

AIM

- Attention in the here and now, with touch and emotions.
- Letting go of demands on the product.
- Awareness of underlying schemas, modes, and needs.

Connection to healthy ego functions

- Personality integration and the formation of a self-image.
- Healthy emotion regulation.
- Contact with one's own feelings/needs and those of others.

Materials

Clay, pad, plant sprayer with water, Post-its, and pen or pencil.

Group/pair/individual

- Individually in the group.
- Individually.

Further details

Ensure that the working method can actually be experienced by having it executed with the necessary calmness, paying attention to hands and feeling. Validate experiences positively that these are good. Adjust the number of balls if necessary; ten is the maximum.

This assignment gives good opportunities:

- For clients who find it difficult to allow work pieces to emerge spontaneously.
- For clients who have difficulty accessing their feelings.
- For clients who have high demands on results.

This assignment is not for clients with excessive problems with their hands and/ or have a great aversion to clay.

EVALUATION

- Did you manage to keep your attention on what you were feeling?
- What shapes evoke something in you, give connection?
- Can you link this to any of your schemas or modes?
- What emotions or needs came up during this exercise?
- Was the Free Child or Healthy Adult active, and if so, at what time and how?

2.24 Scratch exercise

Description

Introduction

During this scratch exercise or "scratch dictation," focus attention on yourself: "How do you experience this movement?" "What do you perceive in your body?" and/or "What thoughts arise?" Observe yourself during the exercise; analyzing and interpreting, if necessary, may take place in the follow-up discussion.

Always make a continuous movement, keeping the crayon on the paper. If you really do not like a particular movement, you can stop earlier. In this case, go back to a movement that is comfortable for you.

Exercise

Start with a short attention exercise as a kind of baseline.

Let the clients explore the paper and crayon on their own.

Then start with Assignment 1 (which makes clients break free from their own pattern and start to move). Ask clients to hold each movement for about 15 seconds, then ask them to return to their own preferred movement and give the next instruction.

1. Accelerate your pace, increase the pace until you go as fast as you can.
2. Make your movement as big as possible, from your whole body.
3. Now make your movement as small as possible and feel how this movement feels.
4. Put more and more pressure on your crayon, using as much force as possible.
5. Draw a repetitive pattern.
6. Draw a searching movement.
7. Freeze your crayon (15 seconds) and then get moving again in slow motion.
8. Draw softly.
9. Draw away from the paper (on the table).
10. Close with the most pleasant movement.

AIM

- Emotion regulation skills.
- Listening to body signals.
- Recognizing physical and emotional reactions.

Connection to healthy ego functions

- Personality integration and the formation of a self-image.
- Healthy emotion regulation.
- Contact with one's own feelings/needs and those of others.

Materials

Large drawing sheets (50 × 65 cm), crayons, and painter's tape.

Group/pair/individual

- Individually in the group.
- Individually.

Further details

As a therapist, observe carefully what you see in the participants, which you can then mirror and/or inquire about in the follow-up discussion.

EVALUATION

- What did you experience during the exercise?
- What struck you the most?
- Which movement did you like and which one did you not like?
- What does the paper look like? What do you notice about it?
- How can you relate your experiences to what you know about yourself?
- What movement would you like to explore further?

2.25 Land grabbing

Description

The materials have already been set up by the therapist when the clients enter. The explanation follows: "We are going to have a contest! Choose a color of paint, and put a large blob of this on your palette. As I count down from 3 to 0, we are both going to paint on this sheet as quickly as possible with our 'own' color. When no more white (paper) is visible, the contest is over, and whoever has 'grabbed' the largest surface with his color has won. 3... 2.... 1... Go!"

AIM

- Being able to play.
- Connecting with the other person(s) in a playful way.
- Being able to take up space, to become visible.

Connection to healthy ego functions

- Contact with one's own feelings/needs and those of others.
- Testing reality and assessing situations, conflicts, and relationships.
- Seeking enjoyment and fulfillment in a mature way.

Materials

Several bottles of gouache, all of the same size, fairly thick brushes, palettes, one sheet of paper (A3 size) for two people or a large sheet for a group.

Group/pair/individual

- Group.

- Subgroups/twos or threes.
- Individually.

Further details

By setting up the materials, the therapist does not invoke coping modes or modified parent modes in preparation for the working method, and the client can get started immediately. The client is challenged by the game element to engage in quick, free, and active competition.

The therapist can participate himself. The therapist's enthusiasm and energy can be contagious; for example, playfully indicate that you are quite competitive and not a nice therapist for a while. That your "true nature" also comes out when working in the medium, and therefore it will be a "man to man" battle. This can cause the client to be less aware of the therapist/client relationship for a while, which may make him freer.

As a therapist do pay attention to your choice of paint color. If the other person chooses a dominant color (black, dark), deliberately choose a light vulnerable color. How does the other person handle this unfair contest? Where on the sheet do you begin to paint? Your own corner or under the other person's nose? Sneak up on the other person's paint, cheat! Does the client notice this? How does he react? Making a mess on the table is allowed and as a therapist you should set the example in behavior (*modeling*).

This working method is suitable for clients who have little or no motivation for treatment, as is often the case in a forced setting.

Whereas during the game the Happy Child is primarily addressed, in the follow-up talk the therapist appeals more to the Healthy Adult.

EVALUATION

- Invite the client to have a follow-up discussion of "the contest," similar to that in soccer, for example:
- How was it started?
- How was it played?
- Who did what?
- What were key moments and who won?

With this, you invite the client to contemplatively name his own behavior.

For example, "I waited to see which way the wind blew at first but when you went over my color ... yes, then I started the attack too!" Or "I started and immediately made sure you had no chance! Attack is the best defense!"

Repeat, summarizing the client's words in which he names his own behavior and ask him whether he knows this behavior of himself. If so, invite the client to name the advantages and disadvantages of this behavior in everyday situations. If the answer is no, explore how this behavior was evoked in this form of work anyway, and how the client normally acts differently. In this case too, you can try to have the client name the advantages and disadvantages of this behavior (shown or not shown).

- Can you make a link to the problems you experience in your living environment?
- What influences/functions does your behavior have then?
- What modes do you recognize and what function do they have?
- Was this working method a free, playful form for looking at your own actions together without judgment?
- What have you noticed in yourself in this?

2.26 Examining materials

Description

The therapist starts with the following instruction: "We are going to do an assignment in which you can get acquainted with your feelings, in the sense of touching, sensory experience of materials. Walk through the art space and select different materials, such as wire, fabric, wood, plastic, cork ... materials with different surfaces."

On a large sheet, make an arrangement of the materials you have collected. What feels good and/or what you want to be close to you, you put close by. You put anything that feels unpleasant or bad at the back of the sheet. The important thing is not how it looks, but how it feels. Take time to feel each material with your hand or other parts with your skin. You can close your eyes.

Tape the materials to the sheet. If you like, you can write down associations with each material or some of the materials.

Next:

From the pleasant material, create a pleasant spot or a free assignment.

Or just make a piece of work with the unpleasant materials. If the client himself has no idea, a theme can be suggested, for example, tree, animal, or landscape.

AIM

- Awareness of bodily sensations and experience.
- Getting to know one's own likes and dislikes.

Connection to healthy ego functions

- Contact with one's own feelings/needs and those of others.
- Testing reality and assessing situations, conflicts, and relationships.
- Seeking enjoyment and fulfillment in a mature way.

Materials

Various art materials and "found" materials or materials from nature such as twigs, stones, leaves, and shells.

Group/pair/individual

- Group.
- Individually in the group.
- Individually.

Further details

This assignment is appropriate for people who overcontrol in a rational way, who are not in touch with their feelings, and who avoid experience during therapy.

The exercise is clear because the confrontation with the material is short and the client is in control. An arrangement can be made too, which appeals to autonomy and makes the client retain a sense of control. Nevertheless, this assignment can evoke memories and also trigger the creative process.

The working method provides opportunities to work with material in a creative process in which the meaning may still remain dormant, "in the medium."

EVALUATION

During the discussion the therapist again emphasizes feeling:

- What materials did you choose and why?
- How do you like the feel of these materials?
- What feels nice and what does not feel nice?
- What associations do you have with this?

By running his hand over the material himself, the therapist can experience the same as the client, while questioning the client to give words to his experience and hear the associations. The therapist thereby follows the client's highest energy/arousal. The therapist can also probe what may have been meant by using his own words.

In the follow-up:

- Did you continue working with your preferred material or the material you disliked?
- What did you do with this?
- What insight did you gain in the process?

Modes can be discussed if necessary.

2.27 My Healthy Self-Soother

Description

Choose a material that you feel comfortable with, for example, one that feels pleasant to touch and that you can handle well. What appeals to you today? Think, for example, rubbing with pastels, big strokes with paint, applying force to clay? Try different actions, apply a lot of force or very little, try to make the movement big or small....

What colors do you choose today, which ones please you? Find a material and colors that calm you, that cause you to unwind.

Observe which movement makes you feel good. What shapes do you like to allow to emerge? What happens spontaneously and what is pleasant? Connect to your body and notice what the movement and seeing the colors do to you. Observe your breathing, your muscle tension, your heartbeat. Often, there is repetition in the movement; feel free to take advantage of that. Repeat the movement. Experiment a little with making this movement bigger and smaller. Take occasional breaks too, to experience what it does to you. You may want to close your eyes from time to time on the repetition of the movement.

AIM

- Increasing body awareness.
- Making a healthy equivalent for addictive behavior.
- Gaining confidence in artwork in preparation for trauma therapy.

Connection to healthy ego functions

- Personality integration and the formation of a self-image.
- Healthy emotion regulation.
- Contact with one's own emotions/needs and those of others.
- Seeking enjoyment and fulfillment in a mature way.

Materials

A wide choice of materials with different appeal values and expression possibilities, think of pastel crayons, oil crayons, colored pencils, markers, (finger) paint and brushes, clay, fabric, wood and nails, saw, sandpaper. Materials that allow you to perform repetitive movements or invite tactile experience, with opposite opportunities for applying force while working.

Group/pair/individual

- Group.
- Individually in the group.
- Individually.

Further details

This assignment helps people realize that they can regulate their emotion. Often, they do not know that emotion regulation plays an important role in their psychological functioning. They only know the extremes: the state of being cut off (Detached Protector) or of an openness that is boundless and means engulfment, of which they are very afraid. Often, they have destructive ways of regulating emotion such as addiction, self-harm, or compulsion.

By becoming aware of the direct effect of the expressive action on body, emotion, and mood, they increase the Healthy Adult with respect to safety, autonomy, and self-expression. More space is created for experiencing pleasure and for a willingness to explore the origin of their schemas.

This instruction can be given indirectly, for example, when the therapist sees someone performing a calming action. The client may feel caught out: "I'm just doing something, I don't know what I'm doing," "I'm avoiding." Practice shows that clients are relieved then and feel understood by the explanation that trauma work, for example, is not possible until you know how to regulate your emotions as well. As a follow-up, tasks such as depicting a trauma or nightmare are appropriate. Often, clients like to have their Healthy Self-Soother work next to them to switch to its calming movement when the emotion gets too high.

EVALUATION

- Show the group what material, color, and movement or action you have chosen. What symbolic meaning do you give to the chosen material or to the movement that is in the artwork?
- What did you feel in your body while modeling?

- Were you able to make a connection between the movement and your body reactions? What did you notice?
- What do you gain from it for your daily life? How does this knowledge about yourself and your body help build your Healthy Adult?
- For example, how might you use this if you are afraid of being overwhelmed by feelings, or are there similar actions in your daily life that you can use then?
- How might you use this Healthy Self-Soother as you set out on work about your past?

2.28 Body-oriented name drawing

Description

Draw your name! Use the letters of your name to create a piece of work. You can paint, draw, chalk, or work with other materials.

Your name was given to you by your parents, but you may have multiple names, pet names, abbreviations, a name given to you by your friends, or you yourself have changed your name at some point. You have a first name and a last name.

Choose what name you want to make this piece of work about. You can also design the background/environment of the letters by placing them in a landscape, for example, or putting symbols next to them.

AIM

- Coming to self-expression.
- Portraying self-image.

Connection to healthy ego functions

- Personality integration and the formation of a self-image.
- Contact with one's own feelings/needs and those of others.
- Healthy internal dialogue.

Materials

Drawing and painting materials as the initial selection, but in principle all art materials are appropriate.

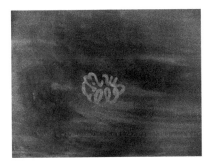

Name drawing of "Mees."

Group/pair/individual

- Group.
- Individually in the group.
- Individually.

Further details

This assignment offers a lot of structure and is accessible. Clients who think they are not creative can deal with this; it is also suitable as a first introduction. Some people find the assignment "childish." Here it helps to explain that childish things actually have a place within schema therapy and that it is worth trying.

Putting down one's own name visually can reveal how someone thinks about and looks at himself. Different modes can also become visible, for example, the Vulnerable Child mode, the coping mode, or the Free Child mode.

EVALUATION

The client can talk about his work himself if he wants to.

- How did you depict your name?
- What is the significance of your piece of work?

However, sometimes people are unable to give a meaning to their work, or are quickly done with it. Then, it is interesting to give it a body-oriented dimension.

- What movement did you use to depict your name?
- Did you use force or did you not use force at all?
- How did this feel? (Physically)

The therapist can also take the lead in this process. In this case, he can start with a phenomenological description of the material used, the shapes and colors that can be seen. He also describes the relationship between the letters or between letter and background, for instance, the letter stands firmly, your name seems to float, is curled together, your name is hidden/not legible. With hands or posture, the therapist depicts the movement dimension of the letters or the name. Through this translation from image to gesture, he opens a new access for the client, showing how he understands the drawing. The therapist checks to see if the client recognizes this in the drawing and can then open the conversation as to whether he himself is like this in life, who he is hiding from, for example, where he felt solid or just curled up.

2.29 Parental home

Description

Create a piece of work with the theme "parental home." This includes the garden, the street/neighborhood, the route to school, or what happened at school. Did you always live in the same house, or did you move? Did you have your own room? You can approach it in different ways: for example, draw a floor plan, an important object from the house, a room, or a certain (repeating) scene. Which room did you often use, where did you never use? Where did you feel well, where did you not? What did you do or what did the other people in the house do? What was the atmosphere like? You can portray atmosphere, for example, with colors that you find pleasant or unpleasant.

AIM

- Getting in touch with/becoming aware of the origin of the primary schemas, the Vulnerable Child mode.
- Getting in touch with/becoming aware of needs as a basis for building the Healthy Adult.
- Sharing one's own history.

Connection to healthy ego functions

- Personality integration and the formation of a self-image.
- Healthy emotion regulation.
- Contact with one's own feelings/needs and those of others.

Materials

Free choice.

Group/pair/individual

- Individually in the group.
- Individually.

Further details

This assignment is about the origin of schemas in the client's past. Here, we deliberately choose a concrete place rather than a psychological starting point: the house. This offers the opportunity to freely associate and to get in touch with the reality in which one found oneself as a child.

This working method is also suitable for people who say they have no memories of the past or have difficulty picturing imaginary rescripting.

The therapist constantly monitors the client's artwork and bodily signals and starts talking to him when tension builds or the client seems to get bogged down in coping (think of drawing the wall brick by brick or wanting to draw the rooms to scale with a ruler). On the other hand, some degree of coping is indeed necessary to achieve a design and provides the necessary safety to approach an emotional piece.

The therapist verbally mirrors what he sees and looks for solutions, suggesting, for example, working in series or other practical and creative solutions.

EVALUATION

The therapist discusses the identified coping:

- "This coloring of the brickshow long do you think that is going to take? Could there be avoidant coping underlying it? Is that helpful and pleasant here or should you actually stop it and get on with what really matters?" This reinforces the development of the Healthy Adult's autonomy. Or validate the Vulnerable Child's anxiety: "I understand you want to work toward it slowly because there is so much feeling behind it, just take your time."

The therapist discusses practical bottlenecks and variation options:

- You can also make more pieces of work for different ages or different houses.

The therapist invites the client to tell the story of what has been depicted and uses his own art observations to make the story more complete. For example:

- I see that all the rooms are green but this one is red, does that color mean anything?
- How did you notice it was dangerous there, do you notice it now (body reaction)?
- What sounds were there?
- What coping did you learn here?
- What may repeat itself in interaction with others?
- Is this where your schema ... originated? What did you miss as a child/ what should have been there?

Step to rescripting: Create a piece of work in which your needs are taken care of, an ideal home, an Ideal Parent.

2.30 Window work

Description

In this group assignment, we use the window as a work surface. On it, we will create a transparent collage together.

Each of you will choose your own color of kite paper. With this, we are going to fill the window together by taking turns adding a piece.

When it is your turn, tear off a piece and add it. We work in silence as much as possible. You can always ask for a time-out.

AIM

- Becoming visible and taking up space.
- Connecting with oneself and others.
- Becoming aware of schemas and modes.

Connection to healthy ego functions

- Personality integration and the formation of a self-image.
- Contact with one's own feelings/needs and those of others.
- Testing reality and assessing situations, conflicts, and relationships.

Materials

A fairly large window, several colors of kite paper (quarter of a large sheet), tape.

Group/pair/individual

- Group.
- Subgroups/twos or threes.

Further details

This working method can create a lot of tension. If necessary, make it safer by agreeing on certain rules and/or insert a time-out option to discuss needs and emotions. Validate repeatedly.

Do not use this working method at the beginning of a group process.

Take plenty of time for the follow-up talk and, if necessary, do a relaxation exercise afterward.

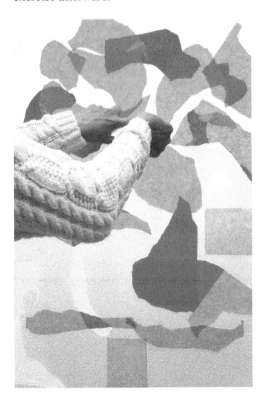

EVALUATION

- Were you touched in this exercise and if so, when?
- Can you link this to a schema or mode?
- How did/do you deal with that?
- Were there times when you were able to experience your Free Child/ Healthy Adult?
- How do you experience the piece of work and your part in it?

2.31 Life-size self-portrait

Description

Make a life-size portrait of yourself, in a powerful posture. Before you begin, stand in the pose you are thinking about and feel how it feels.

You can try different postures. When you have found an appropriate posture in which you feel strong and powerful, try painting it life-size. Start with the outline.

It is an option for the client to let himself be outlined by standing in front of a large piece of paper on the wall or by lying on the paper on the floor so that a silhouette can be drawn. In this case, always ask who can outline. After all, it comes very close.

After this, look at the picture. How does it feel? What image would you give the piece and what clothes do you feel strongest in? Paint these into the portrait as well or keep it more abstract.

You can paint, paste, or write things in the background that fit your powerful self, what you like, what you feel happy about, and what makes you feel good and strong.

AIM

- Positive self-image.
- Focusing on oneself and one's own strengths.

Connection to healthy ego functions

- Personality integration and the formation of a self-image.

Materials

Roll of paper, preferably an available wall to paint on, acrylic paint, pencil, eraser, water, brushes, collage materials, or personal photos of the client.

Group/pair/individual

- Individually in the group.
- Individually.

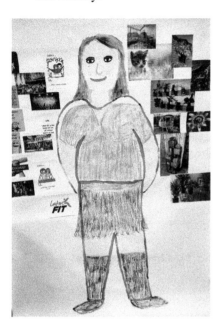

Further details

When starting the exercise, it is advisable to try out the postures together with the client and possibly mirror them so that the client can feel not only what the posture feels like, but also what it looks like and whether it is the desired image.

Usually, the exercise is confronting at the start. As the client progresses through the exercise, it is often nicer to work on the picture and the client begins to identify with it more. Several sessions can be used for this.

If necessary, qualities can also be added when working on the background.

EVALUATION

First evaluation after the outline is complete:

- How is this posture image for you? Does it indeed feel like a strong posture?
- What image did you want to give to the piece of work?

Second evaluation after having painted the whole portrait:

- How does it feel looking at this picture?
- What do you recognize of yourself in the portrait?
- How does it feel to face a life-size portrait of yourself like that?

Final evaluation after making the background:

- How does the portrait feel now?
- What did you notice in yourself as you worked on this portrait? Were schemas activated and, if so, which ones?
- In what mode can you now look at the work?
- Do you notice a difference from the start of the exercise in how you looked at the piece then and how you can look at it now?
- What can you do in your daily life to look at yourself more from this strong, Healthy Adult attitude too?

2.32 Schema boat with crew (two to three sessions)

Description

Step 1

As a group, paint a large boat. Do not deliberate in advance but you may do this as you go.

Step 2

In the second session, each group member will make a symbol for himself that can be placed somewhere on the boat. Everyone then considers where he would like to see himself on the boat and in what way, possibly what function he has there, and then goes on to make it. There is no consultation with each other about this.

Step 3

In the third session, each person places the symbol on the boat (or in the imme-diate vicinity of the boat). Each person looks at the position chosen, why this choice was made, and whether it was done from the Healthy Adult or from a mode. If it was done from a mode, what mode is examined and what underlying schema was activated. The latter can be done with the whole group so that there is a mutual connection with each other and a group process starts per person in which the client can again make a choice from the Healthy Adult. This choice then connects well with a need or something one would like to work toward. Once the new position is chosen, a question is asked how this is; Is it okay or is another mode then actively linked to a schema? Through Good Parent messages from the group, permission is given that it is really okay. In doing so, the person in question closes and it is the next person's turn.

AIM

- Becoming aware of and discussing the different roles and positions in the group.
- Awareness of whether your choice is made from a mode with underlying schema.
- Gaining insight into own patterns and schemas that are thereby confirmed.
- Breaking a schema by expressing need.

Connection to healthy ego functions

- Personality integration and the formation of a self-image.
- Contact with one's own feelings/needs and those of others.
- Healthy internal dialogue.

Materials

Table-sized paper from a roll (approximately 90 × 1.80 cm), paints (preferably acrylic), palettes, brushes, sponges, and tape for attaching paper.
    Materials for the symbol (flat surface or spatial).

Group/pair/individual

- Group.

Further details

In between, the process is stopped so that everyone can see if a mode and related schema(s) are active during the work.
    If a schema is active, we look at how to break it so that the client's needs are met.
    It is determined for each client what he will practice in order to break the schema.

For the follow-up discussion, a starting situation is defined with the symbols in the form of a photograph.

Everyone is discussed individually looking at the symbol and the way it was placed (mode related to or from the Healthy Adult).

After each discussion, the starting position is taken up again and the next client is discussed.

EVALUATION

Making the boat:

- How did you experience making a boat with the group?
- Who had which role?
- What modes have you encountered?
- What was your need that activated the mode?
- Could you detect the underlying schema?
- What did you do to break the schema?
- What were your actions?
- What was the result, how did the group respond to your change?

Creating a symbol:

- What symbol did you make?
- What does it stand for?
- What does it say about you?

Placing the symbol:

- Why did you put your symbol in that position?
- Did you do this from a mode? Or from the Healthy Adult?
- What modes have you encountered?
- What was your need that activated the mode?
- Were you able to detect the underlying schema?
- How could you break the schema?
- Which position would you choose then?
- If the position is occupied, what do you do now (breaking through is asking the other person if you can stand in that position, for example, at the helm).
- Just move your symbol to that position.
- What is it like to be in this position?
- If this is completely okay, the process is complete.
- If another mode is active, for example, the Punitive Parent, the process repeats itself by again looking at how it can be broken.

2.33 Expressive glossy paper

Description

The therapist gives the following instruction:

- To break free from your high standards, today we will do a working method in which the materials and tools are deliberately limited. Take a 50 × 70 cm white sheet of paper or half of it. Choose two or three colors of glossy paper.
- Tear up to three rough shapes per color off this paper. Do not try to make recognizable shapes with this.
- Move the shapes around on your white sheet to try out different options. You do not have to use all the pieces in this process. In between, you can use your cell phone to take pictures of your creations if you like.

Challenge yourself to experiment. Ask for help from the therapist if you find that you get stuck.

- Finally, glue the shapes to your sheet. If required, further elaborate the image using other materials.
- Write down what you have encountered in yourself in this working method. List the points of pride and improvement, your needs, and questions that come to mind.

AIM

- Discovering where your high standards affect play and experimentation.
- Becoming aware of (basic) needs.
- Letting go of high standards and developing fun.

Connection to healthy ego functions

- Personality integration and the formation of a self-image.
- Healthy internal dialogue.
- Seeking enjoyment and fulfillment in a mature way.

Materials

Sheets of solid white drawing paper (70 × 50 cm or half of it), colored glossy paper, glue or glue stick. For further elaboration, various drawing and painting materials.

Paper/logbook and pen to take notes. Possibly clients' own cell phones to take pictures.

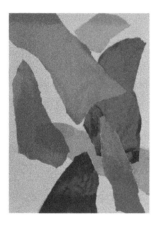

Group/pair/individual

- Individually in the group.
- Individually.

Further details

Try to keep this working method especially stimulating and light-hearted. Ask people to focus on their own work; to avoid distraction, do not talk to each other.

Pay attention to which clients need more or less challenge, keep in touch where needed, be available.

Have clients write down experiences and points of improvement and pride.

EVALUATION

- What did you notice about yourself during this working method?
- How did you come across your schemas or modes?
- What was your need?
- How did you deal with this?
- Did you experience freedom/pleasure?
- How do you experience your piece of work?
- What are points of pride and improvement?

2.34 Mirror assignment

Description

Sit facing each other on the short side of a large piece of paper. Tape the paper to the table with painter's tape.

You are going to mirror each other. The center of the paper is the mirror.

You do the exercise twice, once in the role of leader (the one in front of the mirror) and then in the role of follower (the one mirroring).

Mirroring each other means that if the leader leads with the right, the follower follows with the left. During the exercise, keep the crayon on the paper (mirroring in the air is difficult). What is drawn does not have to represent anything, it can be just lines. Really try to draw at the same time, as if you are the mirror image. Consult with each other who starts leading and who starts following. Between the first and second exercise, there is room for a brief exchange (see Evaluation).

After the evaluation there is an opportunity to repeat the exercise, with the same or a different partner. Practice different ways of doing things based on the new insights.

AIM

- Developing adaptive skills in collaboration.
- Distinguishing between what belongs to you and what belongs to the other person.
- Staying in touch with yourself while being in touch with the other person (e.g., expressing desires and boundaries).

Connection to healthy ego functions

- Personality integration and the formation of a self-image.
- Contact with one's own feelings/needs and those of others.
- Testing reality and assessing situations, conflicts, and relationships.

Materials

Large drawing sheets (50 × 65 cm), crayons, and painter's tape.

Group/pair/individual

- Subgroups/pairs.

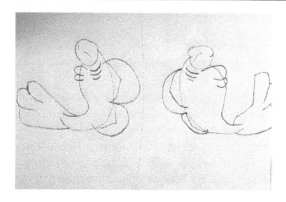

Further details

The follower is responsible for following and the leader for leading. They need each other to make a success of it. The follower is not the same as the Compliant Surrender mode. In the role of the follower, he remains equal and he can indicate from the Healthy Adult what he needs to carry out this role in a pleasant and good way. And the leader is only responsible for his leadership role. What does he need to carry out his role pleasantly and well?

EVALUATION

For both intermediate and final evaluations:

- How was the consultation process in choosing the roles?
- What did you experience in the exercise?
- What did you do when things didn't go the way you wanted?
- Who was responsible for the course of the exercise?
- Which role do you prefer?
- How could you make collaboration better and more pleasant?

2.35 Objections to the Critical Parent

Description

Create a full-screen portrait of your Critical/Demanding Parent as you experience him. How does the design best fit this mode?

Then, write messages on Post-it notes that the Critical/Demanding Parent keeps giving you. Write one message per Post-it. Stick these on and around the portrait.

Briefly discuss this in the group.

Everyone then works on thinking of and writing down positive objections, again one per Post-it (of a different color from the one in the first round). Keep these with you until the follow-up discussion.

AIM

- Dwelling on defining, critical, and demanding messages.
- Formulating objections and putting them first.

Connection to healthy ego functions

- Personality integration and the formation of a self-image.
- Contact with one's own feelings/needs and those of others.
- Healthy internal dialogue.

Materials

Pastel crayons, charcoal, oil pastel crayons, painting materials, paper (50 × 65 cm), Post-its in two colors, e.g., orange/pink for the Critical/Demanding Parent and green/yellow for positive objections.

Group/pair/individual

- Individually in the group.

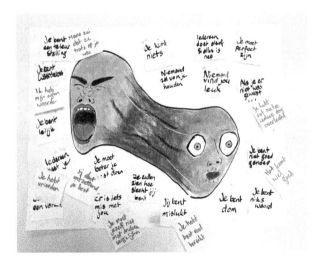

Critical/Demanding Parent mode messages and positive objections.

Further details

Explain and implement this working method step by step.

EVALUATION

Intermediate discussion (briefly):

- What messages does the Critical/Demanding Parent keep giving you? Read these aloud. (This is often confronting, ask if the client dares to do this.)

Follow-up discussion (longer):

- How did you portray your Critical/Demanding Parent?
- What does this show about how you experience him?
- What positive objections have you been able to come up with?
- Stick these near/on the portrait over the negative messages.
- How does it feel to look at the image now?
- Involve group members.

2.36 Drawing threads

Description

We are going to make some pieces of work together as part of the Free/ Happy Child using thread and ecoline.

Everyone chooses a color of ecoline and carefully dips part of a (rinsed) cotton thread into it, keeping at least 20 cm clean. Everyone drapes the thread on one and the same large sheet of paper, making sure the clean piece of thread sticks out.

When all the threads are on the paper, cover the sheet together with another sheet of paper.

Then, you use one hand to take hold of your piece of thread and one hand to press the two sheets of paper together. Then you pull your thread toward you. Keep the paper pressed closed until the last thread is out.

Then remove the top sheet together.

Repeat this several times and experiment together; stay in touch with each other.

AIM

- Experiencing fun in experimenting and play.
- Feeling connected to others.

Connection to healthy ego functions

- Healthy emotion regulation.
- Contact with one's own feelings/needs and those of others.
- Seeking enjoyment and fulfillment in a mature way.

Materials

Large sheets of solid white drawing paper, different colors of ecoline, cotton knitting yarn or string up to 120 cm long (rinsed out so it can absorb color well).

Group/pair/individual

- Group.
- Subgroups/twos or threes.

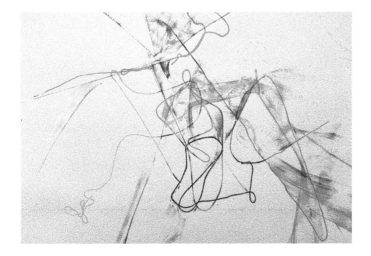

Further details

In this working method, good organization is important. This means that the therapist warns against staining and recommends the use of aprons. Do not make the strings longer than the specified length; this prevents a lot of mess. Pour the ecoline into cups in advance, diluted if necessary. Work standing at a table so that everyone can stand equally close to the paper.

Occupying a place and a close proximity can be tense, encourage and keep it light-hearted and playful.

EVALUATION

- How did this working method go?
- What did you come across in it?
- Could you experience the Free/Happy Child?
- What do you think of the resulting work and your role in it?

2.37 Resilience assignment

Description

This working method consists of a number of steps. These are explained step by step.

Step 1

Fill the entire sheet with colors and shapes that you associate with happy/pleasant/cheerful and so on.

The crayon/oil pastel can be applied thickly (if necessary, the therapist can briefly illustrate this on another drawing sheet). The white of the surface should no longer be visible. The work may be illustrative, realistic, or abstract.

Step 2

Take a black crayon and use it to apply a black layer over the entire image; so you will be chalking over your own drawing. The bottom layer should no longer be visible.

Step 3

Now use a scratch pen or another sharp-pointed tool. When you go over the black layer with the scratch pen, the colors underneath will reappear. Use these colors for your final step. You are free to make of it what you like.

AIM

- Gaining insight into dealing with adversity and into which modes are then activated.
- Gaining insight into degree of resilience (Healthy Adult).

Connection to healthy ego functions

- Personality integration and the formation of a self-image.
- Healthy emotion regulation.
- Healthy internal dialogue.

Materials

Solid quality drawing and/or watercolor paper (A5 or A4 size), oil pastel/crayon, scratch pen. The black chalk might be replaced with black acrylic paint.

Group/pair/individual

- Individually (in the group).

Further details

It is advised not to mention the title of the working method beforehand, as this may appeal to resilience in advance. For maximum experience, it is important to guide the client through the working method step by step.

The choice to have the black layer applied with acrylic paint can be made if a "faster" and less labor-intensive option is desired.

The choice to have it done with crayon/oil pastel can be made to reinforce the "trigger" in that it takes more time, energy, and resilience to make the entire image disappear.

Step 2 is often about dealing with setbacks and unexpected situations such as loss. Step 3 is about resilience: the ability to rebuild after setbacks. This working method is based on the analogous process. Therefore, it is important to make the link with daily life: What does the client recognize from this working method in other situations?

EVALUATION

- Discuss this working method afterward step by step.
- What was it like doing this working method?

- What picture did you make in the first step?
- What choices did you make in terms of colors and image?
- What emotional connection did you feel with the work you created?
- How was the instruction to black out the image received by you?
- How did you experience this?
- What choices have you made?
- How did you carry out this instruction? Think of pace/destructiveness and so on.
- Did you black out parts first or last and what was the reason?
- Did you/did you not indicate boundaries in the face of resistance?
- What modes became active during this working method?
- What choices did you make in Step 3 and what do these choices say about you?
- In what ways has your Healthy Adult side played a role?
- What does your chosen image say about your Healthy Adult?
- What do you recognize of this working method in your daily life?
- What do you take away from this working method into everyday life?

2.38 Safety for the Vulnerable Child

Description

Imagine yourself as a child. What did you look like? What were you like? What did you feel? What did you think at the time? What was your attitude? What were your fears?

Model this into an image as you see fit.

Then, make something for the child of that time, that is, for yourself, something you want to give to the child. Figure out what helps the child to feel safe. This could be a place or it could be an object or a person. Make a picture of this in a form that you yourself like.

AIM

- Experiencing that you can give yourself security and love from your Adult Self.
- Being gentle and caring for yourself.

Connection to healthy ego functions

- Contact with one's own feelings/needs and those of others.
- Healthy internal dialogue.

Materials

Free choice, for example, clay, paint, colored pencil, pastel crayon, or a wide range of three-dimensional materials.

Group/pair/individual

- Individually in the group.
- Individually.

Further details

In this working method, the client is challenged to take charge of his own safety. What does he need? And how can he provide this?

Safety is experienced by everyone in a personal way, so meeting this need requires a personal approach.

As a Healthy Adult, it is important to recognize and know one's own needs regarding safety and to be able to take care of oneself in that regard.

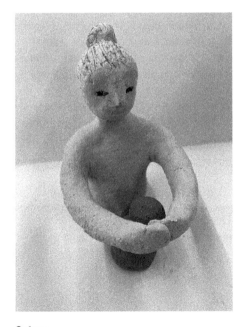

Safety.

EVALUATION

- How did you picture yourself as a child?
- What does the image show about how you were, what you felt and thought?
- How is the child's attitude?
- What did you add to make the child of that time feel safe?
- Is this an existing something or someone?
- In what ways does this or this person provide safety?
- What feeling does the image evoke in you? (Also ask group members.)
- Is anything more or anything else needed?

2.39 Who is your Healthy Adult?

Description

A brief introduction reflecting on the role of the Healthy Adult is the starting point.

If necessary, ask each group member about this position and brainstorm with each other.

What does the Healthy Adult do? What function does he have? Consider whether and how you recognize the Healthy Adult in yourself or in another person.

What might your Healthy Adult look like? Think about how you see the Healthy Adult and what image he has. Choose what material would match this aspect.

Sometimes it works better to get an image through another person; someone the Healthy Adult can be projected on to. This can also be a symbolic Healthy Adult, such as an animal with certain characteristics.

Create a picture of your Healthy Adult and possibly add any elements to the piece of work that fit the characteristics you think match with your (future) Healthy Adult.

AIM

- Self-reflection concerning the Healthy Adult position.
- Exploring, picturing, and gaining insight into one's own image of the Healthy Adult.

Connection to healthy ego functions

- Personality integration and the formation of a self-image.
- Healthy internal dialogue.

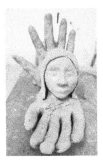

Materials

Free choice, think of clay, collage, paint, and so on. A well-equipped therapy room offers plenty of choices of materials.

Group/pair/individual

- Individually in the group.
- Individually.

Further details

The Healthy Adult acknowledges one's own vulnerability and supports the state of mind of the Vulnerable Child. The Healthy Adult corrects the unhealthy state of mind and takes care of what is normal for an adult: work, taking responsibility, and engaging in connection. The Healthy Adult strives for balance between pleasant adult activities, intellectual, cultural, and sports activities on the one hand and social obligations on the other.

The assignment can be done in the group with everyone creating their own version of the Healthy Adult, or working together on one piece of work to which everyone adds their own elements creating a unified image.

This task is too difficult at the beginning of treatment. It is important that the client already has a concept and has already practiced with what a Healthy Adult can mean before he can shape it.

EVALUATION

- What does your image of your Healthy Adult look like?
- What do you notice when you look at your piece of work?
- What elements did you consciously incorporate into the work as matching with your (future) Healthy Adult?
- What elements ended up in the work more unconsciously?
- What did you discover while making this piece of work?
- What characteristics of the Healthy Adult do group members find recognizable (to themselves or the creator)?
- What characteristics of your (future) Healthy Adult do you already recognize in who you are now?

2.40 Exploring the Happy Child

Description

Stand as a pair, each on one side of the table, facing each other. The sheet of paper is between you.

Part 1

Get a marker each. Both put a dot in front of you on the paper.

Now try to go across the paper with your marker and touch the dot of the person facing you with your color, while at the same time defending your own dot. Keep the marker on the paper. Repeat this a few times on new sheets of paper, and in different pairs.

Part 2

All kinds of sheets with lines on them were created while you were doing this. Look at what you see in the lines and make a picture of them. Or fill in the white pieces on the paper with other colors. This can be done individually or in pairs. Maybe you can cut out the most beautiful piece and make a 3D object with it.

AIM

- Spontaneity and play.
- Having fun together.
- Exploring the Happy Child.

Connection to healthy ego functions

- Contact with one's own feelings/needs and those of others.
- Seeking pleasure in a mature way and needing fulfillment.

Materials

Sheets of paper (50 × 65 cm), felt tip pens, pastel crayons, and oil pastel crayons.
For the sequel: Acrylic paint, crayons, scissors, and glue.

Group/pair/individual

- Subgroups/twos or threes.
- Individually in the group.

Further details

The first part of the working method is about being able to play together. The sequel can be done individually or in pairs.

EVALUATION

- What was it like trying to hit the other person's dot while defending your own dot?
- What did this evoke in you in terms of behavior, thoughts, and feelings?
- Did you notice any physical reactions?
- How did you build on the interplay of lines and what did you make of it?
- How was the work process/cooperation in this?
- How are you feeling now?
- Can you use what you have discovered in this working method in terms of play at other times outside of therapy?

2.41 Fulfilling missed basic needs

Description

The therapist briefly explains the five basic needs based on schema therapy (safety and attachment, autonomy, self-expression, spontaneity and play, and realistic boundaries). Put these on a writing board or on paper for the client to look at during the session. Do this while the client is offered the clay and is already allowed to knead it.

The client is asked about the experience of kneading the clay. Did it feel wet/dry/hard/soft/cold/warm?

While the client is kneading, the therapist asks him about his childhood and his experience of it. To give preliminary direction for the clay assignment, the therapist asks questions such as:

- Did you miss anything in your childhood?
- What image did people have of you and were there sides that were not so visible to others?
- How did you really feel and were others allowed to see that?

The therapist then asks the client to create an image of himself as a child in a pose that expresses the potentially unmet basic need. When this image is completed, what it expresses and what the creator's intention was are discussed.

Finally, the art therapist asks the client to depict the fulfillment of his needs or his own Healthy Adult in clay in response to the previously created image. What does the clay figure need? How can you put these two images in relation to each other to reinforce the fulfillment of the basic need?

AIM

- Recognizing one's own missed basic needs.
- Reinforcing the Healthy Adult vision of fulfilling one's own basic needs.

Connection to healthy ego functions

- Contact with one's own feelings/needs and those of others.
- Healthy internal dialogue.

Materials

Soft chamotte clay, clay board, and clay tools.

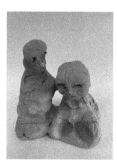 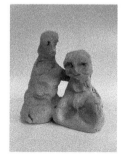

Group/pair/individual

• Individually.

Further details

The working method can be varied as follows: when the client has not yet developed a sufficient Healthy Adult mode, the therapist fills in the missed basic need of the clay work piece.

To increase the emotional connection to one's own piece of work, the client is asked to work with his hands as much as possible, without attributes/aid materials. Only later can the client use tools for detail work to finish his work.

EVALUATION

• What was it like to do this?
• What basic need does the figurine express?
• What strikes you?
• How did you depict the fulfillment of your needs in response to the earlier image?
• Are the two clay figurines in good proportion to each other? Make an adjustment if necessary.
• Do you still miss a need in the "here and now"?
• How can you deal with this now? What do you need?

2.42 Taking care of the basic needs of the other person's Vulnerable Child

Description

Step 1

A situation in which clients recently felt vulnerable is reflected upon through an image:

"Sit firmly in your chair with your feet on the ground. Put your hands gently on your lap and close your eyes. Feel the chair under your buttocks and the ground under your feet. Focus your attention on your breathing and notice how this feels right now. Take several deep breaths, in and out.

"Now go back to a time when you felt vulnerable. When you were not completely safe. How does your body feel? What colors or shapes do you see? Try to form an image of this moment in your mind. After this, open your eyes slowly."

Now make a picture of what you have just experienced. The choice of materials is free. (20 minutes)

Step 2

When the clients have finished making their picture, they put down their materials. They then tell each other in pairs about the picture they have made. (six minutes)

The basic needs on paper hang on the wall (with subtitles):

- Safety: "I'm here for you, you can count on me."
- Connection: "I see you, I notice you."
- Autonomy: "I am confident that you can do it."
- Self-esteem: "I think you are important."
- Realistic boundaries: "I give you direction and make sure you understand why."
- Self-expression: "I want to know what's going on inside you."
- Spontaneity and play: "Come, let's relax, let's enjoy ourselves together."

Everyone has now heard another person's story and chooses one of the basic needs he feel fits the other person's image and corresponding story. What did the other person need at that time?

Then, everyone creates an image in response to the other person's work, using the chosen basic need as the theme. (20 minutes)

AIM

- Increasing perspective.
- Recognition and acknowledgment of basic needs, focusing on a healthy way of fulfilling these needs.
- Developing and discovering the Healthy Adult.
- Being able to accept care.

Connection to healthy ego functions

- Healthy emotion regulation.
- Contact with one's own feelings/needs and those of others.
- Testing reality and assessing situations, conflicts, and relationships.

Materials

Free choice, think of paints, pencils, clay, collage materials, and so on. Printed A4 sheets with the basic needs and subtitles.

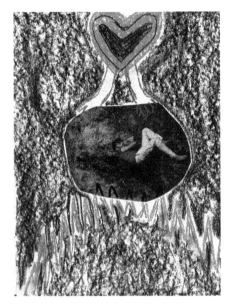

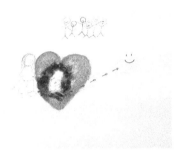

Art responses based on basic needs from others.

Group/pair/individual

- Group.
- Subgroups/twos or threes.

Further details

This working method can offer clients a new perspective on what they need. It often generates special and nice pieces of work for someone else. This is a positive experience for the group as a whole, and for the individual.

The starting point of this exercise is to develop the Healthy Adult and the experience that it is often easier to fulfill through caring for others than in caring for oneself. In this exercise, clients can experience that they can use their Healthy Adult and also what it is like when their Vulnerable Child is cared for starting from the Healthy Adult.

Possible variation/addition:

- A pictorial flashcard (helping image) with helping text can be created in response to the care that emerges from the paper to encourage Healthy Adult self-care.
- Passing on group assignment, which involves first making a Vulnerable Child drawing on large format paper. This drawing is then passed on to the

person sitting next to the client. The person with the paper in front of him is asked to now draw for the other person something from his own Healthy Adult that he thinks the Vulnerable Child of his groupmate needs. Every few minutes, the sheet is passed on again and everyone adds a drawing based on the care of his own Healthy Adult, until the sheet is back with the first client.

EVALUATION

- What did you make about the moment you recently felt vulnerable?
- What is it like for you to see what someone else has made for you?
- Do you recognize the basic need that the other person has chosen?
- How might you yourself apply/seek out this need fulfillment in your daily life?
- What basic need did you choose for the other person?
- Can you tell something about the work you did for the other person?
- What was it like for you to care for someone else based on your Healthy Adult?
- What do you take away from the exercise/drawing in how you yourself can use your Healthy Adult more in everyday life?

Extra, in the variation "passing on group assignment."

- What do you see and what do you experience when you finally see your drawing again?
- How do you think your Vulnerable Child has been taken care of? What do you see in the picture?
- How does the Vulnerable Child feel as a result?

2.43 Walk through the modes

Description

Part 1: Destructive modes in image

Picture three modes: a child mode, a parent mode, and a coping mode.

You can do this in one session or over several sessions. Also, take a look at your previous work to see if you have already depicted the modes somewhere, then just get them. You can also first think of a situation in which you believe several modes played a role. Choose a sentence for each mode. What does this mode say?

With clay, the modes can arise on the spot. Write the sentence on a note and put it next to your work. Then put the modes in relationship to each other. For other arts and body-based therapy disciplines: choose symbols in the room that match the modes. Also pay attention to the action you can perform with objects (e.g., boxing glove, percussion) or are hidden in the symbol (e.g., spider, bird). Group members can enter the role of modes here, then no notes are needed.

Part 2: Step to the Healthy Adult

The therapist or a group member reads the phrases of the different modes aloud; the client responds to these statements from the Healthy Adult mode.

What are you saying? Do you want to put the mode somewhere else? How do you want to change the image?

Part 3: Imagining the Healthy Adult

Would you also like to picture the Healthy Adult? (For this, you may also do an imagination first.) The therapist provides materials that match the Healthy Adult mode, such as fabric when cherishing or firm material when support is needed.

AIM

- Strengthening the Healthy Adult.
- Fulfilling the needs of the Vulnerable Child.

Connection to healthy ego functions

- Personality integration and the formation of a self-image.
- Contact with one's own feelings/needs and those of others.
- Healthy internal dialogue.

Materials

Clay, symbols such as wooden blocks, plastic figures, objects from nature, or other free symbols/three-dimensional materials. In Psychomotor Therapy (PMT), drama or dance: various materials/objects from the therapy room.

Group/pair/individual

- Individually.

Further details

This assignment is an adaptation of the "walking through modes" assignment by Farrell and Shaw (2015). It takes place imaginatively. This working method is appropriate for clients who already have insight into their modes and want to reinforce the Healthy Adult. Making the modes visible gives the client more control.

The therapist looks at the forms and discusses the literal functions of the various forms and whether they are connected to the right modes (sometimes a protection or support function has crept into the parent mode form; in that case, it is good to split them up).

Then, the therapist discusses the relationship between the different modes: What does coping do to the child, to the parent? The parent with the child? and so on. See if the forms and sentences are congruent with each other (corresponding verbally and non-verbally).

Make sure the client chooses the child's perspective. To do this, the therapist mirrors the client's body responses and discusses the need of the Vulnerable Child.

The Healthy Adult can also be given a form/symbol, but the client can just as well enter the scene himself as a Healthy Adult. The therapist demonstrates or complements when things become difficult (combination *reparenting* with reinforcing the client's Healthy Adult).

The parent mode is recognized and/or pushed aside or ignored through anger.

- The coping mode is validated, thanked, and asked to now give space for contact with the Vulnerable Child.
- The Vulnerable Child mode is noticed and needs are pointed out.
- The Healthy Adult expresses that he will take care of the Vulnerable Child's needs and explains how he will do that.

The picture/scene might be created in which a Healthy Adult figure fulfills the Vulnerable Child's needs. The Healthy Adult is also given one or more sentences that are written down.

The client can bring a picture of this scene as a flashcard.

If it is too difficult, the therapist readjusts on the spot and does a rescripting that does not call upon the Healthy Adult. Instead, an Ideal Parent comes into the picture in a scene at a certain age.

EVALUATION

The evaluation will not take place until the next session.

- How did this help you? Were you able to retain your Healthy Adult even outside of therapy? How did it work out?
- What else do you need?
- Have you felt any needs other than these?

The therapist discusses that it is okay that the coping mode still wants to intervene, that the client still hears the parent mode voice. A delay or a reduction in destructive modes is also progress. The therapist describes where the Healthy Adult was present and compliments the client on the effort.

Also discuss that not everything can be solved alone and that asking for help or protection is also a Healthy Adult response (humans are social animals).

2.44 Clay throwing contest

Description

Everyone can make an "aiming board" on a large piece of cardboard. This can be a kind of dart board with circles to be hit with points in them, or other things (worries, insecurities, agonizing thoughts of the Critical/Punitive Parent modes). They can be written on it.

The point is to create a playing field on the sheet that everyone would like to throw at.

Each person gets to knead five balls of clay that are nice to hold and have a nice size. The sheet is attached (firmly) to a straight wall that one can stand in front of at a distance.

Define a boundary line on the floor from which to throw. Clearly agree on what rules of play or agreements you will use together. In this way, you guard the safety and boundaries within which the client can safely let himself go completely. Decide in advance when the game will finish and when there will be a winner.

Then, the game of throwing clay on the game board can begin. Everyone takes their turn five times, then removes his clay from the board and when this client is behind the boundary line again, it is the therapist's (or another client's) turn.

From the removed pieces of clay, balls are kneaded again and can be used until the game is over.

AIM

- Collaborating and playing within a safe context.
- Being released responsibly.
- Getting in touch with one's own body signals.

Connection to healthy ego functions

- Healthy emotion regulation.
- Seeking enjoyment and fulfillment in a mature way.

Materials

Large sheets of solid cardboard paper (A2 or A1 size). Thick markers in different colors. A *tacker*, thumbtacks, or solid tape for hanging (the clay will be heavy against the sheet, so the sheet may tear or come off the wall). Soft chamotte clay.

Group/pair/individual

- Group.
- Subgroups/two or threesomes e.g. individually with therapist

Further details

Make sure the sheet is hung in a place where there is fairly little that can go wrong, even if the client misses (no vulnerable objects around). This is to prevent the client from breaking something, which evokes all sorts of modes in both the therapist and the client that get in the way of the Happy Child experiences.

Create safety and freedom for the client, he cannot do anything wrong (in the Happy Child mode). In case of mess, clay splatters flying around, mistakes, misses, a torn sheet, noise: reassure the client.

Anything goes within the set context, and the parent modes do not participate in this working method! In this working method, the enthusiasm of the therapist is often contagious. Set a good example by activating your own Happy Child as well *(modeling)*.

When tensions rise too high, the therapist intervenes. Help regulate, limit, maintain, make sure the client is noticed. This also provides safety in a working method that can feel like a loss of control for the client. To show that the client is noticed, one can point out which body signals are visible in the client.

It may be useful to let colleagues in adjoining rooms know that there will be noise, so that they are informed and do not come to see what is going on. Contraindications include sensitivity to noise (due to trauma for example) and a treatment relationship that is still not safe enough.

When this working method is carried out with clients with Cluster B issues, the goal may also be to release/regulate in a safe way, more than appealing to the Happy Child. This may also depend on what mode the client is in.

EVALUATION

- What was it like to do this?
- What body signals did you notice in yourself while playing?
- Were you fanatical as a child? How is this now?
- Did any modes come up during the working method that got in the way of the Happy Child?
- How did you deal with this, and can you translate this to other situations?

2.45 Circle exercise

Description

Draw a circle on your sheet of paper using a pastel crayon. Then make a spiral movement with a pastel crayon from the outside of the circle to the center. Be sure to move slowly and to keep your attention on the movement. Feel what it is like to make this movement. You can repeat this movement over and over again, with the option of using a different color crayon. As a second step, you can make the movement again, but this time by using your fingers to trace over the spiral shape you made, wiping out the pastel crayon.

AIM

- Learning to connect with oneself and one's own emotions.
- Learning to focus inward.
- Discovering what emotional blockades are present, if any.

Connection to healthy ego functions

- Healthy emotion regulation.
- Contact with one's own feelings/needs and those of others.

Materials

Sheet of paper (at least A3 size), pastel crayons, tape to attach the sheet to the table.

Group/pair/individual

- Individually in the group.
- Individually.

Further details

As a variation, the movement could also be done the other way around, from the center to the outer edge of the circle. This involves turning the focus back outward, for example, when a client experiences being too overwhelmed emotionally when turning his attention more inward.

When experiencing resistance spots in the circle, the focus may get to be more on this; in this case, a client can, for example, primarily make smaller movements around the resistance spots in order to discover in this way what emotions underlie the resistance.

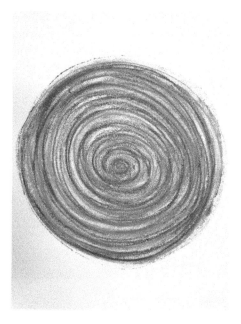

EVALUATION

For both follow-up talk and intermediate evaluation:

- What did you notice when doing the exercise?
- Does the circle feel the same throughout or are there points where you experience change?
- What emotions did you encounter?
- Where did these emotions come from/what triggered them?

2.46 Angry!

Description

Start with a brief imagination.

After attention has been paid to breathing and being firmly based, these questions are asked: "Let your thoughts go back to a moment last week, a week and a half when you felt angry or irritated. Dwell on this moment. What happened that made you angry, irritated you? Was anyone with you? If so, who was with you? What was happening? When you have this image in mind, take an imaginary picture of it. Then come back into this room with your attention."

1. Depict this moment in a symbolic way. (20 minutes)
2. Depict the moment again but now in an abstract way working from movement and from senses (motor and sensory). You can do this in your very own way. You can make a mess/smear, tear, break. As long as it contributes to expressing this feeling. (15 minutes)
3. Reflect on what messages you have to yourself while creating this image. Write these messages on a separate sheet and/or use these texts in the picture.
4. Lastly, create a Healthy Adult art response to the last piece of work. From that angle, what do you want to do with it or add to it? (15 minutes)

AIM

- Contacting and exploring feelings of anger.
- Creating self-insight.
- Exploring and gaining more control in handling a more Healthy Adult interaction with oneself.

Connection to healthy ego functions

- Personality integration and the formation of a self-image.
- Healthy emotion regulation.
- Contact with one's own feelings/needs and those of others.
- Healthy internal dialogue.

Materials

Three or four sheets of paper (50 × 65 cm) per person. Drawing and painting materials.

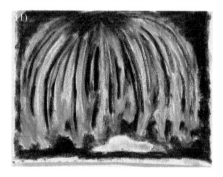

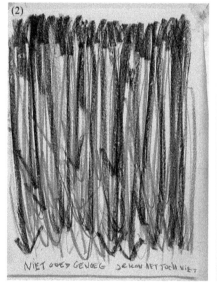

NIET GOED GENOEG   JE KON HET TOCH NIET

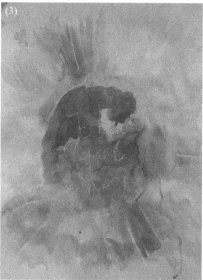

Feeling angry: symbolic (1), abstract (2) and picturing a Healthy Adult response (3).

Group/pair/individual

- Individually in the group.
- Individually.

Further details

A variation could be to perform this working method in clay. In that case, a warm-up is desirable in which force is used, for example, throwing clay on the table, kneading hard, making a lot of noise together.

Be alert to the client's reactions to himself. Does it tend toward Critical Parent messages that interfere during the steps? If so, help him take the next step and possibly use his thoughts during implementation (for Steps 1–3).

Sometimes there is a coping reaction in the first image, at other times a child reaction or a Critical Parent mode. The point is that through the different steps, deeper layers are reached in behavior and perception. Thus, the connection between the modes can be explored.

EVALUATION

- What situation occurred to you during the imagination in which you were angry/irritated?
- What were you angry about?
- How did you depict this symbolically?
- How did you abstractly depict this from movement and from senses?
- Was there a difference between working symbolically and abstractly?
- Where in your body did you feel it?
- What did you do that connected appropriately to your need?
- In doing so, what reactions/messages did you have to yourself?
- What was your Healthy Adult response to that? How did you shape that/what in the picture is important?
- How might you use this response in your daily life?

2.47 Symbols and "Good Parent" messages

Description

Session 1: Making symbols and writing down Good Parent messages

Make at least three 3D clay symbols that help you get or stay in Healthy Adult mode. They are small symbols that you can carry with you and hold. They can be a fantasy shape or an existing shape.

These symbols represent three different maladaptive schemas.

To do this, use the schema domains (see notes) to focus on three different needs that are most prevalent to you that are not being met. As a result, there may be a mode active and underlying a negative schema. For each need, write down the mode and underlying schema.

Think of three Good Parent messages/permissions for each symbol that are helpful in breaking the negative schema. Write these messages on a 50 × 65 cm sheet of paper.

Session 2: Painting symbols and recording Good Parent messages

In this session, the symbols are painted and then an audio recording is made for each client on his own cell phone.

- Everyone now has his own sheet with nine Good Parent messages (created in Session 1), and these are hung on the wall.
- Each client gets an audio recording of his own messages. Group members record a Good Parenting message on the cell phone of the person whose turn it is. When a Good Parent message has been recorded, the phone is passed to the next person who also records a message and passes this on until all nine messages have been recorded.
- It is important that the group sits in a circle so that the cell phone is easily passed around in a fluid motion. The client thus receives an audio recording of his own Good Parent messages, recorded by the group.
- The Good Parent message becomes extra powerful when the client's name is used with it, but this is not necessary with every message. The Good Parent message is heard by the client when recorded, which has an intense effect when first heard.

AIM

- Becoming aware of needs.
- Learning to receive Good Parent messages.
- Preparing for difficult moments.
- Becoming aware of modes and schema activation.

Connection to healthy ego functions

- Personality integration and the formation of a self-image.
- Healthy emotion regulation.
- Contact with one's own feelings/needs and those of others.
- Healthy internal dialogue.

Materials

Clay (e.g., Darwi clay), clay tools, paint (preferably acrylic), palette, brushes/sponges, sheets of paper (50 × 65 cm), tape for attaching paper to the wall.

Group/pair/individual

- Individually in the group.

Further details

Some clients find it difficult to come up with Good Parenting messages, in which case the group can be used to provide an impetus. For privacy reasons, one's own cell phone is used. Endorse a Good Parent message with the name. As a therapist(s), join in the recording.

Check carefully in the follow-up talk how the messages affected the client and/or if a mode was activated.

Make use of the overview of schema domains and dysfunctional schemas (Arntz & Jacob, 2012; Young et al., 2003) in Table 2.1.

Table 2.1 Overview of schema domains and dysfunctional schemas

Schema domains	Schemas
Disconnection and rejection	· Abandonment/instability · Distrust/abuse · Emotional neglect · Inferiority/shame · Social isolation/alienation
Weakened autonomy and weakened performance	· Dependency/incompetence · Vulnerability to illness and danger · Entanglement/jumble · Failure
Weakened borders	· Appropriating rights · Lack of self-control/self-discipline
Focusing on the other person	· Submission · Self-sacrifice · Seeking approval and recognition
Excessive vigilance and inhibition	· Negativity and pessimism · Emotional inhibition · Relentless standards/overly critical · Punitive attitude

EVALUATION

Session 1

- What symbols did you create?
- Did you manage to discover a schema or mode for the need that is not met?
- What Good Parenting/Healthy Adult messages have you formulated?
- Do you think you can use them during difficult moments?

Session 2

- How did you experience hearing your message uttered by the others?
- Were you able to receive the messages?
- Are there any situations now in which you think you will use the audio recording?

References

Arntz, A., & Jacob, G.A. (2012). *Schema therapy in practice: An introductory guide to the schema mode approach*. Wiley-Blackwell.

Farrell, J.M., & Shaw, I. A. (2015). *Schematherapy in clinical practice*. Nieuwezijds B.V. Publishers.

Haeyen, S. (2018). *Art therapy and emotion regulation problems: Theory and workbook*. Palgrave Macmillan.

Young, J.E., Klosko, J.S., & Weishaar, M.E. (2003). *Schema therapy: A practitioner's guide*. Guilford Press.

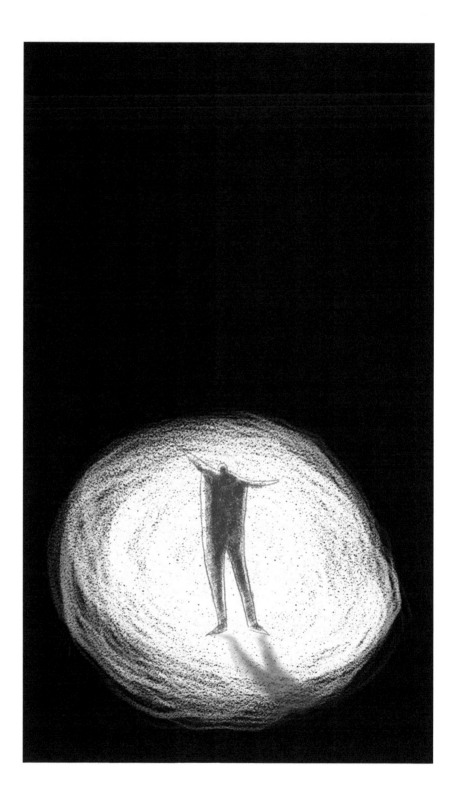

Chapter 3

Dance therapy working methods

Summary

Through body, movement, and dance, dance therapy focuses on initiating change and integrating emotional, social, cognitive, and physical processes. Dance can connect, express what goes on within us, consciously and unconsciously, and be an artistic product. Using practice-based dance and movement methods such as improvisation, composition, play, synchronization, relaxation, and the use of metaphors, the client learns, among other things, to experience and express himself authentically and give meaning to this.

DOI: 10.4324/9781003456988-3

3.1 Blind Free Child dance

Description

"Make pairs. One of you (A) is about to dance with his eyes closed."

"Do whatever you feel like doing at the moment. You have your palms against each other." The other person (B) ensures that A is and remains safe and free to do as he pleases.

"You do this only through non-verbal signals through the movement of the hands, without agreeing in advance what something means."

The therapist indicates when this section is completed and roles are switched.

So it is up to B to be caring and protect the partner: "Make sure he doesn't bump into anything, so A can do whatever he feels like doing without limits."

Then there is a brief reflection in pairs in which experiences are shared with the partner.

In doing so, the dancer (A) is the first to talk from his experience and only then is it the other person's (B) turn. "What do you like? What do you not like?"

Then, switch roles and repeat the working method. Next, there is another short reflection in pairs: "Which role did you like better?"

A moment of reflection on the modes then takes place in the group.

Repeat the working method. "Switch roles again and repeat, but now we take better care of ourselves."

Brief reflection in pairs.

Switch roles and repeat.

Brief reflection in pairs.

Another moment of reflection on the modes takes place in the group.

AIM

- Awareness of coping.
- Awareness of child needs.
- Non-verbal communication.
- Alignment.

Connection to healthy ego functions

- Contact with one's own emotions/needs and those of others.
- Testing reality and assessing situations, conflicts, and relationships.
- Seeking enjoyment and fulfillment in a mature manner.

Materials

Music.

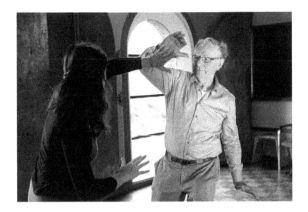

Group/pair/individual

- Group.
- Subgroups/twos or threes, for example.
- Individually in the group.
- Individually.

Further details

A physical warm-up is desirable to prepare muscles and joints for unexpected exertion, to prevent injury. If necessary, a body-oriented mindfulness exercise can be done beforehand so that clients make contact with themselves and with their need of the moment and become less lost in the interaction.

The repetition in this intervention would allow the partners to keep better and better track of their need. They can also take better care of the other person and communicate (non-verbally) to thus become attuned to each other. In this way, corrective experiences arise.

There are many variations and options in leading and following. This intervention involves multiple layers and could serve multiple purposes. This intervention deals primarily with Laban's Modes of Shape Change category, which means it is about body shape and shape changes. What is the relationship to his environment or how does he interact with or is in accordance with it?

In this case, it can symbolize a parent–child relationship (A child, B parent). A, the child, is the protagonist here. While A (the child) goes for his own needs, he allows himself to be protected and B (the parent) is at his disposal whereby he (A) does watch his own limits, and has to say "stop." Both have to communicate (non-)verbally for this.

This intervention requires non-verbal communication, cooperation, and courage to trust. Preparatory interventions to this could serve goals related to schema Distrust, Emotional Deficit, or Abandonment/Instability and, for example, Detached Protector mode.

Music can be not only supportive, but alsodirecting and therefore limiting. If music is used, it should be chosen intentionally. Music can be used to support a safe atmosphere. A few options:

- To support the Impulsive Child: Beyond Midnight—Brent Lewis.
- To support the Vulnerable Child: Run Cried the Crawling—Agnes Obel.
- To support the Enraged Child: Tsunami Lyrical—Gabrielle Roth and The Mirrors.

As a therapist, be a helping Ideal Parent and help keep it safe. In addition, support the child to dance freely: motivate and applaud. Give the Free Children enough time to get into their roles and solve "problems."

Communication is non-verbal. Yet, it can be healthy behavior to also talk, indicate what you need when you are not understood, or take a break when emotions run high.

The working method based on schemas, modes, and basic needs: A, the Free Child, goes for his own needs and is protected, which helps with the basic need Safety and Self-Expression. In doing so, he is matched in his needs. This might trigger, for example, the schema Self-Sacrifice or Submission.

If B assumes the child role, there may be parentification. This can be rescripted by actually allowing B to become A.

Variations

- To complement the intervention, a historical scene could be imaginatively rescripted where necessary by creating an affect bridge.
- By repeating everything with another partner, the process can be repeated and new experiences can be gained, corrective or perpetuating.
- A (continued) variation of the intervention could be that B, the parent, takes the leading role. The attention, emphasis, and reflection are then on him. Then, the goals change to applying healthy adult behavior: taking care of oneself; listening to one's own physical and movement needs and taking care of the other person; adjusting, helping, protecting, limiting. Could he still continue to take care of himself as well?
- On repetition, the child could be asked to deliberately engage another child mode. What then do you ask of B, the parent?
- As a conclusion, you could do another intervention with opposing movements. So, independently or in the group, with eyes open and uncontrolled and fast, for example.

EVALUATION

Modes reflection in the group:

Child mode:

- Did you do what you wanted to do yourself?
- What modes became active?

As a therapist also question what you think you have seen.

- Child mode, were you well taken care of?
- What did your "Good Parent" do? What made you feel safe(er)?
- When would you have needed this? At what age, what situation? (A rescripting with roles may be a follow-up.)

Parent modes:

- Did you also take care of yourself and how?
- Or how could you do this?

3.2 Healthy Self-Soother in dance

Description

"Walk criss-cross through the room at the pace you like at the moment."
"Find a spot in the room where you feel comfortable. Close to a wall, in the middle, close to others, or away from others."
"Where do you feel most comfortable right now?"
"Look for movements that make you feel comfortable. Movements that soothe you or make you feel calm."
"What parts of your body do you move? What feels nice in your body and is pleasant to do? For example, rubbing your hands, swinging your arms wide, or kicking your legs vigorously?"
"Try different actions: use a lot of force or very little, try to make the movement large or small."
"Find movements that soothe you, that calm you down."
"Observe which movement makes you feel good. What arises? What might happen spontaneously and what is pleasant? Connect with your body and notice/ feel what the movement does to you: observe your breathing, muscle tension, and heartbeat. There is often repetition in the movement; feel free to make use of it. Repeat the movement. You may find that your movement changes along the way."
"Let it happen."

"Experiment a little with making that movement bigger and smaller. What makes you calmer: Bigger or smaller? Fast or slow? Hard or soft?"

"Also, take occasional breaks and feel. You may want to close your eyes occasionally as you repeat the movement to experience the quiet even more consciously."

"Meanwhile, I'm going to put on music, continue your research quietly. Observe what that music does to your movement."

AIM

- Increasing body awareness.
- Emotion regulation.
- Gaining confidence in dance work in preparation for trauma processing.

Connection to healthy ego functions

- Personality integration and the formation of a self-image.
- Healthy emotion regulation.
- Contact with one's own emotions/needs and those of others.
- Healthy internal dialogue.

Materials

(Indulging) music.

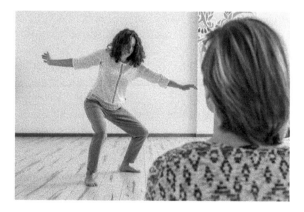

Group/pair/individual

- Group.
- Individually in the group.
- Individually.

Further details

The alternation of expression and impression of and with movement can make clients realize that they can regulate their emotion.

Often, clients do not know that emotion regulation plays an important part in their psychological functioning. They know only the extremes, such as the Detached Protector: closed off, or the Vulnerable Child: overwhelmed. Often, they have destructive ways of regulating emotion such as addiction, self-harm, or compulsion.

By becoming aware of the direct effect of movement on body, emotion,and mood, they increase the Healthy Adult with respect to safety, autonomy, and self-expression. More space is created for experiencing pleasure and for the willingness to explore the origin of their schemas.

Showing it to the group is, at the same time, an "exposure": practice and application.

Walking your own path, walking at your own pace, and choosing a nice place are interventions that can already be used to practice and/or explain body awareness and emotion regulation.

Music can be not only supportive, but also directing and therefore limiting. To support the calming, self-soothing effect, music of an indulging quality can be used.

When someone says, "I don't know what to do or I'm avoiding," provide an explanation and background for that, for example, working on trauma is not possible until you know how to regulate your emotions as well. Clients may feel relieved and understood by the explanation that trauma work, for example, is not possible until you know how to regulate your emotions as well.

As a follow-up, an intervention might be done focused on symbolizing a trauma or nightmare in movement.

Often, clients enjoy repeating and being allowed to do their Healthy Self-Soother movement on a regular basis. For example, when emotions get too high, switching to the calming movement.

Other arts and body-based therapy disciplines can also apply this intervention after adaptation.

Reflection and evaluation need not always be verbal; it can also be done in movement.

EVALUATION

- Show the group which movements you chose. What symbolic meaning do you give to the chosen movements?
- What did you feel in your body while modeling ?
- Were you able to make a connection between the movement and your body responses? What did you notice?
- What do you gain from it for your life? How does this knowledge about yourself and your body help build your Healthy Adult?
- For example, how might you use this when you are afraid of being overwhelmed by feelings or are there similar actions in your daily life that you can use then?
- Could you use this Healthy Self-Soother as you embark on work about your past?

3.3 Part of the whole

Description

Ask the group to form a circle.

Ask the group to choose four body parts together, determine a sequence in them, and memorize them. As a therapist, make a movement sentence out of these body parts as a memory aid to remember the order.

Then, ask the group to collectively choose a final line-up: a row, circle, small hole, pyramid, and so on. Explain: Your dance will start in this line-up. Each person improvises independently (moving) with the first body part. Everyone stops when, where, and how he wants. When everyone has stopped, you can start improvising with the second body part, and so on. The dance is over when you stop improvising with the fourth body part in your chosen final line-up.

Briefly repeat the explanation and let the group start.

AIM

- Following one's own need in the Healthy Adult way without overdoing it and taking into account the group and the assignment.
- Increasing self-awareness.
- Strengthening regulation, autonomy, and spontaneity.

Connection to healthy ego functions

• Contact with one's own emotions/needs and those of others.
• Testing reality and assessing situations, conflicts, and relationships.
• Seeking enjoyment and fulfillment in a mature manner.

Materials

None.

Group/pair/individual

• Group.

Further details

As a preparation, interventions focused on concentration, learning to improvise with different body parts, space division: line-ups and collaboration, and action–reaction might be done.

If necessary, a body-oriented mindfulness exercise can be done beforehand so that clients connect with themselves and become less lost in the interaction.

The therapist keeps a primarily verbal distance but is non-verbally present as a silent witness. The therapist intervenes when a harmful situation threatens to arise.

Repeat if necessary with new starting and ending line-ups and new body parts, to make acquired experiences take root or to adapt them.

Or the whole thing may be repeated with a halved group, allowing the other half to watch, to consider things from a different perspective. This group dynamic micro-intervention involves multiple layers and serves multiple purposes.

This intervention deals primarily with Laban's category of Space, which means it deals with how the client relates to general space, others, and his personal use of space. Where does he place himself?

Several modes can be activated in this working method, for example, the Compliant Surrender: the client behaves in a submissive manner, only following the others, not standing up for his own needs. Or, on the contrary, the Self-Aggrandizer: the client does not pay attention to the other person and therefore sets the pace.

The Healthy Adult learns to follow his own needs, without overdoing this, while still being considerate of the group. To complement the intervention, by creating an affect bridge a historical scene for one of the clients could be rescripted into dance, either imaginary or experiential.

EVALUATION

- How did you experience this?
- How do you know, where did you feel this and what did you feel? (This helps the Healthy Adult with self-awareness and regulation.)
- What was better than expected? What was disappointing? And how did you handle it? (This helps the Healthy Adult with the basic need for autonomy: evaluating yourself.)
- What would you like to do differently on repetition? (This helps the Healthy Adult with the basic need for spontaneity: being allowed to repeat, to learn, and, for example, contradicting extremely high demands.)
- What did you see in the others? (Facts, not opinions.)
- What did watching this do to you?
- How do you know, where did you feel this, what exactly did you feel? (This helps the Healthy Adult with self-awareness and regulation.)

3.4 Setting the pace together

Description

"All of you will be criss-crossing the room at the same time, setting the pace together. So, everyone walks his own path and each one of you is responsible for an equal pace. If someone speeds up, then everyone speeds up."

"If someone slows down, everyone slows down. If someone stops, everyone stops, if someone starts, everyone starts, and so on."

Emphasize at the beginning that the pace should be exactly the same: you do not have to walk starting with the same foot or in the same direction, as long as it is the same speed.

Wait until all the clients stop the exercise and the concentration is broken by everyone.

Repeat the intervention after reflection.

AIM

- Taking and assuming responsibilities; taking initiative and following.
- Promoting assertive behavior; standing up for one's own needs without overdoing it; learning to limit.
- Attuning to the other.

Connection to healthy ego functions

- Healthy emotion regulation.
- Contact with one's own emotions/needs and those of others.
- Testing reality and assessing situations, conflicts, and relationships.
- Seeking enjoyment and fulfillment in a mature manner.

Materials

None.

Group/pair/individual

- Group.
- Individually in the group.

Further details

Clients already need to have a basis of a Healthy Adult to benefit from this assignment, and the group must be safe. The assignment is intense and evocative, so it is best that the group is not too large: a maximum of eight people.

As preparation, interventions focused on concentration, body control, space allocation, starting and stopping, speeding up and slowing down could be done. If necessary, a body-oriented mindfulness exercise can be done beforehand so that clients make contact with themselves and disappear less into the interaction.

The therapist may repeat the task again during the exercise: "Keep the same pace!" This may involve the therapist stepping into the role of a Demanding Parent. It is important to explain this at the end and "step out of the role" for the clients.

Give clients plenty of time. Let what happens happen. Meanwhile, be supportive and encouraging in what is happening: smile along, also react with surprise, and so on.

Sometimes, long silences occur; do not intervene. Watch the reactions and how the clients deal with the silence or confusion. Observe what feeling you yourself as therapist get at different moments. See what happens in the group. See who responds to whom and how, and who does not. What modes become active? Sometimes, movements other than walking arise. Let it happen.

Do not predefine how or when the assignment ends. If you do, a pause or silence could quickly be interpreted as an end. Someone or some clients may break concentration early on, for example, out of discomfort. Wait and see how the group reacts. Perhaps the rest will continue, and the assignment will continue as before. Perhaps others will not dare to continue, and so on. What modes do you see? This all provides material for discussion.

There are many variations and options in leading and following. This intervention relates mainly to Laban's (1947) category of Effort (factor Time), which means it is about personal commitment. What is the inner attitude (toward time)?

The group dynamic intervention involves multiple layers and could serve multiple purposes. In this case, the clients experience the contradictions in basic needs. It could symbolize the family, in which balance is constantly sought to meet different needs and pleasure and fulfillment. In this, concentration and body control are also needed, which could serve goals related to (emotion) regulation and so, for example, the Impulsive Child mode.

The working method can promote cooperation, expose group dynamics, or advance the feeling of belonging to a group (and the feeling of belonging) to break the schema of Social Isolation or to connect with the Vulnerable Child. Different factors (e.g., group dynamics and process) determine the emphasis the dance therapist places with (non-)verbal interventions and attitude, and how the growth process is supported.

The working method from schemas, modes, and basic needs: in this working method, clients experience the opposites in the basic needs: for example, Connectedness versus Autonomy and Realistic Boundaries versus Self-expression or Play. This plays out in the interaction as well as in the internal dialogue: "Do I want to connect or choose my own form? Do I move with the other person, or do I take the risk that no one imitates me, and I remain alone?"

When repeating the intervention, motivate clients who are focused only on themselves to now also be mindful of others, to care for each other, without losing themselves in it. For example, clients with the schema Isolation, Distrust, and Emotional Deficiency. Motivate those clients who are only focused on the other person to connect with what they want for themselves. For example, clients with the schema Self-Sacrifice, Submission, Dependence, Entanglement, or indeed Distrust or Emotional Deficiency from overcompensation.

The Compliant Surrender mode (constantly following) and the Self-Aggrandizing mode (constantly leading) are clearly challenged here. But, we also see many parent modes ("I'm not doing it right"), Angry or Detached Protector ("Stupid assignment/makes no difference to me anyway").

In conclusion, a working method could be done with opposite movements. For example, let everyone determine his own direction and pace, eventually quieting down in his own spot, to come to himself again.

With modifications this intervention can also serve other purposes. By following up with opposite tempos or movements, a client with the Submission schema may choose the "Standing Up for Your Rights" schema or the Self-Aggrandizing mode as overcompensation.

You may also challenge the clients to stay in the same or opposite height layer (in terms of mode) in pairs, which in that case is more often about feelings of power and power relations. This is to combat, for example, the schema Submission or the Demanding Parent.

EVALUATION

- Does everyone agree that this is the end?
- Who would like to respond to it?
- What specifically happened at various times during the assignment?
- What was the consequence of the interaction? What did you feel and think?
- What modes play a part here?

The therapist makes sure that the opposites in basic needs become clear to the clients, as in any group and family. There is ease and discomfort at the same time. Balance is constantly sought to meet different needs and pleasure and fulfillment.

The Healthy Adult can live with this continuous dynamic and even experience pleasure in doing so.

But it does mean that sometimes we have to endure discomfort, get angry, or feel abandoned.

3.5 Mirroring

Description

"Pick a partner. Find a spot together in the room where you want to work. You are going to mirror in a moment. One person (A) will do movements for you and the other one (B) will do the same as best he can in the same moment. Like looking in the mirror."

If necessary, show what you mean briefly with one of the participants. Emphasize that it must be exactly the same in the same moment.

"Choose who will be mirrored and who will mirror. I will tell you when to switch roles."

See what happens. Help if the clients have not yet mastered the concept of mirror image. Give them plenty of time. Emphasize that the therapist indicates when they will switch roles.

"Okay, a short break. Just briefly exchange a first reaction with each other. (...) And we're going to switch roles now, so the other person (B) shows what to do, A mirrors. This time without verbal explanation or help.... I will again tell you when to switch roles."

Pause, give time to briefly exchange a first reaction with each other and reflect with the group, "What works and what doesn't?"

You might explain the Healthy Adult and the balance between taking care of oneself and consideration for others. In this, A represents the Healthy Adult and B the child that mirrors.

Repeat: A shows, B imitates. This time shorter and with music.

You might challenge clients to vary more with different body parts, then with changes in direction and perhaps even moves.

Change roles without stopping:

"Go ahead and while you're at it, you're going to switch roles, so the other person (B) now shows what to do and the first one (A) imitates."

Repeat, "Continue and switch roles."

Repeat, "Switch roles."

Repeat, "Change."

Make the time between switches shorter and shorter.

AIM

- Taking care of oneself as a Healthy Adult and taking care of others.
- Awareness of coping.
- Awareness of child needs.
- Non-verbal communication.
- Alignment.

Connection to healthy ego functions

- Personality integration and the formation of a self-image.
- Healthy emotion regulation.
- Contact with one's own emotions/needs and those of others.
- Testing reality and assessing situations, conflicts, and relationships.

Materials

Music.

Group/pair/individual

- Group.
- Subgroups/twos or threes, for example.
- Individually in the group.
- Individually.

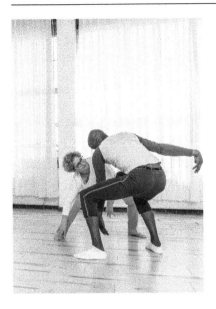

Further details

If necessary, a body-oriented mindfulness exercise can be done beforehand, so that clients make contact with themselves and their need of the moment and become less lost in the interaction.

Music can be supportive, but it can also be directing and therefore even limiting. Add music initially as soon as there is some calm and concentration. For example: Philip Glass—Houston Skyline. Repeating with different music may actually support or challenge clients to a greater or lesser degree to stay with their own needs.

As a therapist be a helping Ideal Parent and help keep it safe. Support the Parent/Healthy Adult. Allow the clients enough time to come into their role and solve "problems." Step in when harm is about to occur.

There are many variations and options in leading and following. This intervention relates primarily to Laban's (1947) category of Effort, which means it is about personal effort. What is the inner attitude?

In this case, this intervention may symbolize a parent–child relationship (A parent, B child). A, the parent, is the protagonist with the goal of applying healthy adult behavior. While A (the parent) leads his own life and also takes care of the other person, B (the child) mirrors him.

Mirroring involves multiple layers and could serve multiple purposes. The repetition would allow the partners (A+B) to increasingly fulfill their need and take care of the other person, thereby becoming attuned to each other, gaining corrective experiences.

This working method from the perspective of schemas, modes, and basic needs: for A, the parent and thus the Healthy Adult, the conflict becomes palpable. On the one hand, he goes for his own needs, which helps with the basic need Self-expression. On the other hand, he has to think carefully about what B, the child, can mirror, which involves realistic boundaries (schema Self-sacrifice or Submission). Meanwhile, B (the child) is noticed.

If A is acting from a Dysfunctional Child mode, this quickly becomes apparent in the process. Slow, controlled movements with faces toward each other are easier than quick, sudden, uncontrolled movements and when turning or moving away from each other, resulting in B's needs not being noticed.

Raise awareness of coping where necessary. Then, the Healthy Adult can once again find a balance between following his own (movement) needs and consideration for others.

Extensions/additions

- A rescripting of a historical scene imaginary can be done by creating an affect bridge.
- By repeating everything with another partner the process can be repeated and new experiences, corrective or perpetuating, can be gained.
- Both clients mirror in the Healthy Adult parent role. Both are in charge and must follow each other.
- Next, the pair can be expanded where the group mirroring each other gradually grows larger and larger. In this, the contrasts in basic needs become clear.
- If necessary, an intervention with opposing movements can be done as a conclusion, for example, individually or as a group uncontrolled and fast.

EVALUATION

- What coping did you deploy? Or what mode became active?
- Why is coping necessary? Where or when did you learn this protective behavior?
- At what age? In what situation?
- Where necessary raising awareness of coping, connecting to the past and rescripting.
- Have you also taken care of yourself, and how? Or how could you? (Parent role)
- Did you feel noticed? (Child role)
- Were you well taken care of?
- What did you notice?
- How did you feel? What caused this?
- Do you recognize this from your childhood? When would you have needed this (rescript if necessary)?

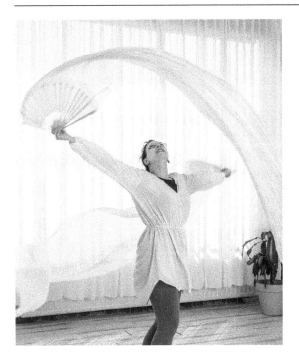

3.6 Dance improvisation with materials

Description

Depending on how safe and free the group members feel, the therapist offers each client one piece of the material that is central in this session (e.g., balls, ropes, chairs, cloths, sticks, balloons, or stones), or the therapist distributes enough items throughout the room.

Let clients play freely, explore what is possible: "Go ahead, see what you can do with the stuff."

Do this first without and later with the movement quality support music present.

Should it not arise, after a while encourage playing, working, and dancing together.

Depending on the situation, you encourage (collectively) creating an appropriate ending/completion for (interim) reflection.

AIM

- Free play.
- Making your own choices, being allowed to be independent.
- Expressing spontaneity and fun.
- Being able to express needs and emotions.

Connection to healthy ego functions

- Personality integration and the formation of a self-image.
- Healthy emotion regulation.
- Contact with one's own emotions/needs and those of others.
- Seeking enjoyment and fulfillment in a mature manner.

Materials

Balls, ropes, chairs, cloths, sticks, balloons, stones, totaling the same number as the number of clients.

Music that supports the movement quality of the moment.

Group/pair/individual

- Group.
- Individually.

Further details

In preparation for or as a follow-up to this micro-intervention, interventions can be done aimed at experiencing various qualities. For example, one can dance as different materials:

- The therapist moves the materials, and the clients mirror them.
- What kind of materials are they? Dance like this yourself: round, straight, hard, soft, light, heavy.
- Improvise as the object with music that supports the movement quality of the material.

As therapist: Repeat the basic rules, for example: do not break anything and do not hurt anyone, including yourself. The therapist is the Positive Parent and provides a safe environment and atmosphere in which to be allowed to play. Watch what happens, with an inviting and complimentary attitude. Point out what you see, also as an inspiration to others.

The therapist may also need to be there for the Vulnerable Child mode, limiting and neutralizing unadjusted coping modes.

This intervention runs over several sessions and can be offered as a module. The structure remains the same. The content is determined by the clients in the moment itself. At the end of this series of sessions, which always focus on one type of material, a session can be offered in which different materials are danced with. Memories can be retrieved, and both the fun of the Free Child and the success of the Healthy Adult can be celebrated.

This intervention relates primarily to Laban's (1947) category of Effort, which means it is about how, with what intention/effort or attitude the client moves. A broad idiom in this provides more opportunities for expression, for example, but also for attunement. Here, clients can practice not only expressing themselves but also keeping it safe, regulating impulses and emotions in contact with each other.

This intervention involves multiple layers and could serve multiple purposes. Different modes and schemas can be activated. To complement the intervention, by creating an affect bridge, a historical scene for one of the clients could be rescripted into dance, imaginatively or experimentally. Another variation is, for example, to challenge the Healthy Adult skills in dealing with scarcity, tuning in and playing together, by each time asking another participant to give you his material, so that in the end there is only one item left to play with (together).

EVALUATION

In the clients' Free Child experience, one hardly needs to reflect.

Applaud them for what they did, celebrate the mood, and so on. If necessary, ask briefly what they liked and/or what schema was broken. You might evoke any nice, special, Happy/Free Child memories.

Do make room for the other modes. Preferably not in a problemizing way, but at the client's request:

- What happened? What was this like? What mode did you find yourself in?
- Was there anything else that bothered you?
- What could help with this?
- When would you have needed this? At what age? In what situation? (A rescripting could be a follow-up.)
- What was a nice moment for you?
- Reflect only in between games if verbal interventions during play do not work.

3.7 Interpersonal dialogue between Healthy Adult and Vulnerable Child

Description

This working method consists of a group dance improvisation and a writing and drawing reflection.

This exercise can be done after a warm-up and/or an individual dance exploration of schemas and/or modes.

Step 1

"The field in which you will move today for this dance movement exploration is this field: show on the floor a large square field with enough space for the whole group to move freely. Use objects or tape to clearly indicate the field."

"Around the main field is a safe space/frame. This space is there to be able to step out of the exploration field to return to yourself, reset, breathe, regulate, orient yourself, and observe the experience and choices of others."

Step 2

"Half of the group (Group A) will embody and explore the Healthy Adult mode, while the other half of the group (Group B) will embody and explore a child mode. It is up to you to choose the child mode that attracts you the most. You can also choose to play with different child modes during the exploration. The exploration lasts 15 minutes."

Step 3

"During dance exploration, your task is to connect with other movers and communicate through dance and movement from your mode. You are free to connect with both movers in child mode and Healthy Adult mode."

Step 4

"After 15 minutes of dance exploration, you step out of the field and have 10 minutes to reflect on your exploration by writing and/or drawing on a piece of paper."

Step 5

"After these 10 minutes (without verbal exchange—no talking), we switch roles: Group A embodies a child mode and Group B embodies the Healthy Adult mode."

Step 6

"After movement (15 minutes) and writing/drawing (10 minutes), we will meet in a circle for the follow-up discussion, where you will have room to reflect on the experience and share your writing and drawing with the group."

Step 7

Still any questions? I will guide you through this structure step by step.

AIM

- Embodying mode and connecting with another person.
- Regulating emotions in contact with others.
- Experiencing self-esteem.

Connection to healthy ego functions

- Personality integration and the formation of a self-image.
- Healthy emotion regulation.
- Contact with one's own emotions/needs and those of others.
- Healthy internal dialogue.

Materials

Paper and writing and drawing materials.
   Optionally music: Providing structure and/or a source of inspiration during improvisation.

Group/pair/individual

- Group.

Further details

This working method is appropriate after a warm-up in which the client has already made a connection with the body, his emotional state, the room, and the other group members.
   It is an exercise to offer to a group that has a basic idea of dance therapy.
   The safe space is designed for clients to practice getting in and out of the space, feeling and setting their boundaries, practicing their ability to regulate and orient emotions.

When offering this exercise, many different interrelational dynamics take place non-verbally and it is interesting to have the clients use the safe space to observe each other. It is also important during the exercise to encourage group members to stay connected to their bodies and emotions.

The child modes are the Vulnerable, Angry, Enraged, Impulsive, or Undisciplined Child as well as the Happy/Free Child.

The Healthy Adult can be substituted by the Demanding or Punitive Parent to gain more insight into unhealthy dynamics, if the group and client feel safe enough to address this.

EVALUATION

- What did you experience when you embodied the Healthy Adult in contact with someone who was in a child mode or Healthy Adult mode (and vice versa)?
- What were the differences between the roles for you?
- What did you perceive emotionally, physically, and mentally?
- Could you connect with another person?
- In what way did you make contact?
- What succeeded and what did not in contact?
- What affected or confronted you?
- What were your triggers?
- Where did you feel resistance?
- Where did you experience tension or overwhelming emotions?
- Did you step out of the exploration field/have you used the safe space?
- If so, why did you get out and what did you experience there?

3.8 Internal dialogue between Healthy Adult and Vulnerable Child

Description

Step 1

"Walk quietly through the room and ask your body where it wants to begin movement exploration. Find your safe spot in the room. Starting from this spot, you have 10 minutes to explore and discover your Healthy Adult and Vulnerable Child through dance improvisation. Without spending too much time thinking about what it might look like, ask your body during dance improvisation and movement exploration how the Healthy Adult feels in your body, how it moves, and how it expresses itself. The same with the Vulnerable Child; ask your body how it experiences this and how it feels inside. And as you go further in this exploration, see how and if they can communicate internally with each other. How does your

Healthy Adult communicate with your Vulnerable Child? How does this communication and connection manifest itself in movement and dance?"

"The most important thing is to let your body and emotions guide you through the experience."

"You can use movement, gestures, and postures, open and closed eyes, and keep your attention on yourself—try not to be distracted by others. Be guided by your body and emotions as you explore. You can use the space around you, different dynamics and forms." Instructions while moving: "stay connected to your body, try to keep moving. If moving is difficult, use postures or gestures."

Step 2

"Now you get 10 minutes to create a short movement sequence/choreography based on your dance improvisation in which you explore the relationship between your Healthy Adult and your Vulnerable Child. Stay close to your exploration and emotions and use these movements to create a short choreography. Use a minimum of five movements for the Healthy Adult and five movements for the Vulnerable Child. Here, the therapist can give an example of how to use improvisation in a fixed movement (choreography), how to repeat it, and how to stay close to the emotional charge behind the movement."

Step 3

"One by one, you will show your choreography to the group. Choose the spot and position in the room where you want to start moving and where the group should stand or sit. Who will go first?"

Step 4

"Now that all of you have shared your choreography, we can come back to the circle and share your personal experience about the session with each other" (follow-up discussion: 20 minutes minimum).

AIM

- Enduring one's own vulnerability.
- Emotion regulation and being able to mentalize.
- Creating meaning from emotional states.
- Being able to shape and express mental, emotional, and physical tensions in relation to vulnerability and self-care.

Connection to healthy ego functions

- Personality integration and the formation of a self-image.
- Healthy emotion regulation.
- Healthy internal dialogue.
- Seeking enjoyment and fulfillment in a mature manner.

Materials

Possibly music as structure and/or a source of inspiration.

Group/pair/individual

- Individually in the group.
- Individually.

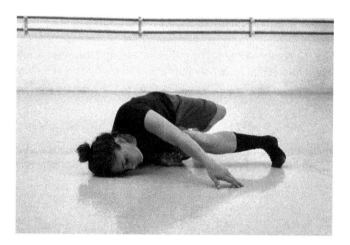

Further details

This working method is appropriate after a warm-up in which the client has already made a connection with his body, his emotional state, the room, and the other group members.

It is an exercise to offer to a group of clients who have a basic idea of dance therapy, who know how to bring attention inward and how to listen to body sensations and emotions, and who are able to keep moving on their own for 10 minutes.

During the exercise there may be clients who are not yet able to register their emotions and who go into hyper- or hypo arousal; in other words, they get outside the "window of tolerance." Depending on the situation, general or individual instructions can be given to orient (return to the here and now), keep moving, and alternate between inner and outer focus.

The Vulnerable Child mode can be interchanged with all other child modes, such as the Angry, Enraged, Impulsive, Undisciplined Child mode. But also, with the Happy Child mode. The Healthy Adult mode can be substituted by the Demanding Parent or Punitive Parent mode to gain more insight into unhealthy dynamics, if the group and client feel safe enough to address this.

EVALUATION

- What did you experience when you embodied the Healthy Adult and/ or the Vulnerable Child?
- What affected or confronted you?
- When you embodied these two modes, could you allow yourself to feel the emotions and turn them into movement?
- If not, what prevented you?
- Were you able to perceive and/or what did you perceive in your physical, emotional, behavioral, and thinking patterns as you embodied the two modes?
- Do you recognize these mechanisms in your daily life?
- Have you gained new perspectives on your patterns?
- Which emotions were more difficult to regulate?
- Could you stay in the window of tolerance?
- Did you recognize other modes that came up?
- Could you remain present, caring, and compassionate to yourself when you feel vulnerable?
- What do you take away from these experiences and what do you want to leave behind here?

3.9 Battle of Protectors

Description

"Choose a protector that bothers you. For example, the Detached Protector, Angry Protector, Over-Controller, Self-Soother, Compliant Surrenderer, Perfectionist, Bully and Attack mode."

Protector visualization (two minutes): "Close your eyes and think of situations in which this protector was active. How do you feel, talk, move, and behave? Imagine it as clearly as you can."

Imagining modes (five minutes): "Create some movements that symbolize this side of you. How would you represent this side of you with gestures and body language? You can think of silent movies with exaggerated actors or pantomime. Try out some movements (about two minutes)."

"How would you portray this side of you without words? Is this side of you fast or slow? Does it feel heavy or light? What body parts do you use? Exaggerate a little, it's okay! (About two minutes of neutral music.) Keep moving and exploring in order to further internalize these movements; embody this part of you."

Modes model imagining: "Now two volunteers are needed. One will play the Healthy Adult and the other will play the Vulnerable Child. After this, you will play the protector again, so remember the moves you just made."

The therapist explains the following: "The Vulnerable Child sits down in this corner of the room, all sad, anxious, alone. The protectors are standing around the Vulnerable Child. The Healthy Adult stands on the other side of the protectors' wall. When I turn on the music, the Vulnerable Child starts trying to ask for help, attention, and love from the Healthy Adult."

"The protectors block the Healthy Adult with their movements and bodies. Do your best, protectors." (See Figure 3.1.)

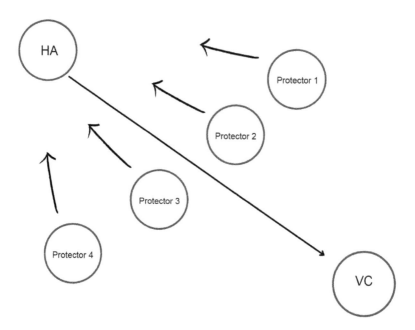

Figure 3.1 The protectors in action.

"The Healthy Adult wants to reach the Vulnerable Child and goes out of his way to break through all the protectors to meet the emotional needs of the Vulnerable Child."

"When the Healthy Adult has reached the Vulnerable Child, the protectors stop protecting."

"The Healthy Adult and the Vulnerable Child remain together for a moment. For example, the Healthy Adult may compliment the Vulnerable Child, hold his hand, give attention, stay with him, make eye contact. The Healthy Adult checks carefully what feels comfortable for the Vulnerable Child—maybe physical contact is too frightening but maybe not, ask what feels right."

"The Healthy Adult can ask, 'what do you need?' Only when the Vulnerable Child's need is met, is the exercise completed."

The therapist takes care of the music and encourages participants. If the protectors are too soft, the therapist asks for more opposition or vice versa.

If necessary, the therapist also coaches the encounter between the Healthy Adult and the Vulnerable Child.

"Well done!"

"Now we're going to switch roles!"

AIM

- Becoming aware of protectors and survival mechanisms.
- Asking for and receiving help.
- Developing the Healthy Adult.

Connection to healthy ego functions

- Personality integration and the formation of a self-image.
- Contact with one's own emotions/needs and those of others.
- Testing reality and assessing situations, conflicts, and relationships.

Materials

Music. Possibly masks.

Group/pair/individual

- Group.

Further details

The therapist can choose to share the experiences in plenary, in pairs, or have them written down.

Not everyone has to play the Vulnerable Child or the Healthy Adult. The therapist can decide how often the roles are switched. Given the available time, two or three times would be ideal.

The working method might also be carried out using masks designed in the likeness of the various protectors.

EVALUATION

- What was it like doing the exercise? Experiences?
- What was it like to portray the protector? What did you find difficult about it?
- As a Healthy Adult, what was it like to offer the child attention and help?
- How do you do this with your own emotional needs?
- And as a Vulnerable Child, what was it like to ask for and receive help?
- How do you do this in your daily life?

3.10 Happy Child plays freely

Description

Step 1: Visualization (about seven or eight minutes)

"We begin by closing our eyes, or you can leave them half-open if you prefer."

"Use a mindfulness exercise of your choice, for example, body scan, breathing exercise, short progressive relaxation, bubble."

"Let images of your Happy Child surface (…). Moments in your childhood when you could feel free, playful, and spontaneous (…). When you could be totally absorbed in a game, or you were enjoying nature, friends (…). If your childhood was very tough and you have trouble getting an image, create it yourself. Create an image yourself of your Happy Child playing, safe. Now try to evoke this child in you, bring it into the here and now, so to speak (…). Slowly open your eyes."

Step 2: Balloon Phase I (maximum 10 minutes)

"As you can see, we have a balloon here, a balloon that can fly, but should not touch the floor. I will turn on the music and you will keep the balloon in the air.

When I stop the music, you will freeze and one of you can hold the balloon. When the music continues, you will continue moving (music on, with random pauses)."

Suddenly, the therapist throws a second balloon. Without instructions, they will understand that this one must not touch the floor either. Their adaptability is put to the test.

Then, the therapist throws another one, and another one, until the number of balloons equals the number of participants. Also continue to pause the music occasionally for relaxation and regulation.

Step 3: Balloons Phase II (five minutes, also with music)

"Without stopping moving, you choose a balloon for yourself. Now you start playing on your own. You can dance with your balloon, or you can transform the balloon into an animal or something else with your imagination. You can do whatever you want, together with your Happy Child and your balloon."

"You are free to do what you normally wouldn't dare to do, you can go crazy, no one is going to criticize or punish you."

Slowly find a way to wrap up the exercise. Leave the balloon on the floor, stretch and take a deep breath.

AIM

- Allowing fun.
- Experiencing spontaneity and play.
- Experiencing barriers of punishment and criticism.

Connection to healthy ego functions

- Healthy emotion regulation.
- Seeking enjoyment and fulfillment in a mature manner.

Materials

Balloons.

Group/pair/individual

- Group.
- Subgroups/twos or threes, for example.

Further details

In the phase with the balloons, there may be many different possible reactions from clients: not feeling like doing this, being critical or punitive, shame, a Detached Protector mode, and so on. The therapist can point this out, for example, "I see a lot of Detached Protectors here."

If the energy is too low, the therapist can join in and do things in a more playful or energetic way. If the energy is too high, the therapist can save the balloons in a calmer way (modeling).

EVALUATION

Take a moment to write down your experience.

- How did you experience the exercise?
- Did you suffer from your critical side at times?
- How did you respond to that?
- Do you notice this happening outside of therapy as well?
- How does this hinder you?
- Can you lose yourself in the activity?
- In what situations in your life can you experience pleasure?
- Choose an activity you can do next week, something you can experience the Happy Child with.
- Be specific and also write it down in your notebook. Discuss the chosen activity in pairs.

3.11 Anger is allowed

Description

Start with the following introduction:

"A Healthy Adult is also allowed to be angry at times; anger is an important emotion we need to indicate our boundaries and desires. We like to express anger in a non-explosive way, as in the Angry Child; or not in a hurtful way, as in the Bully and Attack mode. We do not want to swallow the anger either, as in the Compliant Surrender side or be passively aggressive as in our Angry Protector side."

"In this exercise, we will experience and express anger in a safe way. Take a piece of paper and write on it one or two words that summarize what bothers, irritates, frustrates, or angers you. It can be something small or something bigger (therapist gives examples). Do not choose a very traumatic memory or anger directed at yourself."

Step 1: Initial phase

"Choose a spot in the room where you have enough space and put the piece of paper in front of you on the floor. We are going to do various movements with our arms and legs."

In the beginning, the client can follow the therapist and later he can seek out his own speed and intensity. The therapist chooses one or two songs from the table, or another song with equal tempo and power, for example, rock or percussion:

Artist Song	Song
Meute	Rej
Moderat	A New Error
Dover	Cherry Lee
Joy	Division Disorder
Zombie Nation	Kernkraft
The Cure	Forest
Ludovico Einaudi	Taranta
Tribal Dance	Gathering
Rage against the Machine	Killing in the Name

Step 2: The construction phase

"We start with our arms, move them slowly, push forward with our palms up. Think about the subject you have written about."

"Keep moving, feel the strength in your body. We follow the rhythm of the music. Take occasional five-second breaks to rest your arms and breathe."

"We now go a little faster; you can make fists with your hands" (the therapist's voice also becomes more intense, louder).

"Follow your breath, hitting the air with each exhalation. Now use your legs and kick forward."

"Feel the strength in your whole body. Let your Angry Child be complete for a moment."

"For another 20 seconds, give everything you have, throw everything out, maximum intensity!"

Step 3: Regulation phase (music off)

This stage is essential—so do not skip it.

"Stay standing, relax your arms, shoulders, neck, and legs. Feel your feet on the ground. Let the tension and emotion sink in slowly. Take a deep breath. Look around you calmly and observe the colors and sounds of the room. Walk around and take a sip of water if you like."

AIM

- Experiencing anger in a healthy and safe way.
- Reducing fear of overwhelming emotions.

Connection to healthy ego functions

- Healthy emotion regulation.
- Contact with one's own emotions/needs and those of others.

Materials

Music system, Post-its, or paper and pen.

Group/pair/individual

- Group.
- Individually.

Further details

In some people the Angry Child is too uninhibited and impulsive. In that case, it is especially important to be able to set limits on our anger. For others, on the other hand, it would be a good thing if they expressed their anger more often.

Try to avoid (to have) too much tension on the shoulders and neck, the movement should come from the center of the body, legs bent and powerful.

People may shut down (affect phobia) during the exercise. Pay attention to this in the evaluation.

EVALUATION

Discuss the following questions in pairs (the therapist writes the questions on the board).

- How can you set boundaries to your Angry Child next time?
- How could you do this exercise at home if you are too high in frustration? For example, jumping, climbing stairs before responding.
- Ask your Healthy Adult, "What can I do now to express my anger in a healthy way?" (The therapist may explain simple assertiveness skills.)
- Do you want to discuss anything with someone? Set boundaries?
- How can you make sure you do not swallow your anger next time?

3.12 Emotion circles

Description

"We will work with three emotions today. Choose two from anger, fear, sadness, and shame. Joy will be used to conclude the exercise."

"Write each emotion on a piece of paper."

"Now choose a spot in the room for each emotion and put the corresponding piece of paper there."

"First, we all stand in a neutral space. Take a deep breath, observe your bodily sensations. We will now enter Emotion 1."

"Take a step and close your eyes or leave them half-open if you feel restless."

Phase I: Observation

- "Let memories and images come up that evoke this emotion." (30 seconds of silence)
- "Take your time."
- "What are you scared/angry/sad/ashamed of/about?" (30 second pause)
- "Let the images grow or develop, observe your thoughts." (Pause)
- "Now observe your bodily sensations. Do you feel anything in your body?" (Pause)
- "If you don't notice anything, that is okay too."

Phase II: Gesture

- "Keep your eyes closed."
- "If your hands expressed this emotion, if your hands communicated how you feel, what would they do?"
- "Try to find a gesture that can express your emotion and show this gesture. Leave out the demanding side, anything goes. Everything is okay. No one is judging you."
- "Remember this gesture, hold on to it."
- "Take a slow, deep breath, release the gesture and open your eyes. Take a step back to the neutral space."

Repeat this step with Emotion 2 and then with Emotion 3 joy. Between each emotion there is a moment of rest in the neutral space to be able to release and regulate the previous emotion.

Phase III: Merging emotions into a dance

Share the gestures in pairs and find a way to transform the gesture to a movement using the whole body.

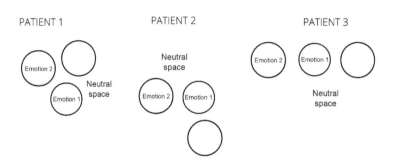

Figure 3.2 Emotional circles.

The therapist puts on quiet music and allows five minutes for this.

Now try to create a complete dance, with all three emotion movements. Leave out the demanding part and give your Happy/Free Child space to play and explore in the creative process. (Quiet music plays and clients have seven minutes to do this.)

"Finally, we will present the dance. We make a circle and each of us will share the little dance of the emotions. It may be confronting, but we practice leaving the critical voice aside. We are here to support each other."

"You are allowed to show your vulnerability. We are not going to judge or compare."

AIM

- Getting in touch with your own emotions.
- Regulating and sharing emotions.
- Developing creativity.

3.12.2 Connection to healthy ego functions

- Healthy emotion regulation.
- Contact with one's own emotions/needs and those of others.
- Healthy internal dialogue.

Materials

Possibly circles/hoops to symbolize each emotion.

Group/pair/individual

- Group.
- Subgroups/twos or threes, for example.
- Individually.

Further details

If time is short, you can omit Phase III.
   The exercise can also be done in individual therapy.

EVALUATION

- How did you experience the exercise?
- What was the easiest and the hardest step?
- In which emotion did you feel more comfortable, in which one less comfortable?
- What helped you regulate emotion at the beginning?
- If you didn't feel anything, what could be the reason?
- What helped you overcome the tension at the end of the exercise?
- Our Happy Child can play and be spontaneous without thinking much; what was the creative process like for you?
- Have you noticed things that also occur in your daily life?

3.13 Discarding critical pebbles

Description

Introduction

"Today we will work on the critical voice. Almost everyone suffers from a negative and judgmental voice in his head. If it is too present, it becomes difficult to let the Healthy Adult grow and even more difficult to give space to the Happy Child."

   "It can be a demanding, punishing, or guilt-inducing voice. Do you have any examples?"

   The therapist writes these on the board.

"Today, we will try to become more aware of our internal dialogue. Here is a bag of pebbles, take a handful and put them in your own pocket. Then put the container on the floor in the middle of the room."

Step 1: Warm-up (five minutes)

"We will physically warm up without music. During the warm-up, the idea is to observe if any critical thoughts come into your mind. If so, throw a pebble in the container right away. 'For example, "Come on! You need to try harder, don't show off!' 'Oh, I'm not agile enough!' 'How poor my condition is, how stupid of me!' 'Pff, it's my own fault because I do not go to the gym.'

You throw away one pebble for each thought. If you have three critical thoughts, throw three pebbles. Every time. As soon as you feel it coming. Are there any questions?"

Step 2: Circle (10 minutes)

We will slowly stand in a circle, and I will turn on the music and start leading (Chacian Circle). I will do simple dance steps or movements, and you will try to follow me. Without words. And when I call your name, you become the leader and the rest will follow your movements. Then you call someone else's name to pass on the turn.

It is important to adapt to your abilities and not push yourself to do everything, you do not have to do exactly the same thing 100%. It is totally okay to adjust the movement.

We are going to use the pebbles again. Every critical thought (even when you are leading) you throw into the container. For example: "I'm really not creative, I can't think of anything," "She is much better than me, I'm really useless." Also, when criticizing the exercise itself, this can sometimes be a sign of avoidance: "What a stupid exercise," "What are we doing this for?" "I don't really feel like doing this." Then you too throw a pebble in the container.

3.14 Guessing game

Description

This is a warm-up exercise.

Everyone stands in a circle (Chacian circle) to create equality, connection, visibility, and support/holding. The group has already done a bottom-up (from feet to head) warm-up of the muscles and joints and is ready to begin this exercise.

We are going to play a game, still in the circle, and the goal is to guess the mode that the person in the middle of the circle embodies/expresses. The person who guesses correctly is the next to step to the center and to embody a mode. You can use dance, movement, gestures, and postures. Follow your instinct and your body. Keep moving until the correct mode is mentioned in the group. If no one guesses correctly, try changing your movement form or perspective, think creatively and connect with the other group members so that you get the clients to follow your movements.

Here you (as therapist) may give an example of choosing a mode, make/ embody a movement of it and have the whole group mirror it. "Who wants to start?"

I invite you to move and feel along with the person standing in the middle as you try to guess what mode that person is in.

We will continue until everyone has stood in the middle at least once.

AIM

- Exploring modes.
- Experiencing pleasure and connection.
- Contact with bodily sensations.

Connection to healthy ego functions

- Contact with one's own emotions/needs and those of others.
- Testing reality and assessing situations, conflicts, and relationships.
- Seeking enjoyment and fulfillment in a mature manner.

Materials

Possibly music.

Group/pair/individual

- Group.
- Individually in the group.

Further details

Asking a client to stand in the center of the circle often causes tension. Being seen and watched is often a trigger and stressor. It takes some courage to step in, but once the group gets into a flow, the tension and pressure drop.

It is possible to break the circle and use a different arrangement, such as a line, half a circle, or scattered around the room. You can do the exercise with or without music.

A point might be given for each correct guess. Thus, a winner might be desig-nated at the end of the exercise. This all depends on the intention of the exercise and the stage in the group therapy.

EVALUATION

Brief follow-up talk (it is, after all, a warm-up):

- Did you experience any triggers or tensions during the exercise?
- Can you name and describe them?
- Do you recognize this reaction in your daily life, or can you link it to your past?
- In which modes did you feel resistance?
- Where does the resistance come from?

3.15 Being empathetic and moving along

Description

Round 1: Embodying the Healthy Adult

- "Find a partner and decide together who is A and who is B."
- "For five minutes, A will move from the Healthy Adult side while B moves along. In moving along, you are freer than in exact mirroring. So, watch how you decide to move along with the other person. A, your job is to stay true to the Healthy Adult side, and B, your job is to be as aware as possible of your way of moving along with A's movement. Try to keep observing yourself as you move."
- "After the first round, A and B take two minutes to verbally reflect on the experience. A begins to share, B listens without response or feedback to A's story."
- "Then B gets two minutes to share about the experience of moving along, while A listens. Again, continue to observe your internal reaction and tendency."
- Switch roles and repeat this entire exercise (moving and follow-up talk).

Round 2: Embodying a chosen child mode

- We do this exercise again, but this time embodying a child mode in which you are most affected or triggered (Vulnerable, Angry, Enraged, Impulsive, Undisciplined).

Round 3: Change of partner(s)

- Go through Rounds 1 and 2 again but this time with a new partner.

AIM

- Empathizing with the other person while staying connected to oneself.
- Setting boundaries.
- Observing internal dialogue.

Connection to healthy ego functions

- Personality integration and the formation of a self-image.
- Contact with one's own emotions/needs and those of others.
- Healthy internal dialogue.

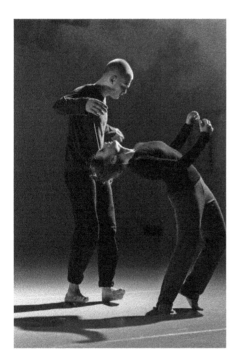

Materials

None.

Group/pair/individual

- Subgroups/twos or threes, for example.

Further details

The distinction between mirroring and moving along is that when you mirror, you try to imitate the other person's movement as exactly as possible, whereas when you move along, you are freer in how you decide to move along with the other person.

Moving along creates the opportunity to experience/create matches and mismatches during movement exploration. This creates different interactional dynamics and generates different emotions, which can be observed and reflected upon.

During the short follow-up talk, there is one speaker and one listener. This is intended to train both verbal self-expression and the ability to listen without having to take up space. Listening without saying a word can be challenging and is an interesting topic to talk about during the follow-up discussion with the group.

It is recommended that each client does the exercise with as many different people as possible to experience the difference in exchange and contact.

The difference in experience is an interesting topic to discuss during the follow-up group discussion.

This working method is about creating an empathetic bond while maintaining self-esteem.

EVALUATION

- Did you experience any triggers or tensions during the exercise? Can you name and describe them? Do you recognize this reaction in your daily life, or can you link it to your past?
- In which modes did you feel resistance? Where did the resistance come from?
- As a mover (A): What did you experience while moving? What did you feel? How did you experience the connection or contact with B? Did your mode change while moving?
- As a co-mover (B): What modes did you get into?
- In the short talk during the exercise, did you manage not to interrupt the other person? If not, why did you interrupt the other person? Was it difficult to just listen? What exactly did you find difficult?
- Could you empathize with your partner during the movement? What did you feel?
- What were your coping mechanisms as a mover and co-mover?
- Do you recognize these patterns also outside of therapy, in your private life?

3.16 Warm-up: Embodying modes

3.16.1 Description

"Everyone stands in a circle (Chacian circle) to create equality, connection, visibility, and support/holding. The group has already done a bottom-up (from feet to head) warm-up of the muscles and joints and is ready to begin this exercise."

"In the center of the circle, you will see pieces of paper with different modes written on them. Take the time to read them all and ask questions if a term is unclear."

"One person begins by choosing one mode written on the piece of paper and makes it into a (dance) movement in the circle and to music. At the same time the rest of the group mirrors/moves along with the movement that is presented. Once everyone has picked up your movement and has repeated it a few times, you pass the lead on to someone else. Instructions while moving: stay connected to your body, try to keep moving. If moving is difficult, use postures or gestures."

Here, you as therapist may give an example of choosing a mode and making/embodying a movement and have the whole group mirror it.

Continue in this way until everyone has had the lead at least three times.

AIM

- Experiencing modes from an embodied perspective.
- Becoming aware of and using emotions.
- Experiencing empathy and connection with each other.
- Emotion regulation.

3.16.2 Connection to healthy ego functions

- Healthy emotion regulation.
- Contact with one's own emotions/needs and those of others.
- Seeking pleasure in a mature way and needing fulfillment.

3.16.3 Materials

Music, cards with modes written on them.

3.16.4 Group/pair/individual

- Group.
- Subgroups/twos or threes, for example.
- Individually in the group.
- Individually.

3.16.5 Further details

This working method introduces clients to the various modes and how to put them into motion. By mirroring each other, clients learn new movements and learn to physically empathize with each other and the modes. Therefore, it is important that the structure of the exercise is clear and that clients are encouraged to take the time to let the body instinctively find the movement most appropriate to the modes.

Both the amount and repetition and ways of passing the lead on can be adjusted.

Rhythmic music helps create structure and grip during the exercise.

Emotion regulation takes place through dancing together, repetition, and rhythm.

EVALUATION

- Did you experience any triggers or tensions during the exercise?
- Can you name and describe them?
- Do you recognize this reaction in your daily life or can you link it to your past?
- In which modes did you feel resistance?
- Where does the resistance come from?

Reference

Laban, R., & Lawrence, F.C. (1947). *Effort*. MacDonald & Evans.

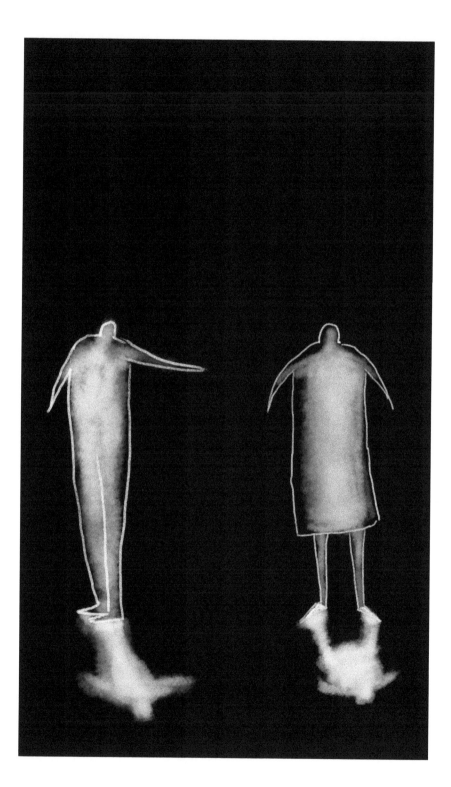

Chapter 4

Drama therapy working methods

Summary

Drama therapy involves working methodically with a fictional reality. This can be done by using the imagination to create distance from the client's issues, or by working with realistic situations to foster recognition. During the therapy, clients gain insight into their thoughts and feelings, and how these influence their functioning. Drama therapy thus contributes to the expression and management of emotions, the capacity for reflection, the expansion of the role repertoire, and the development of a more positive self-image or interpersonal and communication skills. Experiential techniques derived from drama therapy are also applied in verbal forms of psychotherapy and psychodrama, such as schema therapy.

DOI: 10.4324/9781003456988-4

4.1 Somebody at the door

Description

The clients stand in a circle. One client approaches another and pretends to ring the doorbell.

The person opens the door and the client tries to enter while playing a certain role or expressing a particular emotion. When the client is let in, the scene stops and it is the next person's turn. In general, all clients get one turn.

AIM

- Have fun.
- Connect with others.
- Assess a situation and set boundaries.

Connection to healthy ego functions

- Healthy emotion regulation.
- Contact with one's own emotions/needs and those of others.
- Testing reality and assessing situations, conflicts, and relationships.
- Seeking enjoyment and exploring needs in a mature manner.

Materials

Optional: Dress-up clothes such as hats, jackets, etc.

Group/pair/individual

- Group.
- Subgroups of two or three.
- Individually.

Further details

If clients struggle to think of a role or repeatedly choose the same type of role, cards can be used that describe a role or situation. The various schema modes can also serve as roles. For example, the client opening the door can play the role of the Punitive or Demanding Parent. Often this leads to nobody being let in; the theme of loneliness can then be discussed in the evaluation.

EVALUATION

- Did you manage to get into your role?
- Was it realistic to let someone in or out? (Schemas: safety and boundaries)
- Did you assess the situation appropriately?
- Were you able to act on the basis of your Healthy Adult? For example, were you abscle to listen to your own needs?
- How easy or difficult do you find it to let someone in?

4.2 Doing what mother does

Description

The group members walk around the space. One is given a hat; this is the "mother." The others imitate the mother as best they can, doing whatever she does. The mother can also put the hat on the head of another group member, at which point that person becomes the mother.

The therapist encourages the "mother" to do whatever she feels like doing in order to practice self-reliance and independence. The other group members can be instructed, depending on the purpose of the session, to mimic the mother's actions (an appeal to the fulfillment of the basic need of security) or, conversely, to disobey the mother in order to draw out the different modes.

This exercise is intended as a 10-minute warm-up, but it can be prolonged if group members benefit from connecting with the different modes and their protective or limiting effects.

AIM

- Experience fun.
- Practice leading.
- Practice following.
- Connect with basic needs.
- Connect with personal modes.

Connection to healthy ego functions

- Personality integration and the formation of a self-image.
- Contact with one's own emotions/needs and those of others.
- Testing reality and assessing situations, conflicts, and relationships.
- Seeking enjoyment and fulfillment in a mature manner.

Materials

A hat.

Group/pair/individual

- Group.
- Subgroups of two or three.

Further details

When a group member opts to disobey, it is important for the therapist to support the "mother," so that she can cope with the different modes and permit the group members to express them.

This exercise can be repeated with the different variants and evaluated in terms of its effect on each person.

EVALUATION

- Do you dare to take charge and move around, make noises, and vary the exercise (independently, spontaneously)?
- Are you willing to follow?
- What modes does this exercise draw out, and are they helpful or unhelpful?
- Do you dare to have fun (make strange/comical movements or noises, vary the tempo)?
- Do you dare to do whatever you feel like doing (Happy Child mode)?
- What were you like as a child? Were you obedient or not?

4.3 Cluedo

Description

Three clients leave the room. Quietly (so the clients outside do not hear), the rest of the group—the "audience"—comes up with an occupation, a location, and a murder weapon for the fourth client, who remains in the room. The therapist makes sure that the group accepts the first thing that is mentioned, unless it is offensive or disrespectful. This keeps the pace and spontaneity high and prevents the group from deliberating over how they can make it more difficult for the clients who are going to guess.

The first of the three clients in the hallway is called in. Through sounds, gestures, and movement, the fourth client tries to act out the occupation, location, and murder weapon (in that order, so the client knows which category is being acted out). Sounds are permitted, but no recognizable words. When it comes to the murder weapon, the actor pretends to kill the client.

When the client is ready to guess, he/she shakes the actor's hand.

Then the next client waiting outside is called in, and the process is repeated until all three clients have had their turn.

All of this must be done within two minutes per client. An audience member keeps track of the time and blows a horn to stop the game. This keeps the pace high and prevents clients from thinking instead of doing.

Generally, this exercise is used as a warm-up.

AIM

- Experience having fun.
- Permit mistakes (this leads to comedy!).
- Do, rather than think.

Connection to healthy ego functions

- Seeking enjoyment and fulfillment in a mature manner.

Materials

- Stopwatch, horn, or someone imitating a horn.

Group/pair/individual

- Group.
- Subgroups of two or three.

Further details

This exercise should be done at a high tempo. The point is to get clients to do rather than think. Make sure the occupation, location, and murder weapon are not too difficult. Consider giving each team a name and keeping score.

From the sidelines, the therapist offers encouragement and (silent, through, for example, gestures) coaching if someone gets stuck. It is important for the experience as a whole to be a positive one.

EVALUATION

- Did you have fun?
- Did you get in touch with your Happy Child mode?
- Did you manage not to overthink things and, when in doubt, to say yes (and to shake hands) anyway?
- What did you find helpful? The smiles or laughter of the other clients when you guessed correctly? The fast pace?

4.4 The basic needs store

Description

Ask clients what basic need of theirs was not met last week/weekend. What happened? What did they miss or need in that situation?

An imagination assignment may prove helpful.

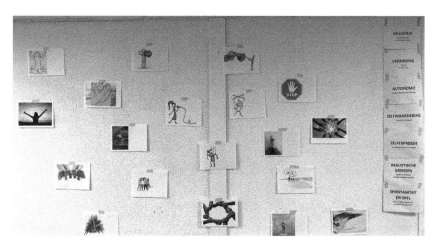

On a wall in the therapy room, use masking tape to hang up sheets of A4 paper identifying the basic needs: safety, connection, autonomy, self-esteem, self-expression, realistic boundaries, and spontaneity and play. Add sheets with pictures that represent these needs:

- Safety: Mother holding child; "protective" hands.
- Connection: Arms around each other; multiple hands in a circle holding each other.

- Autonomy: Puppet that cuts strings.
- Self-esteem: Person holding a heart; person patting themselves on the back.
- Self-expression: Colorful artwork with splashes of paint; singer with microphone.
- Realistic boundaries: Person with a stop sign; line drawn in the sand.
- Spontaneity and play: A child jumping in a puddle; a person in fancy dress.

The therapist—the "shopkeeper"—tells the group that she has a store full of basic needs and invites the first client to look around and see what he needs. "Good morning, sir. How nice to see you. Please feel free to look around and see what takes your fancy." If needed, the shopkeeper provides an explanation.

When the "customer" makes his choice, the shopkeeper asks, "What appeals to you about this image? What basic need does it portray? What exactly were you lacking last weekend? What was going on/What was the situation?"

The shopkeeper can point out another image that fits the basic need mentioned by the customer, or suggest a different basic need that the therapist believes fits the situation better or is more dominant in the client's mode model. It is up to the client to stand up for his need or choose a different picture.

The shopkeeper can make it easier or harder: "I understand that you really want this picture—it's very special/valuable, after all—but I only have one of these, and I'm expecting lots of customers today."

When the shopkeeper is persuaded, she removes the image from the wall and gives it to the customer.

As the game goes on, fewer and fewer pictures will be left on the wall. Clients will have figured out which one they want and be eagerly awaiting their turn. Two or three may want the same picture. Encourage them to negotiate, to stand up for themselves, to come up with better and better arguments—perhaps the shop-keeper can find an extra copy in the warehouse (read: photocopier) somewhere?

Clients may take the picture home and hang it up somewhere, as a reminder to stand up for their own needs, or they can put it in their therapy folder.

AIM

- Raise awareness of different basic needs.
- Consider your own basic needs and identify the strongest.
- Practice standing up for your basic needs as a Healthy Adult.

Connection to healthy ego functions

- Personality integration and the formation of a self-image.
- Contact with one's own emotions/needs and those of others.
- Seeking enjoyment and fulfillment in a mature manner.

Materials

- A4 sheets naming the basic needs
- A4 sheets with pictures that match the different basic needs (approx. four per need).
- Tape to stick the sheets to a wall.

Group/pair/individual

- Group.
- Subgroups of two or three.
- Individual work in a group setting.
- Individually.

Further details

Depending on the stage of therapy, clients receive more or less help from the therapist and group members, and the therapist/shopkeeper makes it easier or harder for them.

In the initial phase of therapy, the therapist helps clients explore which basic needs they lack, and the group members contribute ideas for how they can "persuade" the shopkeeper. For clients in the final phase, the therapist expresses confidence that they will succeed in standing up for their basic needs and persuading the shopkeeper themselves.

This exercise gives clients a better sense of what basic needs are and which of their own needs have gone unmet. The pictures make the words more meaningful.

EVALUATION

- What was this like to do?
- What are you satisfied with, for example, when you consider how you dealt with the shopkeeper?
- Was there another picture you also considered? What do you think about that now?
- What would you do differently next time?

You now know which basic needs are important to you. As a Healthy Adult, it is important to keep these needs in mind and be able to stand up for them. You practiced doing so during this exercise.

- How will you stand up for your own needs in the coming week? Set some concrete intentions and revisit the issue next week.

4.5 The invisible leader

Description

One client (A) turns around and the others point to a client who will play the role of leader (B). Now client (A) can turn around again. As the group members move around the room, the leader subtly changes something in their own movement. The others copy this movement.

Client (A) is tasked with identifying the leader. This exercise appeals to the basic needs. The leader enjoys decision-making authority and freedom of expression. Together, the group members try to follow the leader as well and as quickly as possible. This engenders spontaneity and fun, and creates a safe bond among clients.

AIM

- Experience having fun.
- Observe.

Connection to healthy ego functions

- Contact with one's own emotions/needs and those of others.
- Testing reality and assessing situations, conflicts, and relationships.
- Seeking enjoyment and fulfillment in a mature manner.

Materials

None.

Group/pair/individual

- Group.

Further details

If needed, two clients can turn around so they can confer together.

EVALUATION

- Could you handle the tension?
- Could you modify your own movements without giving the leader away?

- As leader, could you keep changing the movement without giving yourself away?
- Did the exercise trigger other modes/schemas for you, for example, failure or disconnection?
- Did you get in touch with your Happy Child mode?
- Did you feel a sense of safety and security within the group? What basic need was met for you?

4.6 A place of one's own

Description

Group members each find a spot in the room and create a space for themselves, such as a little hut.

When everyone has set up their own spot, the therapist asks if they are comfortable or want to make any final changes. Once everyone is finished, they stay in that spot for two to three minutes. Then, everybody moves to another spot in the room.

The therapist times the changes, ensuring that all group members spend a set number of minutes in each spot. Calculate in advance how long the session is in order to allow enough time for everyone to sit in each spot and for debriefing.

At the end, the group members return to their own spot for a few minutes, then sit in a circle to discuss the exercise.

AIM

- Create a comfortable place for yourself.
- Discover what somebody else considers a nice place.
- Experience how it feels to relinquish your own place to somebody else and hear what others thought of your place.

Connection to healthy ego functions

- Contact with one's own emotions/needs and those of others.
- Testing reality and assessing situations, conflicts, and relationships.
- Seeking enjoyment and fulfillment in a mature manner.

Materials

Chairs, tables, rags, sticks, pegs, etc., plus a clock/stopwatch.

Group/pair/individual

- Subgroups of two or three.
- Individually.

Further details

This exercise can also be done outside. All group members find a nice, safe place and sit there for a while, returning to the room at an agreed time. Then, the group walks together to all the spots, pausing for a while in each one. In this case, the debriefing is best done at those spots.

EVALUATION

- How did it feel to create a safe space for yourself?
- What struck you when in other people's spots?
- What was it like to come back to your own spot?
- How did it feel when others were in your spot?

The therapist explains that it is important for the Healthy Adult to listen to their needs and ensure their own safety; from there, they can begin to fulfill their needs.

- Do you experience this sense of safety in everyday life?
- Did you lack this sense of safety when you were younger? (Vulnerable Child)
- How can you maintain this sense of safety?

4.7 Coping museum

Description

The therapist explains, "In this exercise, you are invited to examine your approach to coping. When I choose you, you step outside for a moment and wait while your groupmates adopt different postures to depict the coping mechanisms they see in you. I will then welcome you into your very own 'museum of coping.' Your groupmates are 'sculptures' which you can turn on and off using an imaginary remote control. I will walk with you through your museum."

Instruction to the group when the client selected is outside:

"We will now take 10 minutes to portray the various coping mechanisms of the person outside (the therapist can demonstrate, for example, 'nervous smoking' or an irritated glance). What coping mechanisms have you seen this person use? How might you portray them, as a group or individually? We'll make explicit agreements on who does what. You might have an idea but not want to portray it yourself—that's fine. Maybe your 'sculpture' is accompanied by text, like 'It doesn't matter,' or maybe you need a prop, like a hat or a cup."

Explain this on a repeating loop (a little practice may be necessary).

AIM

- Understand how the distance created by the coping mode affects the other person.
- Gain insight into how coping modes can keep you lonely and prevent you from getting what you need.

Connection to healthy ego functions

- Personality integration and the formation of a self-image.
- Developing a healthy internal dialogue.
- Testing reality and assessing situations, conflicts, and relationships.

Materials

Optional: Props, musical instruments, or materials from the movement room.

Group/pair/individual

- Group.

Further details

This exercise involves a form of empathic confrontation. In an experimental and group-based way, clients see their own coping behaviors mirrored back at them and learn how to relate to them.

It is important to pay attention to basic safety by clearly instructing the group to remain empathetic in their feedback. If there is a conflict involving a group member that affects the group dynamics, this should be addressed in another way first.

The exercise can enhance the sense of safety and trust among group members. The "museum visitor" feels seen and opens up about their protective mechanisms.

Occasionally, a client remains stuck in a coping mode even during the exercise, putting up a wall instead of opening up. The therapist can point this out and reinforce the exercise by placing a Vulnerable Child "statue" behind one of the coping statues and seeking the Healthy Adult response.

This exercise is also appropriate for other disciplines that use arts and body-based therapies.

EVALUATION

- Did you get a good look at all the statues?
- Which ones would you like to set up and see again?
- Do you see what the sculpture is portraying, or do you have questions?
- Do you recognize the behaviors depicted as coping mechanisms?
- What is it like to be on the other side?
- What did you feel while looking at the statues?

Often the emotion of the Vulnerable Child arises, and the conversation can turn to what the client fears. Through this, they learn that sharing helps, that they can be open and trusting, and that these are the skills of a Healthy Adult.

At the end of the exercise, the other group members can share their own experiences to increase both safety and mutual empathy.

4.8 This is your boundary!

Description

The therapist explains, "This exercise is about how you deal with boundaries. A boundary will literally be taped to the ground in front of you and you will explore how you relate to it."

The clients stand and the therapist sticks a line of masking tape on the floor in front of each person, saying, "This is your boundary." She then guides the clients using questions and prompts. "Look at the tape, at your boundary. How has it come to be there? Is it comfortable, or does it hinder you? What are you experiencing in your body? Are you feeling an emotion, or do particular thoughts arise? Which side of your boundary do you currently feel like you are on? What do you see as being beyond your boundary (a danger, or something you want that you can't reach)?"

"Now step away a little bit. Turn around and feel what it's like to have your back to the boundary."

"Step over the boundary—What does that feel like?"

"Choose your favorite place relative to the boundary. What do you see before you? What situation are you in? What are you alert to? Stay connected to your body—Is there emotion there too?"

AIM

- Explore personal boundaries.
- Explore violations of those boundaries.
- Get in touch with the emotions of the Vulnerable

Connection to healthy ego functions

- Personality integration and the formation of a self-image.
- Contact with one's own emotions/needs and those of others.
- Testing reality and assessing situations, conflicts, and relationships.

Materials

Masking tape.

Group/pair/individual

- Group.
- Individual work in a group setting.
- Individually.

Further details

In this exercise, the client is put in the position of a child facing a literal boundary. This can evoke coping modes that can be explored here.

To provide depth, the therapist initially focuses on eliciting clients' direct experiences and the stories, associations, and scenes that have led to the development of these modes. The modes and schemas can be discussed on a more cognitive level at a later time.

In other arts and body-based therapies, this exercise can be adapted by, for example, drawing a line for each person on a large sheet of paper (visual therapy) or by having clients respond to the boundary through movement (dance therapy).

EVALUATION

Clients discuss their different experiences. Based on these reactions, the therapist points out how basic needs can also be opposites: a boundary can sometimes provide safety and can sometimes be perceived as a limitation.

Clients are given the opportunity to recall times in their lives when a boundary, or lack thereof, has led to the development of schemas.

Evaluation questions:

- Who set this boundary and when?
- When have you needed a boundary that wasn't there?
- Who should have been given a boundary, and by whom?
- Are you still guarding your boundary? What happens if you stop?
- What happens when someone else guards your boundary? What does that offer you?
- How has this boundary affected you?
- What do you see on the other side of the boundary?
- What have you not been able to develop because of this boundary, or lack thereof?

As a follow-up, a client can be chosen to rescript a scene from their past. This can be done with imagery rescripting (IR) in the group or played out with role characters.

4.9 Starring role

Description

One client leaves the room and the others build a set in which they themselves appear, but the lead role is missing. Give the group about three minutes to build the set.

The client returns, looks around the set, and tries to figure out what lead role he/she is playing. When the client starts playing the correct role, the others play along.

The client in the leading role directs the scene and brings it to completion.

AIM

- Experience having fun.
- Take initiative and take charge.
- Assess a situation.

Connection to healthy ego functions

- Personality integration and the formation of a self-image.
- Healthy emotion regulation.
- Contact with one's own emotions/needs and those of others.
- Testing reality and assessing situations, conflicts, and relationships.
- Seeking enjoyment and fulfillment in a mature manner.

Materials

Blocks, cloths, dress-up clothes, props.

Group/pair/individual

- Group.
- Subgroups of two or three.
- Individually.

Further details

Optional: Use cards that display a leading role, for example, an operating theater where the doctor is missing, or a courtroom where the judge is missing. Cards keep clients from thinking too long and also work well with more inexperienced groups. The therapist can assist the client if needed; after all, the idea is to have a positive experience.

A conflict can also be inserted at the moment the scene starts, for example, the patient wakes up on the operating table or the accused starts wailing and expresses regret for the offense committed. Keep in mind the experience of the group and look together at what modes might be triggered.

EVALUATION

- What was it like to come in and see what scene had been created for you?
- Did you dare to give it a try?
- How did you feel when the other players did not respond?
- Were you able to take on the starring role and lead the scene?
- Were you able to act on the basis of your Healthy Adult? Or did you react from a different mode?
- Are you satisfied with the scene?
- Would you like to act out the scene again?

4.10 Favorite role

Description

A client chooses a favorite role; a role he/she would like to play. The group then interviews the client about this role. What is the person's name? What work do they do? What was their childhood like? Is the person in a relationship? Does the person do bad things or great things?

After this, the client pictures a scene in which this person stars. The client describes how the scene should be played and what event, setting, and supporting roles are involved.

The group then plays out the scene, with the client in question playing his/her favorite role. If this fails, it may not be the client's favorite role after all.

The group subsequently evaluates whether the scene was played according to the client's wishes. If the client feels that things should have been done differently, the scene can be staged again.

AIM

- Have a pleasant experience.
- Take charge.
- Cooperate and connect with others.

Connection to healthy ego functions

- Personality integration and the formation of a self-image.
- Contact with one's own emotions/needs and those of others.
- Seeking enjoyment and fulfillment in a mature manner.

Materials

Cloths, clothing, make-up, sound effects, music system, and blackout/lighting options.

Group/pair/individual

- Group.
- Subgroups of two or three.
- Individually.

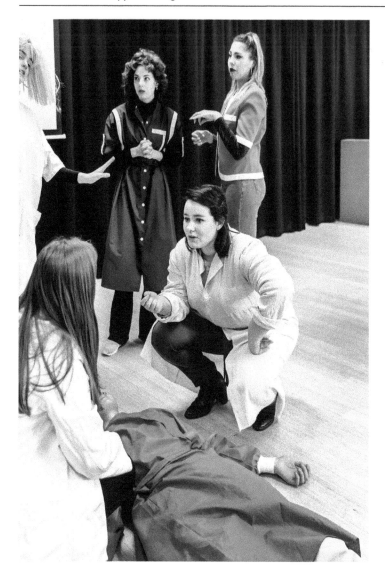

Further details

In organizing the scene, the client has the opportunity to lead the group. He/she may notice that fellow group members are keen to play along in order to give their groupmate an enjoyable experience.

Playing the role brings the client joy and allows him/her to understand its personal significance. After explaining how the role has served him/her or why it is no longer a favorite role, the client can choose a new favorite role. This is how a role career arises.

This exercise sheds light on the client's therapy process: What is important in which treatment phase? What resistance was evident in the initial phase?

EVALUATION

- What was it like to play this role?
- Did you enjoy it?
- Did it strengthen your Happy Child mode?
- How did you experience the collaboration?
- If you didn't enjoy the game, why not? Can it be improved, together with the group? Or are you done with the role?
- What insight have you gained?

If you participated in someone else's scene:

- How did you experience acting alongside the other person?
- What was it like to give your fellow group member this experience?
- Did you play a nice role or a difficult one?
- Were you able to try out new behaviors?
- Did this strengthen your Happy Child and Healthy Adult modes?

4.11 Killer

Description

Everyone sits in a circle and closes their eyes. One client is tapped on the shoulder: this person is the "killer," who can kill people through a wink. When a client is winked at, they wait three seconds and then "die" with a bloodcurdling scream.

If one of the group members catches somebody winking, they point and shout: "You're the killer!" If they are wrong, they die too.

AIM

- Have fun.
- Develop spontaneity.
- Make yourself seen and heard.

Connection to healthy ego functions

- Personality integration and the formation of a self-image.
- Healthy emotion regulation.
- Seeking enjoyment and fulfillment in a mature manner.

Materials

None.

Group/pair/individual

- Group.

Further details

This game is about having fun, being playful, and tolerating tension. Are clients able to let go and get caught up in the game?

Usually, participants get into the game quickly, and even the more inhibited clients show surprising behavior. This exercise draws out a playful and enthusiastic side, and can help the group relax and have fun. There is ample opportunity for the Happy Child to come to the fore and be recognized and discussed.

Variations

- Have the group walk around while playing the game.
- Assign one or two "detectives" to guess who the killer is.

This exercise is also appropriate for other disciplines that use arts and body-based therapies. In music therapy, for example, clients can choose a musical instrument to improvise on while playing the game.

EVALUATION

- Could you bear to watch?
- Could you handle the tension of waiting a while before dropping dead?
- Could you wink subtly without giving yourself away?
- Did you get in touch with your Happy Child mode?
- Do you recognize this kind of Happy Child experience from other situations, for example, from the past?
- What other situations do you know of that offer room for play and spontaneity?

4.12 Red–green game

Description

Each client is given two red and two green cards showing a profession, role, or character type. With four cards in total, each client plays in four scenes.

One client starts by acting out the profession/role/type pictured on a red card. The other clients see if they have a green card that fits with this depiction.

The red card and the green card together form a logical relationship, for example, the strict police officer and the angry crook, or the demanding school teacher and the impulsive child.

Clients who think their own green card fits can jump in. If the card fits, the two clients act out a scene together. If the card is not correct, the client with the red card does not respond, and the others keep looking to see if they have a green card that fits.

This exercise can be made to last the entire session.

Depending on the group's experience level, the therapist can provide structure, such as timing the scenes. A scene can also be replayed with, for example, a different ending.

AIM

- Put yourself "out there."
- Take initiative and take charge.
- Assess a situation.

Connection to healthy ego functions

- Personality integration and the formation of a self-image.
- Contact with one's own emotions/needs and those of others.
- Testing reality and assessing situations, conflicts, and relationships.

Materials

Red and green cards showing a profession, role, or type.
   Optional: Dress-up clothes, such as hats, jackets, and props.

Group/pair/individual

- Group.
- Subgroups of two or three.
- Individually.

Further details

When the scene starts, a conflict linked to the client's history and to schema therapy can be added, for example, allowing the client (as a child) to stand up for their own needs against the demanding school teacher.

EVALUATION

- What was it like to play a role and to be observed?
- Did you dare to give it a try?
- What was it like to receive no response?
- Were you able to act on the basis of your Healthy Adult, or did other modes (protectors) emerge?
- Are you satisfied with the scene?
- Would you like to act out the scene again?

4.13 Fairy tales

Description

A client identifies a fairy tale they enjoyed as a child. A different group member reads the fairy tale aloud, after which the fairy tale is acted out. The first client plays the role of the main character; the others play the supporting roles. Make sure everyone has a role, even if just in the form of a tree.

After the fairy tale has been acted out, the client identifies a part they enjoyed. This part can then be acted out again.

The debriefing revolves around what makes this scene special to the client. Often, it becomes clear that this has been a life script for the client, who now has the opportunity to decide whether this should continue or if the script should be changed.

Finally, the scene can be replayed in the most desirable version for the client.

AIM

- Experience autonomy, connect with others.
- Identify personal schemas.
- Explore the meaning of personal "life script," gain corrective experience.

Connection to healthy ego functions

- Personality integration and the formation of a self-image.
- Contact with one's own emotions/needs and those of others.
- Seeking enjoyment and fulfillment in a mature manner.

Materials

Books of fairy tales, sound clips, lighting and blackout curtains, rags, clothes, hats, face paint, sticks, stones, etc.

Group/pair/individual

- Group.
- Subgroups of two or three.
- Individually.

Further details

The use of fairy tales can be adapted depending on the group process or treatment phase. For example, if a group is distressed about a certain event, the therapist may opt to read one of the group's favorite fairy tales only, in a warm/cozy space they have created in the drama room. This exercise can also be used when a client is already very familiar with the confronting scene of the selected fairy tale and is ready to act it out immediately in a more desirable version (i.e., rescripting an old image).

This exercise highlights to clients the value of jointly acting out a fairy tale that is important to a fellow group member. It allows the client's schemas to be identified and explored. It can also shed light on the client's life script, which can then be rescripted.

The group atmosphere benefits when everyone has a role to play in the fairy tale being acted out. All of this adds to the Happy Child experience.

EVALUATION

- What does the fairy tale evoke in you?
- What thoughts or experiences does this bring up? Experiences from your past? Messages from when you were a child or certain roles that family members played?
- Did you enjoy acting it out? How did the group work together? Could some parts or roles have been played differently? What part of the fairy tale was most special to you?
- Was the scene well acted, and how did it feel to you?
- After replaying the scene, did it feel better this way?

4.14 Comfort chair

Description

The therapist chooses a client and instructs them as follows: "Ask your group-mates to physically form a chair around you on which you can sit, lean, feel supported, and comforted. Give specific instructions for each group member on what posture you want them in, and keep doing this until it feels exactly right for you. Then sit for as long as you want."

AIM

- Request support and comfort.
- Receive support and comfort.
- Work on core needs and have deficits met.

Connection to healthy ego functions

- Personality integration and the formation of a self-image.
- Healthy emotion regulation.
- Contact with one's own emotions/needs and those of others.
- Seeking enjoyment and fulfillment in a mature manner.

Materials

None.

Group/pair/individual

- Group.
- Subgroups of two or three.

Further details

This exercise can also be used in individual therapy; in that case, the therapist receives specific assignments to place pillows, cloths, and blocks around the client.

This exercise is primarily aimed at reinforcing Healthy Adult behaviors.

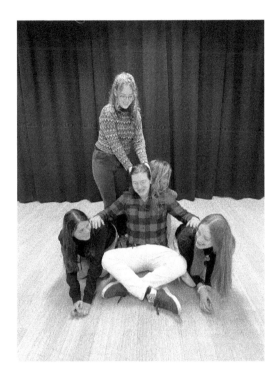

Groupmates may indicate their own limits; for example, they should not be asked to position themselves in such a way that causes pain. Safety and boundaries are ensured at all times.

EVALUATION

- How did you feel about asking and instructing your fellow group members?
- Were you able to act on the basis of your Healthy Adult?
- How did you feel about receiving what you asked for?
- Were you able to relax and give yourself over to the "chair"?
- Were any core needs triggered? If so, which?

4.15 Writing stories

Description

The therapist explains, "I will give you two minutes to choose seven props from the drama room that appeal to you. Place these props in a place in the drama room that you think is appropriate. Then look at the seven props of the group member beside you. What does their composition evoke in you? Write a story about that in a limited number of minutes."

Next, the therapist gives a signal and each client shifts one spot. In other words, they do not write about their own composition of props, but one by one about those of their groupmates. The stories are then read aloud.

After reading, have the clients discuss the stories for each composition; for example, the similarity of the stories with that of the client who made the composition, or the story that appeals most. This story can be subsequently acted out, and what it says about the client examined.

AIM

- Develop intuition and creativity.
- Cooperate with and take interest in others.

Connection to healthy ego functions

- Contact with one's own emotions/needs and those of others.
- Testing reality and assessing situations, conflicts, and relationships.
- Seeking enjoyment and fulfillment in a mature manner.

Materials

Various props, writing paper, and pens.

Group/pair/individual

- Group.
- Subgroups of two or three.

Further details

Decide on the number of writing minutes per composition depending on how much time there is for this exercise. If more depth is needed, the exercise can be spread over multiple sessions. If it has to take place in one session, divide the session length by the number of clients and reserve 30 minutes for reading all the stories and giving feedback.

Clients can photograph their compositions and use the photos to continue their work in the next session. At a later time, the group may choose to act out a story together. Perhaps a story is involved that raises many questions; this can then be clarified through play.

As this exercise involves working with props, using one's imagination, writing, and reading aloud, it is suitable for clients who find play difficult. For example, it may be appropriate for a group that is just starting out or needs guidance to move beyond the superficial.

EVALUATION

- What was it like hearing other people's stories about your own arrangement of props?
- Were you able to listen on the basis of your Healthy Adult mode?
- What was it like to write stories and read them aloud?
- When using your imagination, are you appealing to, for example, your Healthy Adult or your Happy Child?
- If a story was acted: Did you enjoy acting it out? What was it like to see your own story acted?

4.16 Wishful thinking

Description

Three clients sit in a triangle (or two clients sit opposite each other).

One client plays him/herself and tries to imagine what sentence they would like to hear (but have never heard) from their father and from their mother (the "wish sentence"). The client chooses whether to hear the father's or mother's sentence first.

If the client chooses the father, they switch to the "father's chair," putting both feet flat on the floor and inhaling/exhaling steadily. They look at the person sitting on their own chair, identify themselves as their father, and say the sentence confidently.

The client keeps repeating this until the sentence has been uttered satisfactorily.

After this, they switch chairs, and the person now playing the role of the father says the sentence in the same manner. They repeat this until it is uttered with confidence and accepted by the client. The client then thanks the person in the role of the father for saying the sentence.

Optionally, the exercise can be done again with the wish sentence uttered by the other parent.

AIM

- Identify basic needs.
- Explore emotions.

Connection to healthy ego functions

- Personality integration and the formation of a self-image.
- Contact with one's own emotions/needs and those of others.
- Developing a healthy internal dialogue.
- Testing reality and assessing situations, conflicts, and relationships.

Materials

Three chairs.

Group/pair/individual

- Group.
- Subgroups of two or three.
- Individually.

Further details

It is important to assess whether the client can look clearly at the role of the parent and work with the wish sentences as they are uttered. Is the client just playing the game, or really letting the words sink in?

This exercise gives clients the opportunity to identify what they would have liked to hear from one or both parents. They can feel the effect that hearing the sentence has on them.

EVALUATION

- How did it feel to hear the sentence?
- How did it feel to utter the sentence?
- Where in your body did you feel this?
- Can you imagine or accept that although this sentence was never said in real life, it was intended?

4.17 Tableau vivant—memory in pictures

Description

First, the client calls to mind a situation in which their basic needs were not met as a child. Then, the client creates and directs a *tableau vivant* using the other group members as actors. The therapist gives the following instructions: "Translate the scene you imagined to the stage. It can be in *tableau* form, or a smaller scale scene with text and movement. Give your groupmates stage directions by coaching, clapping, replaying the scene, and so on."

Thereafter, the therapist continues to guide the client by asking questions: "Could you put yourself in this space? Think about your posture and facial expressions. What is the other person doing in the scene? How should they be posed?"

Next, the therapist asks the client to choose a stand-in for his/her own role in the scene. This way, the client can view the scene from a distance and verify whether it matches what they had in mind.

Afterwards, the therapist asks the group or client/director: "What is needed in this situation? How can the basic needs of the Vulnerable Child be met? What needs to change in this situation?"

This creates the opportunity for a Healthy Adult (the client or another group member) to jump in and modify the situation to something more desirable, for example, by standing up for the Vulnerable Child and offering comfort.

AIM

- Take direction from the Healthy Adult side.
- Practice distancing.
- Develop (self-)compassion.
- Understand unmet basic needs.
- Identify connections between past and present.

Connection to healthy ego functions

- Personality integration and the formation of a self-image.
- Contact with one's own emotions/needs and those of others.
- Testing reality and assessing situations, conflicts, and relationships.

Materials

Optional.

Group/pair/individual

- Subgroups of two or three.
- Individual work in a group setting.

Further details

This exercise allows the client to practice Healthy Adult behavior in the here and now by assuming the role of director and giving direction to fellow group members in an assertive manner. The client also practices viewing their own situation from a distance and being compassionate toward their own vulnerable side. The exercise provides insight into how past experiences contribute to current symptoms. It can help with a general case conceptualization.

The therapist helps the client to visualize the often painful and/or traumatic memory in such a way that they are not overwhelmed by emotions. If the experience involves violence, an image can also be chosen from just prior to the incident, when the threat was already palpable. This exercise can be used as a prelude to rescripting through play or imagery rescripting.

At all times, the therapist is mindful of the other group members.

Variation

The therapist can also specifically ask clients to picture an image from their childhood that typifies their relationship with their mother or father.

EVALUATION

Questions for the group:

- What do you see happening? What does it evoke for you?
- What does the Vulnerable Child need in this situation?

Questions for the director:

- What was it like to direct your own situation? What does that evoke for you?
- Are you satisfied with how you directed your fellow group members?
- How does it feel to present your own situation in this way?
- What do you feel when doing so?
- What conclusions did you draw about yourself after this situation occurred?
- Do these conclusions still hold?

- What was it like to offer support to the Vulnerable Child in this situation, or to see a groupmate offering support?
- What would it be like if, as in the revised scene, the child's needs were met?
- What would be different now?

4.18 Market merchant

Description

The therapist or an experienced group member plays a market vendor. The therapist creates a stall from which the vendor will "sell" vegetables/fruit, clothing, or another product, while explaining that earlier today, a client bought a bag of apples, a piece of fabric, or some other item from the vendor. On returning home, the client realized that there is something wrong with the purchase: the apples are rotten or there is a stain or tear in the fabric.

The task is to return to the vendor and exchange the product for a new one or get a refund. This allows the client to practice engaging in a discussion on an equal footing in the manner of a Healthy Adult, including raising a problem, explaining the issue, asking questions, and negotiating. The vendor responds in different ways (e.g., different mode roles), thereby challenging the client to employ Healthy Adult behaviors.

AIM

- Stand up for yourself.
- Deal with setbacks.
- Express emotions.

Connection to healthy ego functions

- Personality integration and the formation of a self-image.
- Healthy emotion regulation.
- Contact with one's own emotions/needs and those of others.
- Testing reality and assessing situations, conflicts, and relationships.

Materials

Table or chairs for the market stall, item(s) that can be used as the product to be returned.

Group/pair/individual

• Individual work in a group setting.

Further details

This exercise demonstrates how drama can be used to practice Healthy Adult behavior and potentially also coping styles. Clients can jump in spontaneously to try their hand at the game.

The therapist or a group member can give instructions, such as "Do it again" or "Try something different." A group member can also take over from or coach the client.

EVALUATION

For the client:

• How did you think it went?
• Which side/mode did the exercise trigger in you, during or even before it began (on hearing the instructions)?
• How did you deal with that? Why?
• What did you feel during the exercise?
• What thoughts came to mind?
• Do you recognize Parent sides?
• How were you inclined to behave?
• What do you think we saw in you? Was a coping style triggered?
• Did you feel that your Healthy Adult side came to the fore?
• What else would you like to try out?

For the group:

• What did you think? What went well?
• What did you see? What sides of the group member did you recognize?
• What was/was not Healthy Adult behavior?

4.19 Portray your coping modes

Description

The therapist explains, "In pairs, discuss an encounter you had in the past week when your most common protector took charge and you lapsed into behavior that was not, in your opinion, Healthy Adult behavior. Decide together how to act out these situations for the group. You play the adversary in the other person's situation. Your scene does not have to match the actual encounter exactly. You have five minutes to prepare."

After the debriefing, the scene can be acted out again.

The therapist claps, signaling that the protagonist should now try to recover the desired Healthy Adult behavior during the scene.

AIM

- Understand your own emotion regulation and interaction patterns.
- Stand up for yourself as a Healthy Adult.
- Gain exposure to different behaviors.

Connection to healthy ego functions

- Personality integration and the formation of a self-image.
- Healthy emotion regulation.
- Contact with one's own emotions/needs and those of others.

Materials

Optional: Dress-up clothes or props.

Group/pair/individual

- Group.
- Subgroups of two or three.

Further details

Having the adversary use dress-up clothes/hats or props can help to emphasize that he/she is playing a role. This can make the "critical counterplay" less distressing for the client playing him/herself.

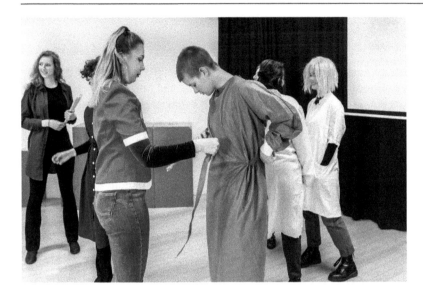

Repeating the scene can, in a playful, experimental way, increase the client's self-awareness. They learn to notice what is happening in their bodies in that moment and to choose different or new behaviors.

EVALUATION

Client:

- What was it like to reenact this scene?
- What did you feel? Where in your body did you feel this?
- What were you thinking? How were you inclined to behave?
- What did you think of the other person?

Adversary:

- How was it for you?
- What did you think and feel?
- How were you inclined to behave?

Group:

- What did you see? What coping style do you recognize, and how?
- What do you recognize from this situation yourself, and how do you deal with it?
- What can you give back to the actors?

4.20 Magic shop

Do away with unnecessary schemas and modes!

Description

The scene takes place in a (swap) store. Each participant reflects on their own schemas and modes. Which of these do you no longer need? What do you have too much of? What are you most bothered by?

The client enters the shop through a revolving door. The shopkeeper (played by the therapist) asks, "How can I help?" The client introduces the trait, schema, or mode being handed in (e.g., "My schema High Standards").

The shopkeeper asks the client to explain, "Why do you want to get rid of it? Where in your body is it?" Having answered these questions, the client is asked to put it on the counter (improvise the shape/size and so on). Encourage the client to exaggerate!

As the shopkeeper/therapist, be very interested and happy to have this schema added to the store inventory. Also validate it by having the client explain how it (having high standards) used to help them—what benefits did it bring? When both the benefits and the burden are clarified, the shopkeeper takes the schema from the client.

Next, the shopkeeper asks what the client would like in its place (e.g., spontaneity). If the client has trouble coming up with something, offer suggestions. The shopkeeper improvises a form in which the new trait can be given to the client (a coat, bracelet, mirror, etc.), and asks the client to try it out.

The Healthy Adult is stimulated most when it is difficult to apply the new trait. If the client again demonstrates, for example, high demands, the shopkeeper can ask the client to hand in some more. Once the client is satisfied with the trait, the client leaves the store.

AIM

- Gain awareness of personal coping modes/schemas that impede growth/the Healthy Adult.
- Practice behavioral alternatives (expand repertoire, foster Healthy Adult behaviors).
- Increase enjoyment of dramatic forms of play.

Connection to healthy ego functions

- Personality integration and the formation of a self-image.
- Developing a healthy internal dialogue.
- Seeking enjoyment and fulfillment in a mature manner.

Materials

None.

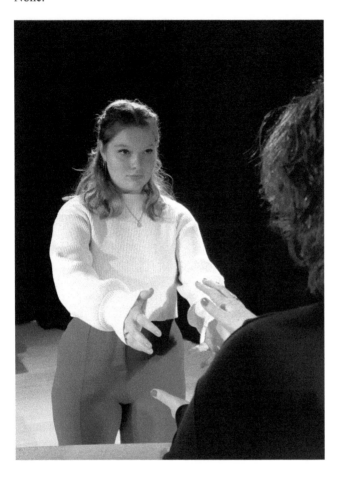

Group/pair/individual

- Group.
- Individual work in a group setting.
- Individually.

Further details

Using distance and a lighthearted approach can often help clients to work on difficult subjects with a light touch.

A key rule is that a client should never hand in him/herself; it should always be a trait, schema, mode, or part.

This exercise is also appropriate for other arts and body-based disciplines. For example, in music therapy, a coping mode can be symbolized by a musical instrument. The therapist plays the role of, say, an ill-informed, naïve, light-hearted, somewhat messy, but good-humored music store owner. The owner fumbles around until the client rings the doorbell to return his/her musical instrument (coping mode). With feigned ignorance, the owner asks the client about the (previous) usefulness of the instrument and why the client wants to get rid of it. The owner asks the client to play the instrument as he/she always has and tries to imitate it. Together, the client and therapist give words to the sounds without literally mentioning the term *coping mode*. Eventually, the owner understands that the instrument used to be but is no longer useful. The client is given a voucher to choose a different instrument from the store. The owner can guide the client in this choice or ask the client to make his/her own choice (stimulating the Healthy Adult). The client can try out different instruments and props, exploring what he/she needs in everyday life.

EVALUATION

- What was it like to openly draw attention to a trait you want to get rid of?
- Were you able to fully relinquish your coping mode (your protectors)?
- Were you able to identify how it (previously) helped you?
- How did you experience the new trait? (Healthy Adult)

4.21 The ten worst ways to...

Description

Participants start in a circle. The therapist mentions something that happens regularly in everyday life (e.g., canceling an appointment). Group members are asked to take turns jumping in and showing a very bad way to approach the situation. A few ways are often enough.

Then switch to another situation, for example, the ten worst ways to:

- end a relationship;
- call in sick for work;
- ensure you get the lead role in the musical;
- avoid washing the dishes;
- explain that you have been given a poor diagnosis;
- leave a group app.

Choose situations that clients can easily picture, and have them come up with their own situations.

AIM

- Have fun, encourage the Happy
- Gain insight into Healthy Adult behavior.

Connection to healthy ego functions

- Contact with one's own emotions/needs and those of others.
- Testing reality and assessing situations, conflicts, and relationships.
- Seeking enjoyment and fulfillment in a mature manner.

Materials

None.

Group/pair/individual

- Group.

Further details

The exercise is about not thinking but doing (improvising), reverse-thinking, and daring to make mistakes. It can often be very funny (activating the Happy Child mode), but also illustrates the opposite of the Healthy Adult mode. In this way, it indirectly evokes the Healthy Adult. Clients gain insight into Healthy Adult solutions and can strengthen their resourcefulness or repertoire. Giving voice to thoughts and actions that are socially unacceptable can also be a lot of fun.

A variation on this is making a "recipe for misery"/"recipe for getting into mischief." For example, discuss what you should do if you definitely want to become depressed or feel bad/guilty, and come up with a recipe together.

In visual therapy, such a recipe can be created as a pictorial description of the ingredients and method, displayed together on a recipe poster.

EVALUATION

- Did you dare to let go and follow your impulses (i.e., release your Happy Child)?
- What did you most enjoy (i.e., when did you most strongly experience the Happy Child)?
- What was the most confrontational moment, and why?

4.22 Angel–devil

Description

Choose a healthy mode (Healthy Adult, Happy Child) and a persistent Protector or Parent mode from which the client suffers (e.g., Punitive Parent or Distant Protector).

The therapist and client stand behind a chair, one to the left and the other to the right. The client starts in the Protector role (devil), the therapist in the Healthy Adult role (angel).

The angel and the devil gossip behind the client's back, as it were. Ask the client to gossip and play the role of Protector or Parent in an exaggerated manner, so there is something to oppose. This gives rise to a dialogue on the different modes.

Then, reverse the roles so that the client can experiment with the angel (Healthy Adult mode).

AIM

- Gain insight into the influence of the Punitive/Protector modes on everyday behavior.
- Practice taking a different perspective

Connection to healthy ego functions

- Personality integration and the formation of a self-image.
- Developing a healthy internal dialogue.

Materials

None.

Group/pair/individual

- Group.
- Individual work in a group setting.
- Individually.

Further details

Consider extending to a court setting with a prosecutor, defense, and public gallery, all in a certain mode.

EVALUATION

- What was it like to play the protector so clearly?
- What was it like to hear the angel, and play it yourself?
- How do the devil and angel influence you in your everyday life?
- Is this influence desirable? If not, what would you like to change?

4.23 Visualizing internal atom in modes

Description

This exercise focuses on the specific dilemma or theme of a group member. The therapist asks who wants to play the protagonist and invites the rest of the group to play along.

The different sides or modes are portrayed by group members, who make statements representing these modes. By viewing these from a distance, the client can see and, ultimately, modify the underlying pattern of their modes.

Example

Anna would like to work on her tendency to procrastinate. She is 34 years old and has started, but not managed to finish, a number of study programs. She has one more exam remaining to complete her current degree, but cannot bring herself to get up on time and study. We visualize her different sides or modes with the help of group members. First is her inner critic, who is given a prominent position beside her and lectures her sternly: "Come on, you have to give 200% or you'll fail." She feels his hot breath on her neck; feels herself becoming small and sad. She places this image of the Vulnerable Child on her other side: "See, let's not even start, it won't work anyway." Immediately, the urge rises to stay in bed and watch films, so she places this Avoidant Protector in front of her.

When she looks at this configuration from a distance (mirroring), she sees the destructiveness of this pattern of modes for her. She grows angry and sends her critic to the corner: "You're not helping me right now, so shut up" (Angry Child).

This gives her more space to consider what she needs. The Healthy Adult in her comforts the Vulnerable Child: "You're allowed to make mistakes and ask for help." During the debriefing, she asks if a fellow group member might send her an email at 7:30 each morning to remind her to get up to study. This system seems to work well: this caring morning email makes her feel seen and acknowledged, which allows her to get to work and gradually develop a gentler side (Doomen, 2018).

AIM

- Express and share feelings of vulnerability or anger.
- Become aware of destructive patterns.
- Fulfill personal needs in a healthier way.

Connection to healthy ego functions

- Personality integration and the formation of a self-image.
- Healthy emotion regulation.
- Contact with one's own emotions/needs and those of others.
- Developing a healthy internal dialogue.
- Testing reality and assessing situations, conflicts, and relationships.
- Seeking enjoyment and fulfillment in a mature manner.

Materials

Blocks, rags.

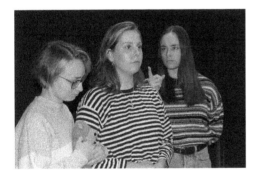

Group/pair/individual

- Group.
- Subgroups of two or three.
- Individual work in a group setting.
- Individually.

Further details

In an internal atom, a client's dilemma is explored intra-psychologically by picturing and acting out different modes. The use of other group members to visualize the modes makes the blockage visible (mirror technique) and tangible.

The therapist has the client switch roles (and thus perspectives) periodically such that he/she can watch from a distance and identify the underlying need. Group members are encouraged throughout the process to give doubles.

This psycho-dramatic exercise is appropriate when the group members are exploring their issues at a deeper level. The client is challenged to shape and share their underlying feelings, needs, and thoughts with others. That other group members often recognize in themselves and share many of the themes that are touched upon can form an additional source of support.

EVALUATION

Questions during the process:

- Which group member/stand-in do you want to choose to play you? Where should they be positioned in this space?
- Which mode comes to mind first when you think about your dilemma?
- Where should your Critic/Demanding or Punitive Parent stand? What does he say?
- What do you experience when you look at and listen to the image of the critic?
- Where do you feel that in your body?
- Who could perform this role for you?
- Is the mode appropriately visualized? What, if anything, is different? Can you demonstrate?
- Can you switch roles with a certain mode yourself?
- If you feel that you are growing angry, what would you like to do?
- If you find it difficult to take on the role of the Healthy Adult, who do you think could do it?
- As a Vulnerable Child, who would you like to comfort you?
- What do you notice when you look at the dynamics of your modes?
- What do you need?
- How could you give shape to that? Who can help you?
- Who recognizes in themselves aspects of what we have now portrayed?

4.24 Yes/no strength exercise

Description

This exercise is aimed at training group members' physical strength and voice volume. Have the group members find a partner of roughly equal size and strength. Demonstrate the exercise with a group member while giving the following instructions:

"We take up a firm stance, facing each other, placing our right foot just slightly in front of the left and the palms of our hands against each other. We decide which one of us will say yes and which will say no. Then we push against one another, at a strength level rising from 0% to as high as possible. At the same time, we take turns saying 'yes' and 'no' ever more loudly. It's important to generate the sound from your belly rather than forcing your voice or shrieking. The idea is to challenge each other in physical strength and voice volume, while also looking out for your partner; make sure you don't push them over! When you both feel you can't go any higher, slowly dial down to 0% without interrupting the exercise."

After the demonstration, the pairs split off to start the first of two rounds. The therapist walks around, offering tips: "Keep going, stay focused, don't laugh it off, step it up a notch," but also watching for any clients who may be overshooting their strength.

In the second round, the therapist coaches group members to increase the intensity. The point here is not to let go at the climax, but rather to hold on and slowly reduce the strength in a controlled manner from, say, 80% to 0%.

AIM

- Discover and harness your own strength.
- Express anger.
- Identify pitfalls when trying to use strength.

Connection to healthy ego functions

- Healthy emotion regulation.
- Contact with one's own emotions/needs and those of others.
- Seeking enjoyment and fulfillment in a mature manner.

Materials

Open space large enough for multiple pairs.

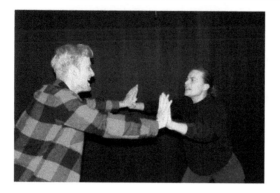

Group/pair/individual

- Group.
- Subgroups of two or three.

Further details

During the demonstration, the clients see the therapist fully engage, but at the same time with an eye for their partner's strengths. This can help them feel invited to engage too.

In this exercise, clients learn to stand firm, use their own physical strength and voice volume, and express anger. They gain insight into what obstacles lie in their way when it comes to finding and using their own power.

Variation

After the first round, clients can be asked to picture a concrete situation from their lives in which they did not feel powerful, set boundaries, or express their anger. With this in mind, they do the exercise again. The therapist decides whether the pairs should do the exercise simultaneously or one at a time to allow more room for coaching. This variation can also precede a psycho-dramatic exercise in which the protagonist practices healthy mental strength.

EVALUATION

After the first round:

- What percentage were you at in terms of physical strength and voice volume?
- What was blocking or holding you back?
- Which coping mode was that?

Often clients discover that their inner pleaser or a sense of overprotectiveness toward the other prevents them from leaning into their own power. Others find it stressful to make physical contact, tolerate closeness, or engage in confrontation. The therapist can say, "Okay, so your pleaser prevented you from leaning into your power; now imagine doing the exercise again from your Healthy Adult or your Angry Child mode. See if you then dare to move toward that 100%. Your partner appreciates it when you offer greater counterforce."

After the second round:

- What was it like doing the exercise this way?
- What was the difference compared to the first round? How did you experience it?

4.25 Late-night talk show

Description

Place the host's (i.e., the therapist's) chair to the left, and three to five chairs beside it. These chairs represent the client's modes (consider using mode cards/materials to symbolize these modes). Ensure that the child mode is closest and the Healthy Adult mode is farthest from the host; the Protective/Parent modes are in between.

While preparing for the exercise, discuss the chairs. The client, with all their modes, is the main guest on the show and may change chairs during it.

To open the show, announce the client and have the group members applaud. The client then enters as him/herself. As the host, interview the client about something mundane. Usually, you will see that the client switches modes. When you observe this, ask briefly as an aside (as if the audience cannot hear), "Are you still in the right chair?"

Usually this works by providing validating responses, listening attentively, and asking for intuitive reflections. Try to respond to each chair according to the need appropriate to that mode.

Then, initiate a role reversal: the client becomes the host (the Healthy Adult) and you as the therapist play the modes. For example, you sit in the Child chair and play the associated feeling (loneliness, sadness, hurt).

The moment you think the client, as host, is truly in Healthy Adult mode, you wrap up the show—with, of course, thunderous applause for all the modes!

AIM

- Strengthen the Healthy Adult.
- Practice switching perspectives.
- Identify personal needs and practice fulfilling them (as a Healthy Adult caring for the child modes).

Connection to healthy ego functions

- Personality integration and the formation of a self-image.
- Contact with one's own emotions/needs and those of others.

Materials

Schema mode cards (homemade or Bernstein's Helpers and Heroes card set: www.schematherapie.nl/professionals/therapiemateriaal).

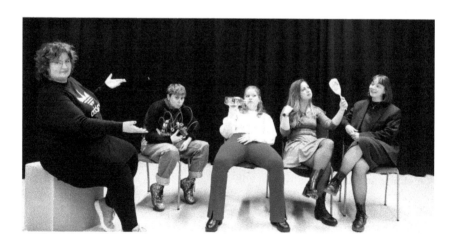

Group/pair/individual

- Individual work in a group setting.
- Individually.

Further details

Group members can be used as protectors/hosts/modes.

EVALUATION

- What was it like to be on this show?
- What did you notice when on the Child chair?
- Could you feel/did you notice any resistance in yourself?
- What was it like to be the host?
- What was it like to be the Healthy Adult for yourself?

4.26 Wimp

Description

Preparation

Set up a "store"/counter and indicate that there are two roles: shopkeeper and customer. Decide together what kind of store it is.

Instruct the client that every sentence spoken, or every question, must be followed by an insult. It can be anything—there are no limits. If necessary, demonstrate this briefly to provide inspiration. It should be as bizarre and unrealistic as possible to maximize laughter. To make it even funnier, tell the clients that they are not supposed to laugh.

Game

Play a scene in a store. Shopkeeper and customer alike use a different insult after each sentence. Neither responds to the insult but simply proceeds to the next sentence. The dialogue may look something like this:

"Good morning, how can I help? Moron!"

"Hello, I'd like half a loaf of whole wheat. Jerk!"

"But of course, anything else? Asshole!"

"Yes, also a few bread rolls, please. Wimp."

The contrast of the cheerful, friendly, everyday conversation is given a strange incongruity by the addition of the insult. Above all, encourage the client to revel in the social undesirability of such a conversation.

AIM

- Have fun, encourage the Happy Child
- Dare to indulge (otherwise repressed) impulses.

Connection to healthy ego functions

- Healthy emotion regulation.
- Contact with one's own emotions/needs and those of others.

Materials

None.

Group/pair/individual

- Individually.

Further details

This exercise depends on the therapist setting an example, especially for clients with inhibitions. So throw yourself into it and encourage the client to join in.

EVALUATION

- What was it like to play this part?
- What did you discover about yourself? What thoughts and feelings?
- Were you able to fully commit to the game (Happy Child)?
- Did you dare to engage in socially undesirable behavior? Did you enjoy acting a bit unhinged?

4.27 Rescripting in psychodrama

Description

Warm up with a short meditation. Follow this with the exercise, which zooms in on painful childhood situations from the past or an abbreviated version of imagery rescripting.

Steps of imagery rescripting

- Begin with a relaxation exercise focusing on breathing and body awareness.

Then continue with the following instructions:

- Imagine yourself in a pleasant situation in the present, in which you feel comfortable and safe. Where are you? Are there others with you? What do you see around you—colors, shapes? Is it hot or cold, are there particular smells? Really absorb this situation with all your senses. Now release it again: rub out the image.

- Now, in your mind, go to an unpleasant situation in the present. What made it unpleasant? Is anyone else present? Who is/are they? Where are you while this situation is taking place? What is happening—is something being said? What do you feel? What do you feel *physically*? Are there other things you notice in this situation? Now rub out the image of this situation, but hold onto the feeling.
- Feeling "bridge": Go back in time to when you were a small child. See if an image pops up with a similar feeling. Don't force it, just let the image arise. Look calmly at where you are, what it looks like there, who you might be with. Feel what all this triggers in you. Look at the situation and what is happening. Focus your attention on the child's feelings and needs.
- Now imagine that you, as the adult you are, walk into this situation. Look at the child. What do you feel? Is there anything you would like to do? What would you do or say to help, comfort, and protect the child? Now imagine actually intervening, addressing the other person. What happens, what is the reaction, what changes in the situation? What do you feel now? Have you said or done everything you would like to?
- Return to the difficult situation in the present. Build a bridge to how you can help yourself in the present with comfort, protection, permission, and intervention. How do you feel right now?
- Now, let go of this situation and rub out the image again. Return to the pleasant situation in the present. Do you remember where you were? Try to recall this situation clearly again, and feel what it does to you.
- Now let go of this situation again slowly and bring your attention back into this space.

Group members are invited to share experiences. Then the therapist asks for a volunteer to work with, for example, the image that arose during the IR.

The therapist guides this protagonist toward a physical staging of the situation in the form of a psychodrama:

1. First, the original, painful situation is acted out. The protagonist plays the child role and chooses group members for the other roles. Group members are invited to support the protagonist at the experience level with a hand on the shoulder, for example, "I feel sad and not seen."
2. Then, a corrective intervention is acted out, where a helping other or the adult protagonist him/herself stands up for the child. Parents can be called to account and given boundaries. A desirable situation is created in which the child's needs can be met.
3. Finally, a scene is acted out in which the protagonist again plays the child role and experiences what it is like to receive protection and comfort from a helping other.

For the therapist, it is important to stay close to the client to offer holding as needed, and invite group members to double (Doomen, 2018).

AIM

- Experience and express repressed feelings and needs.
- Activate Healthy Adult resources.
- Gain insight into the links between current problems and past events.

Connection to healthy ego functions

- Personality integration and the formation of a self-image.
- Healthy emotion regulation.
- Contact with one's own emotions/needs and those of others.

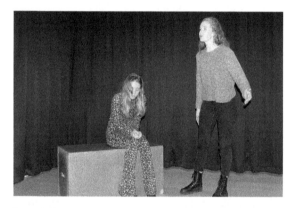

Rescripting: Elise addresses her mother on the basis of her Healthy Adult mode.

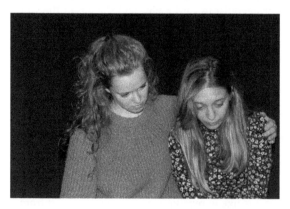

Rescripting: Elise comforts her Vulnerable Child mode.

Materials

Blocks for staging, dress-up clothes, rags, etc.

Group/pair/individual

Group.

Further details

Rescripting in psychodrama is appropriate when clients are ready to work on an underlying trauma. It involves the physical staging of painful situations from the client's past that can be addressed and processed in the group context. It is only advisable when the group has developed an adequate level of trust and openness.

Example

Elise has borderline issues and suffers from separation anxiety and distrust. Her parents are divorced and her mother was punitive and unpredictable. As a child, Elise sought refuge in music; she enjoyed playing the piano. One day, she came home to find that her mother had gotten rid of the piano without discussing this with her; she could no longer stand her "awful plonking."

1. Elise plays herself as an eight-year-old child and a group member plays her mother. She returns from school and is distressed to find that the piano is gone. When her mother responds bluntly and harshly, she clams up. A group member doubles her: "Mommy, you've hurt me!" Elise repeats the lines and cries.
2. Elise wants to try to address her mother as her adult self. She is assisted by a regular double. Another group member plays the child. "Mother, how terribly mean," says the double. "Look at your child, you know very well that that piano meant a lot to little Elise. A mother is supposed to protect and cherish and give love to her child. You are depriving her of the very thing she was passionate about." Elise, strengthened by her double, is increasingly finding her own power.
3. Elise is a child again, comforted by her grandmother or another trusted figure. Elise cries when she receives a genuine hug and is told that she is not a bad child, but that her mother is, unfortunately, unable to give her love.

EVALUATION

After rescripting, the protagonist is first given a moment to gather him/
herself. Group members who played a role give brief feedback based on
that role, for example,

- How did the mother feel during the scene?

After this, they shake off the role (literally by shaking their bodies for a
moment).

Next, group members are invited to share their experiences:

- What did it make you think about/feel?
- What did you recognize in this situation for yourself?

This takes the focus off the protagonist for a while and allows him/her to
feel supported through the recognition and experiences of the others.
    Finally, the protagonist is invited to share his/her insights. It is impor-
tant that this exercise helps the client to experience, identify, and express
his/her needs and feelings. The client should feel empowered and gain a
better understanding of healthy or unhealthy behavior.

- How was it for you?
- What feelings and needs did you experience?
- What was it like to act out the situation again?
- How did it feel to intervene in the situation/when somebody else
  intervened?

4.28 Role-playing with modes

Description

The group sits in a semicircle around the therapist. A "living room" is created,
with a suitcase and an assortment of travel gear. The therapist explains:
    "We're going to do a role-play where the modes keep on changing. Imagine
A has agreed with a friend to go on a five-month trip together around Australia.
The suitcase is packed and the tickets are ready; tomorrow is the big day. Then

the doorbell rings: it's B, the friend A is going traveling with. Enthusiastically, A motions at the suitcase and everything ready for the trip. Suddenly, B says, 'Sorry, I can't go with you. I made a mistake—I don't know if our friendship is safe enough for me to travel with you for so long.'"

Two group members then act out the situation. A draws a card from a stack of mode cards and responds to B based on the mode indicated on the card. The modes are angry, vulnerable, Avoidant Protector, Pleaser, Overcompensator, Demanding Parent, Punitive Parent, and Healthy Adult.

B always plays the scene on the basis of the Healthy Adult mode.

After the scene has been acted out, the group guesses which mode A was playing and gives feedback on whether B successfully stayed in Healthy Adult mode. The therapist asks what the group based their guesses on and what it was like for the actors.

If necessary, the scene can be repeated, with the therapist able to coach both A and B. All group members take turns playing either the A or B role; the situation always remains the same, with B in Healthy Adult mode and A in a new mode. The therapist may also choose a different situation that is easier for the clients to relate to.

AIM

- Recognize modes.
- Identify personal areas for improvement in terms of modes.
- Gain insight into the interactional dynamics of different modes.

Connection to healthy ego functions

- Healthy emotion regulation.
- Testing reality and assessing situations, conflicts, and relationships.
- Seeking enjoyment and fulfillment in a mature manner.

Materials

Blocks to stage a living room, suitcase with travel items, mode cards.

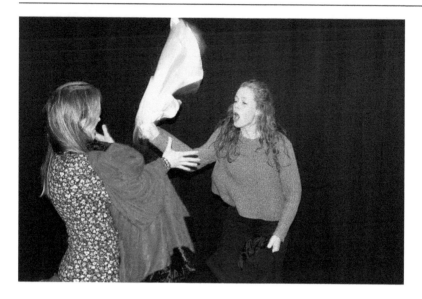

Group/pair/individual

- Group.

Further details

This exercise is particularly suitable for a novice group that wants to gain experience in portraying the different roles. It sheds light for clients on which modes are recognizable and which are challenging. They discover how the different modes influence the dynamics of interaction.

The exercise can be done in more depth if the client knows in advance which mode is challenging and wants to practice it immediately.

Alternatively, a client can suggest a situation of his/her own where the interaction did not go well. This situation is then staged with a group member, and the group indicates which modes are visible. The therapist asks about the client's underlying need, and a mode that might be more desirable is practiced.

EVALUATION

- What mode is being portrayed here? What makes you say that?
- Is this a familiar mode for you?
- Which mode is challenging for you to practice?
- How does this mode affect the other player?

- In what situation do you recognize this pattern of interaction?
- Would you like to practice this situation now?
- What do you need in this situation?
- What effect does the behavior have on the other person?
- What mode evokes anger or fear in you?
- Then what happens to you?

4.29 Theater characters as subpersonalities

Description

The group sits in a circle. The therapist explains, "First we're going to do a guided fantasy to get in touch with subpersonalities. Please close your eyes and picture yourself before the stage exit of a theater. Every evening, a play is staged here that reflects the different sides of a person. So far there's been a clown, a knight, a mean witch, a coward, an angel … Tonight the play is about you. The play has just ended and you are waiting for the actors to emerge. Here comes the first one … closer and closer … you can see them clearly now."

"What kind of character is it? How are they dressed? What else do you notice about this character? The actor is now so close you can talk to each other. What do they say to you? What do you say back? Continue the conversation."

"When you are finished talking, the actor sits down on a bench and the next one now comes out. What does this actor represent? What does the character look like? What do they say? What kind of dialogue develops between the two of you?"

"Then this character sits on the bench too. Finally, the third actor comes out and again a dialogue ensues."

By now you have met all three characters and should have a good picture of them. Have a good stretch and open your eyes."

The therapist lays out drawing paper and felt-tip pens. Each group member takes some supplies and finds a quiet spot. The assignment is to draw all three theater characters and give them a name that reflects the character.

Then, the group members put on dress-up clothes and play the different theater characters, walking around and having brief encounters with one another. The therapist coaches to magnify them for a moment, for example.

Next, the therapist asks for a volunteer to work with the characters in front of the group. This client plays their first character for the group, prompted by questions from the therapist: "Who are you, what do you do, how do you feel, why are you in the client's life?" The client then chooses a group member to take over and play this character, so the client can see what it evokes. Next, the client comes out as the second character. In this way, all the characters are played and the therapist can initiate dialogues between the different subpersonalities. The therapist supports the client in this process.

The exercise is brought to a close with a final image as the client would like it to be in his/her life; if needed, different names can be given to the subpersonalities (Doomen, 2018).

AIM

- Gain insight into yourself.
- Get to know the different sides of yourself.
- Identify blockages, pitfalls, and strengths in your internal dynamics.

Connection to healthy ego functions

- Personality integration and the formation of a self-image.
- Healthy emotion regulation.
- Contact with one's own emotions/needs and those of others.
- Developing a healthy internal dialogue.

Materials

Stage equipment, dress-up clothes, drawing paper, and felt-tip pens.

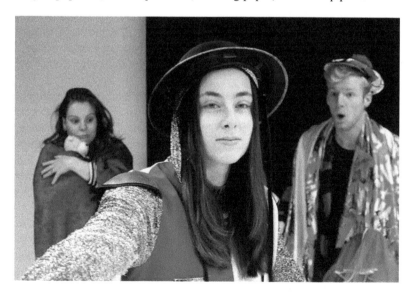

Group/pair/individual

- Group.
- Individual work in a group setting.

Further details

This exercise allows clients to explore their subpersonalities through drama. They gain insight into blockages, pitfalls, and strengths in their own internal dynamics. The use of characters offers a certain distance that enables clients to safely connect with their inner world.

The therapist can use the mirror technique, allowing the client to play a character; however, the client can also watch from a distance when a group member takes over their role.

It is important to activate the group to give doubles at the experiential level so that the client can increasingly connect with and express their underlying emotions. Role reversals help the client take a different perspective and gradually develop a healthier internal dynamic.

EVALUATION

It is important for the therapist to ask questions that demand empathy and force the clients to get under the skin of the character.

- As a clown, what do you do to entertain people?
- Can you show us how that goes?
- What are you as a coward most afraid of?

In a playful manner, it gradually becomes clear which mode is involved: Is it an emotional mode (e.g., the coward), a Protector (e.g., the pleaser or the clown), or a Parental mode (in the form of, for example, a demanding, cold, businesslike character)? Working through these modes and periodically viewing them from a distance help the client to see what he/she needs and ultimately arrive at a healthier dynamic.

4.30 Hints

Description

Create a stack of cards with objects and titles of movies, books, plays, and proverbs. Someone takes a card and acts out what is on the card (either word by word or as a whole). The others try to guess what is being portrayed.

AIM

- Have fun.
- Develop spontaneity.
- Make yourself seen and heard.

Connection to healthy ego functions

- Personality integration and the formation of a self-image.
- Contact with one's own emotions/needs and those of others.
- Seeking enjoyment and fulfillment in a mature manner.

Materials

Cards with different topics.

Group/pair/individual

- Group.
- Subgroups two or three.

Further details

The group can be split into two and a competitive element can be added. Which team can make the most correct guesses in a given time? The game can also be played in pairs if the tension is too much to bear for an individual.

EVALUATION

- Do you dare to let yourself be seen and heard?
- Can you permit the Happy Child in you to emerge? Do you dare to be silly or enlarge your expression?
- What do you feel when the group struggles to guess what you're portraying?
- Do other modes emerge too?
- Are you able to come up with a different approach if the group has trouble guessing? (Healthy Adult)

4.31 Stand up, this is my chair

Description

The therapist explains that this exercise is about coming across as persuasive. Choose somebody in the group (person A) to start and ask with whom they want to do the exercise. This becomes person B. Set up a chair and tell B, "You may sit in this lovely chair. You're comfortable here, and your plan is to stay right where you are."

To A: "This chair that B is sitting on is your chair. You want to sit on it yourself. Walk up to B and say the words, 'Stand up, this is my chair.' Those are the only words you're allowed to use. If it helps, you can think of a reason why it's your chair, but keep this reason to yourself."

To B: "Stand up only if you find A genuinely credible and convincing in tone, facial expression, and posture. If not, remain seated and say, 'No, I'm good here.'"

To A: "Take a moment and decide when you're ready to approach the chair. At that point, the exercise begins."

A may make multiple attempts to get the chair. The therapist provides supporting instructions as needed. B is encouraged to stick to their own plan (I want to stay seated) while at the same time taking on board and responding to what A does.

AIM

- Practice assertiveness.
- Gain insight into personal coping modes that can take over in this exercise.

Connection to healthy ego functions

- Personality integration and the formation of a self-image.
- Contact with one's own emotions/needs and those of others.
- Testing reality and assessing situations, conflicts, and relationships.

Materials

Chair, ideally one that differs from the other chairs in the room.

Group/pair/individual

- Group.
- Individually.

Further details

Variation

As a second step, the exercise can be used to practice putting dysfunctional modes aside, for example, as a Healthy Adult, setting aside a persistent coping mode. In that case, A says, "Stand up, this is my chair now. I'm taking over from you."

B replies: "It's safer if I stay here" (or an alternative claim as appropriate for the coping mode in question).

The exercise is most powerful when the focus is on person A's non-verbal actions. Too many words can form a distraction.

The exercise can also be done one-on-one with the drama therapist.

EVALUATION

Questions for A:

- Were there any moments you found difficult?
- Was there a moment when you went into a coping mode?

Questions for B:

- What convinced you to stand up?
- What made you stay put?

Questions for spectators:

- What stood out to you? What made A come across as convincing/ unconvincing?

4.32 I know a silly walk

Description

The therapist explains, "We're going to do a warm-up exercise to get our bodies moving and awaken our Happy Child. We'll start by criss-crossing the room and filling up the space."

Start walking, and have the group join in. "When I yell, 'I know a silly walk,' your task is to copy me and do exactly what I'm doing."

Then start doing an easy and funny walk—for example, lifting your legs high while walking. The participants should follow suit. After that, anyone can initiate a new, funny way of moving by shouting "I know a silly walk!" which the others then imitate (see also Kapok, 2023).

AIM

- Have fun, connect with the Happy Child and with others.
- Let go (break down the barriers of controlling and avoidant coping modes).
-
- Increase self-expression.

Connection to healthy ego functions

- Contact with one's own emotions/needs and those of others.
- Seeking enjoyment and fulfillment in a mature manner.

Materials

None.

Group/pair/individual

- Group.
- Individually.

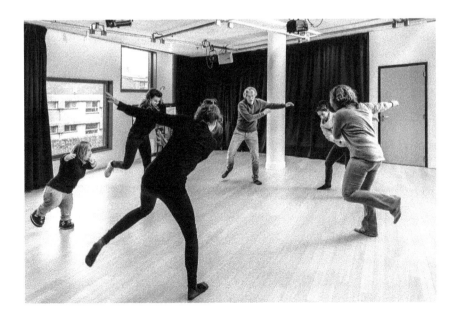

Further details

Keep the pace high by pointing at somebody to initiate a new walk if nobody takes the initiative themselves. Compliment those who do take the initiative.

The therapist can initiate a new walk in order to:

- promote variation of movement;
- end a walk that is physically demanding or difficult;
- encourage a group member by repeating that person's walk or a variation thereof.

Variation

This exercise can also be done one-on-one with the therapist. It can also be set to music.

EVALUATION

The exercise requires no debriefing if it serves as a warm-up.
   Questions may include:

- What was it like to do?
- Which walk brought you closest to your Happy/Free Child?
- Were you inhibited by the Demanding or Punitive Parent modes? If so, how did you deal with that? What helped you make room for your Happy Child mode?

4.33 The Healthy Adult in interaction

Description

The therapist explains that this exercise will help clients to regulate their emotions when a schema is triggered. "Close your eyes and picture a recent situation in which you reacted on the basis of your child mode, making it difficult to interact with another person. Perhaps you reacted in a way that was angrier, sadder, or more stubborn or fearful than was appropriate. Where are you? With whom? What is happening? How do you feel? What are you doing?"

Step 1: Act out the original situation

"We're now going to briefly act out the original situation in a role-play. Make sure the trigger for the schema is clear to the group."

Step 2: Identify the modes

The next step is to figure out which child mode the client was in and how it affected the other person. The therapist asks: "How do you feel? What mode are you in?"

Step 3: Adopt the Healthy Adult mode

"Choose someone as a stand-in to take over your child mode. You yourself now face the situation as a Healthy Adult and try out how you would like to react. In doing so, keep in touch with your child mode, and take note when it speaks up."

Task for the child mode

"Speak up if you feel you are not being properly listened to. If the Healthy Adult says to the other person, 'it doesn't matter,' and you think it does, say so."

The task for the *antagonist* is to listen to what the Healthy Adult says and does and respond to it.

AIM

- Connect with emotions and needs.
- Regulate emotions.
- Practice assertiveness.

Connection to healthy ego functions

- Healthy emotion regulation.
- Contact with one's own emotions/needs and those of others.
- Developing a healthy internal dialogue.

Materials

None.

Group/pair/individual

- Individual work in a group setting.

Further details

This exercise allows clients to seek and find an appropriate response. There is no right or wrong; no "perfect" response. The client practices regulating internal dialogue with the child mode while interacting as a Healthy Adult with the interlocutor. This can be quite a challenge.

If the child mode is strongly triggered, the Healthy Adult may first have to validate the needs of the child, for example, by saying, "I understand that you are hurt because this reminds you of painful experiences in the past, but let me find out what's going on in the here and now." It is also important to be mindful of the possibility of coping modes emerging.

EVALUATION

- At what moments did the child mode make itself heard?
- What stood out?
- When did the child mode settle down again?
- What changed because of the new behavior?
- What stood out about the other person's reaction?
- Was a certain need better met by the new behavior (e.g., safety and connection, autonomy and self-esteem, boundaries, self-expression, play and spontaneity)?

4.34 Echo of the Happy Child

Description

The group stands in a circle. The therapist gives the following instructions: "Imagine we're all children of about six years old. We don't care yet what others think of us; we're just enjoying being free and playful. Now imagine that here before us is a very deep, old well made of stone. When you shout something into the well, the sound comes back as an echo."

"I'm going to shout something into the well and make an accompanying movement. All of you are my echo; you all imitate me at the same time. Try to mirror my exact posture, movement, voice, and facial expressions. Here we go!"

The therapist calls out a sound while making a forward lunge, then encourages the group to follow suit: "And now you!"

Next, the therapist assigns the person to their left to call down into the well, to be "echoed" immediately by the group. See also Kapok (2023).

AIM

- Have fun, connect with Happy Child and with others.
- Let go (break down the barriers of controlling and avoidant coping modes).
- Increase self-expression.

Connection to healthy ego functions

- Contact with one's own emotions/needs and those of others.
- Seeking enjoyment and fulfillment in a mature manner.

Materials

None.

Group/pair/individual

- Group.
- Individually.

Further details

The therapist dictates the turn-taking in such a way as to maintain the pace of the exercise.

Variation

This exercise can also be done one-on-one with the therapist.

The exercise is particularly suited to letting the Angry Child come to the fore. Participants are then instructed to make powerful sounds and gestures.

EVALUATION

The exercise requires no debriefing if it serves as a warm-up.
Questions may include:

- What was it like to do?
- Which movement brought you closest to your Happy/Free Child?
- Were you inhibited by the Demanding or Punitive Parent modes? If so, how did you deal with that? What helped you make room for your Happy Child mode?

References

Doomen, L. (2018). Schemagerichte dramatherapie bij cluster C persoonlijkheidsstoornissen: Een verklaring vanuit neuropsychologische inzichten [Schema focused drama therapy in personality disorders cluster C: A neuropsychological explanation]. *Tijdschrift voor Vaktherapie [Journal of Art Therapy]*, *14*(2):2–1.

Kapok. (2023). Werkvormen.info. www.werkvormen.info/werkvorm/. Accessed 19 October 2023.

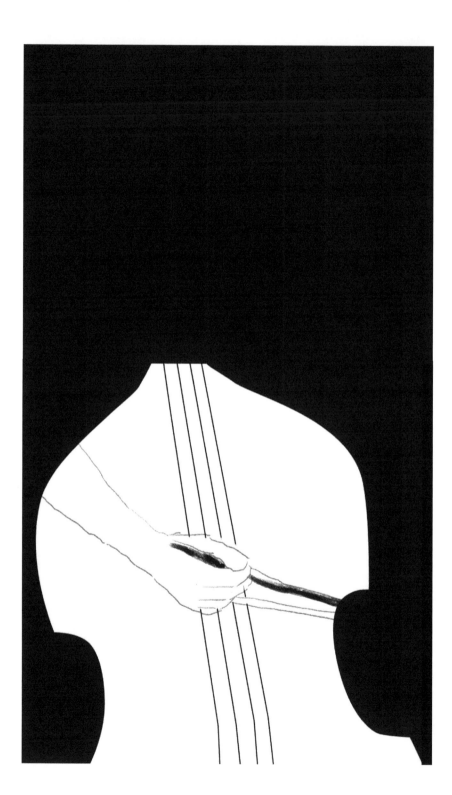

Chapter 5

Music therapy working methods

Summary

Music therapy involves working methodically with the elements of music, such as melody, rhythm, and harmony. This can be passive (listening to music) or active (playing instruments, singing, composing, and improvising). When making music, being attuned to others is essential. As a result, patterns of interaction and communication quickly become apparent. Music therapy can help clients to improve their social and communication skills and learn to recognize and process their emotions. It can also increase self-confidence and coping skills, help with relaxation, and improve concentration. Specific behavioral patterns come to the fore through music therapy, and alternatives can be actively designed and practiced. The music therapy in a group can serve an important function as a sounding board and practice space.

DOI: 10.4324/9781003456988-5

5.1 Base and release: Connection and autonomy

Description

In this exercise, the client is challenged to maintain their own rhythm while playing along with the therapist.

The therapist asks the client to play a simple rhythm on a conga or djembé. This should be something that the client can play without difficulty, such as a continuous beat with alternating strokes using the left and then right hand.

The therapist asks, "Can you feel the contact between your hand and the drum? Try to relax while you play. Find the balance between relaxation and your own strength. Keep the focus on yourself. When I start playing something else, you stick to your own rhythm."

Once the client has control of the beat, the therapist plays something different, exploring how far she can deviate from the rhythm or challenge the client. Does the client maintain their own rhythm even when the therapist plays something more challenging? Eventually, the therapist returns to the client's rhythm.

Optionally, the roles can then be reversed: "Now you can play something different, whatever you like. I'll stick to the basic rhythm."

AIM

- Build trust in your own strength and develop a personal "compass."
- Explore the basic needs of connection and autonomy.
- Encourage the Free Child.

Connection to healthy ego functions

- Healthy emotion regulation.
- Contact with one's own emotions/needs and those of others.
- Testing reality and assessing situations, conflicts, and relationships.
- Seeking enjoyment and fulfillment in a mature manner.

Materials

Percussion instruments that can be played with the hands, preferably a djembé or conga.

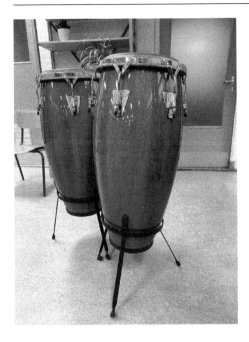

Group/pair/individual

- Group.
- Subgroups of two or three.
- Individual work in a group setting.
- Individually.

Further details

In this exercise, the client is supported in developing autonomy. Maintaining a rhythm different from that of others breaks through the schemas of dependence, self-sacrifice, and submission. It strengthens the client's self-belief when another accepts and complements or follows their basic rhythm. Exercising influence helps to strengthen autonomy.

This exercise is also appropriate within a systemic treatment in which, for example, the parents jointly play a rhythm (do they manage to find and maintain a common rhythm?) and allow the child to improvise.

When this exercise is used as part of rescripting, the therapist or another group member takes on the role of an Ideal Parent figure and musically fulfills the client's need. For example, the need for stability and safety can be met with an even, steady rhythm. Additionally, the Ideal Parent can narrate during the piece: "I am predictable, I provide stability." The client, in the role of the child, can then lean into that rhythm, matching it or improvising freely.

EVALUATION

- What did you enjoy most, playing the basic rhythm or deviating from it? Can you translate this into your everyday life? (Raise awareness of coping modes or basic needs.)
- What was this like for you as a child? Were you rebellious or did you toe the line? (Offer insight into historical influences.)
- What was helpful during the practice? How did you manage to stick to your own rhythm? Could you feel the connection between your hand and the drum?
- Could you feel the connection with the other person even though you were playing something different? (Raise awareness that it is possible to maintain your autonomy while connecting with another person.)
- Did you experience many thoughts while playing? (Identify the voice of the Critical Parent.)
- Could you enjoy improvising? (Encourage Free Child mode.)

5.2 The energy of anger

Description

The music therapist introduces the Angry Child mode and explains how a Healthy Adult can deal with anger. The music therapist explains the role that music can play in this and that the exercise is designed to explore healthy and appropriate ways to express anger while still allowing the client to stay connected.

Ask each group member about the extent to which they experience the Angry Child mode. They can indicate this with numbers (1–10), percentages, or color scales (ideally three to five color gradations). Then have the clients choose a small or large rhythm instrument depending on how much anger or rage they experience in everyday life. Give them the chance to talk about the relationship between their choice of instrument and the salience (number, etc.) of their Angry Child mode and to change their number or instrument accordingly.

After a warm-up activity, the game begins. Clients can experiment with the theme by deviating from or following the therapist's rhythm. The basic rhythm, which a client can fall back on at any time, serves to maintain the connection.

The exercise gives each group member room to express anger. If clients find this difficult, they can be asked to mimic/follow another client to evoke different feelings and tap into their experiences.

Another round can be done where clients once again have the opportunity to experience and experiment with the Angry Child mode.

Finally, the game winds down in volume and tempo, and everyone plays the same rhythm until it comes to a close.

AIM

- Learn to express anger.
- Stay in touch with the music.
- Stay in touch with other participants

Connection to healthy ego functions

- Personality integration and the formation of a self-image.
- Testing reality and assessing situations, conflicts, and relationships.

Materials

Chairs; large rhythm instruments such as congas, djembés, and drum kits; small rhythm instruments such as samba balls, hand drums, woodblocks, cabasas, and tambourines; a whiteboard and whiteboard marker; possibly a notebook and pen.

Group/pair/individual

- Group.
- Subgroups of two or three.

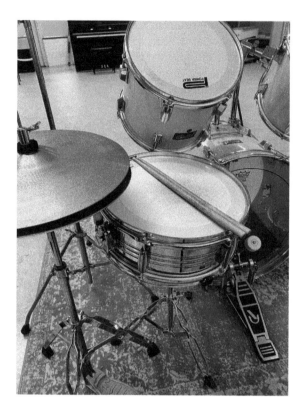

Further details

It is important to determine the extent to which the Angry Child mode is present for each client. For one, it may be a daily occurrence that requires effort to regulate, while for another—for example, a Detached Protector—it may be a rare occurrence.

When delving into a client's situation, it can be helpful to work in pairs where clients take turns to listen; this is often perceived as safer than speaking to the whole group.

When working with anger, other modes may be triggered, such as the Angry Child or Angry Protector. The therapist has a signaling function here, and can use this as a moment of psychoeducation and/or for deepening awareness.

EVALUATION

- What caused you to connect with your Angry Child during this exercise? What style of play is this mode associated with?
- When did you lose (or risk losing) contact with the music and the other participants?
- When did you experience contact with the other participants and feel you were allowed to make yourself heard?
- To what extent was your anger and/or stress reduced (give a number, e.g., from 1 to 10)?
- At what point during the exercise were you able to express yourself and stay connected?
- What schemas did you become aware of during the exercise?

5.3 A song of my mode

Description

Ask clients to choose a song that gives voice to the mode, as if the song was being sung or played from that mode. It could be the lyrics or the sound of the music that expresses the mode.

This exercise can also be done indirectly: in this case, the client is asked to bring their favorite song, or a song that is meaningful to them, or represents their inner selves. During the session, participants together consider which mode or schema this song would fit.

AIM

- Get in touch with the needs of the child mode.
- Raise awareness of the advantages and disadvantages of a coping mode.

Connection to healthy ego functions

- Personality integration and the formation of a self-image.
- Contact with one's own emotions/needs and those of others.
- Developing a healthy internal dialogue.

Materials

Speaker, songs.

Group/pair/individual

- Individual work in a group setting.
- Individually.

Further details

During and after listening to the song, the therapist and client explore the client's physical reactions, associations, and behavioral impulses. For example, while listening to Smoke Weed All Day (chosen for the Detached Self-Soother), a client might notice themselves sighing, sweating, and reaching for the water glass on the table. Different symbols can help to define which mode(s) is/are present.

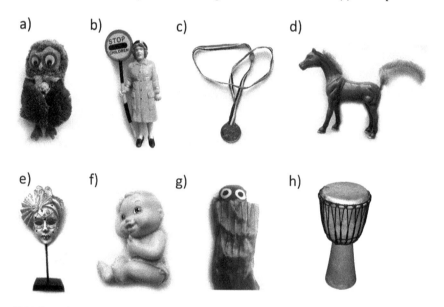

a) b) c) d)

e) f) g) h)

Which mode(s) is/are present? (a) **Healthy Adult**: perceives bodily signals and takes care of one/s own basic needs. Limits coping and Critical Parent mode. (b) **Critical Parent**: "Don't be set up! You're doing it wrong!" (c) **Coping**: The Pleaser: "I take care of the other and ignore my own needs." (d) **Coping**: The Work horse: "I work too hard and forget my limits." (e) **Coping**: The Mask: "I don't show how I feel." (f) **Child mode**: Vulnerable. (g) **Child mode**: Anxious. (h) **Child mode**: Angry.

The therapist discusses the function of the mode, its advantages and disadvantages, and looks to relate it to the music or lyrics. Often, a song chosen for a coping or parenting mode also highlights characteristics of the Vulnerable Child or Healthy Adult modes. This provides opportunities to raise awareness: from here, the conversation can continue to the historical emergence of the mode and its relationship with basic needs.

This exercise is similar to the modes interview in a multiple-chairs technique. The client is able to externalize the mode because somebody else gives voice to the accompanying emotional state, which leads to the realization, "I'm not the only one." The chosen song is usually meaningful to the client, often creating compassion for this side of oneself.

If the chosen song is very negative, causing the client to engage with a Punitive Parent, Angry Protector, or Powerless Child mode, the therapist adopts a reparenting approach and steps into the role of the Healthy Adult, offering interventions that may help the client escape that mode. Such interventions may include using the on/off button for emotion regulation, body-based interventions such as walking around the room while listening, or finding a song that works in opposition to the one that was initially chosen (see also Section 5.6 "Nurture Song").

Eventually, the entire constellation of modes can be depicted musically, resulting in a final product such as a flashcard or a "user manual for myself."

EVALUATION

- What physical reactions do you notice when you listen to this song?
- Is there a set of lyrics from the song that sticks with you? Or a particular sound?
- What emotion does it evoke, and can you connect this to your basic needs?
- Do you notice any behavioral impulses? Does the music prompt certain behaviors in you?
- What thoughts, memories, or associations do you notice?
- Does the song only fit in this mode or does it also tell you something about another personal mode or need?
- Can we together come up with a follow-up step to meet these needs, for example, find/create a follow-up song that speaks to a child mode or offers Healthy Adult messages?

5.4 Recognize your schema

Description

The therapist invites the client to select their own music at home and play it in the session.

Brief exercises can be done at the beginning of the session to allow clients to ground themselves. Consider breathing exercises or physical exercises (e.g., feeling your back, feeling your feet on the ground, stretching).

Remind clients that they were asked to select a song or musical piece that is meaningful to them, and ask them to present their choice. This work is done "in the moment": sometimes, a client may feel that the song they chose is not right after all, in which case, they should have the chance to explore what *is* right, even if this means changing songs (where there is space to work on the Healthy Adult, this is immediately encouraged).

Listen to the music. If the client is having difficulty connecting with their feelings, have them close their eyes and be in the moment.

After listening, allow a moment of silence for reflection. Wait for the client to say something about what they are experiencing, or ask them to do so. Connect feelings/thoughts that align with certain schemas to the music and ask if the client recognizes these (consider showing a list for this purpose). The schemas and modes discussed are noted and can be used in other passive or active (group) sessions.

Draw a conclusion from the notes, ask if it feels right to the client, and, if necessary, answer any further questions the client may have. Then, adjust the notes accordingly.

Finally, the song can be played again and the relevant schemas identified in the music.

AIM

- Identify personal schemas/modes.
- Connect with feelings and emotions.

Connection to healthy ego functions

- Contact with one's own emotions/needs and those of others.
- Developing a healthy internal dialogue.

Materials

Chairs, music system with a source (e.g., iTunes, Spotify, or YouTube) to play music, and a whiteboard with a marker.

Group/pair/individual

- Individually.

Further details

This exercise can be useful for case conceptualization.

When determining the modes, it is important to know how the client listens to their own music: Is it technical, associative, aesthetic, or qualitative?

The therapist has a signaling function, addressing feelings and thoughts evoked by the music and linking these to the theory of schema therapy.

Sometimes, it can be difficult for the client to sit facing the music therapist. An alternative is to sit back to back or facing away from one another while listening.

Modes or schemas can also be revisited in the debriefing. The music therapist can depict schemas for the client and add them to the case conceptualization if necessary.

EVALUATION

- What function does this music serve for you?
- How do you feel about playing this music in this context?
- What does this music say about you?
- What does this music genre mean to you?
- What in this music triggers this schema (e.g., social isolation)?

5.5 Body-based improvisation from basic needs

Description

This exercise starts indirectly, in the music.

The client is invited to improvise on musical instruments with the therapist.

AIM

- Become aware of the basic needs of the Healthy Adult.
- Learn to fulfill those needs in relationships.

Connection to healthy ego functions

- Healthy emotion regulation.
- Contact with one's own emotions/needs and those of others.
- Seeking enjoyment and fulfillment in a mature manner.

Materials

A range of musical instruments.

Group/pair/individual

- Individual work in a group setting.
- Individually.

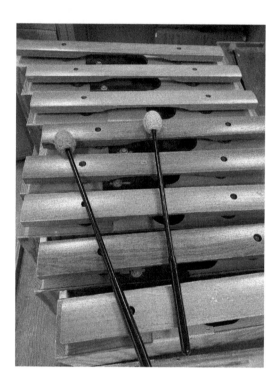

Further details

A musical improvisation takes a free form in which clients are given space to express themselves while connecting with one another. Clients often respond to this openness from specific coping modes. These can be identified in the music they play. The nature of the coping mode and its function can be discussed during the exercise or in the debriefing.

The therapist constantly monitors the client's musical expression and watches for physical cues. Initially the contact between therapist and client is musical and non-verbal (using the improvisation techniques described by Bruscia, 1987).

The therapist then draws links to the client's basic needs (safety, connection, autonomy, boundaries, self-expression, spontaneity, and play).

In a later round, the improvisation can be linked to the client's history and can involve role play so as to contribute to rescripting.

EVALUATION

- What physical sensations did you notice while playing?
- What did you get from playing, and what did you get from the duet with the therapist?
- What does your chosen instrument or the psychomotor actions involved say about you/your feelings?
- What role did the other person/therapist play? For example, were they the one who created the structure (links to basic needs of boundaries and structure), who laid the foundation so you could improvise freely (basic needs of spontaneity and play), or who followed your pace (basic need of autonomy)?
- How was that for you in the past, that is, who should have filled these needs at what age (raise awareness of past experiences)?

To make the step to rescripting, consciously redistribute the roles:

- What do you want to do in the next round of improvisation? For example, will you take on the role of the Healthy Adult, or will you be in child mode while the therapist or a groupmate plays the role of an Ideal Parent (reparenting as an intermediate step en route to doing this yourself)?

If applicable, lyrics could be added, creating a song that explains the origins of—and breaks down—the coping mode.

N.B. Often, it is valuable not to ask too many questions too quickly but rather to allow time to reflect on the musical improvisation or to follow up with a body scan so that the (often new) experiences can sink in.

5.6 Nurture song

Description

When emotions and needs that belong to the client's Vulnerable Child mode become apparent during music therapy, they are identified by the therapist. The therapist sings and plays an improvised song for this Vulnerable Child mode. The client simply listens to the music.

The song acknowledges the client's various emotions (child modes) and connects to their unmet basic needs (reparenting), with reference to the child's age and experiences. While singing, the therapist monitors the client's (non-verbal) reactions and decides on this basis where to go with the song.

AIM

- Connect with emotions and needs of child modes.
- Recognize and acknowledge those emotions/needs; develop compassion for child modes.
- Strengthen the Healthy Adult mode.

Connection to healthy ego functions

- Personality integration and the formation of a self-image.
- Contact with one's own emotions/needs and those of others.
- Developing a healthy internal dialogue.

Materials

Musical instruments, e.g., a piano or guitar, that the therapist plays while singing.

Group/pair/individual

- Individually.

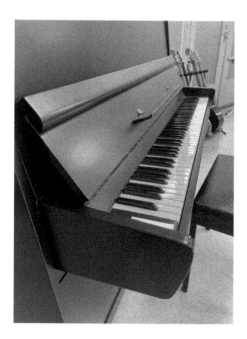

Further details

This assignment falls under reparenting, but it could also be part of rescripting.

The client must be ready to acknowledge their own vulnerability and unmet needs from their child modes. It is also important to check while singing the song that the client is present and not detaching.

For example, if the client leaves their *window of tolerance*, they may not be able to integrate the new experience, may not be open to receiving the song, or may interpret its message negatively. The therapist must be able to spontaneously adapt the lyrics and music in response to their observation of the client's bodily reactions.

If a client is not able to relax into the needs of the Vulnerable Child, the therapist can incorporate the coping side into their lyrics. For example, when the therapist sings, "I needed you so much," the client stiffens. The therapist may continue, "I don't want to know that, I don't want to hear that," and the client relaxes. The therapist sings softly, "but deep down in my heart I admit, very quietly, that I might need you a little bit sometimes."

If the client responds positively to the song, it may be nice to record it so that the client can listen to it at home.

A follow-up to this exercise could be to have the client sing their own song for the Vulnerable Child from the perspective of the Healthy Adult. For this, preferably choose a simple and repetitive melody, such as a mantra, and have the client write their own lyrics.

EVALUATION

It may be nice to be quiet for a while after singing the song and let it sink in, or to perform a short mindfulness exercise or body scan so that the client can connect with their bodily response and identify their needs. It is important to check whether the client can handle this.

It is often good not to discuss the song too much directly after singing it but rather to let it sink in quietly and discuss it further in the next session.

5.7 Multiple-chair music (sculpture)

Description

The client chooses a number of instruments to represent different modes. A guideline for this is to include one child mode, one or two coping modes, and one parent mode. Other modes can be addressed at another time.

The therapist asks, "How do the different instruments sound? Where are they placed in the room? How are they played—hard, soft, fast, in tune with one another?" Provide additional support by asking for clarification, offering suggestions, allowing space for exploration, and so on. Allow the client to substitute instruments and change their placement. The goal is that the client eventually feels that their behaviors, thoughts, and emotions are appropriately represented in the sculpture.

If there are multiple participants, have each of them take a seat behind an instrument. The client decides who sits where. The participants take turns trying to play as directed by the client.

Then the client conducts the "musicians" simultaneously. They may only "turn on" or "turn off" different modes (either in turn or simultaneously). This may provide some insight into how the different modes affect each other.

The idea is to take a moment to contemplate all possible combinations. The therapist might challenge the client to do this, but it is ultimately up to the client to determine when it has been long enough.

After the client shares their experience, the therapist (and the other participants) might ask further questions. The client may also ask questions about the other participants' experience.

Next, the client is asked if any adjustments are needed to make the sculpture more representative of their emotions, feelings, and thoughts. Participants may be asked to change places, instruments may be switched, or instructions regarding the style of play may be modified.

If something is changed, the client begins conducting again. As the therapist, consider whether the client should be given room to experience the Happy/Free Child role (and simply play), or whether they are best served by observing from a distance (i.e., conducting).

Afterward, there will be another round of debriefing.

AIM

- Understand the different modes.
- Connect with personal modes.

Connection to healthy ego functions

- Personality integration and the formation of a self-image.
- Contact with one's own emotions/needs and those of others.

Materials

A range of instruments.

Group/pair/individual

- Individual work in a group setting.
- Individually.

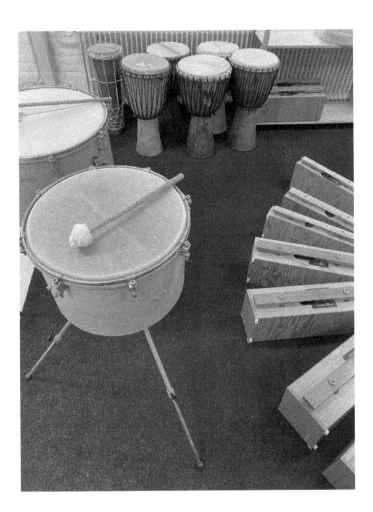

Further details

A possible follow-up to this exercise may be to consider adding a Healthy Adult to the sculpture who meets the child's needs in some way. In this case, the client can play the Healthy Adult themselves at first and later switch roles with the playing child.

The entire exercise can also be performed in a therapeutic duet. In this case, the client and the therapist play the instruments themselves. In one round, the client plays a child mode and the therapist plays the various other modes (as directed by the client). In a second round, this can be reversed.

EVALUATION

- Would you like to share something about what you saw or noticed?
- Did the parent mode impact the (playing) Happy/Free Child?
- Did the coping modes impact the (playing) Happy/Free Child?
- What purpose do the coping modes serve?
- What does the child need at this time?
- What does that look like? Sound like? Where might it be? Shall we add it?

5.8 The playlist

Description

The client is asked to make one (or more) playlist(s).

The music the client listens to and selects for this purpose is arranged according to a theme. Usually, this theme is named after a certain emotion as identified by the client, or it could also be a certain mood or an effect experienced by the client in response to the music.

The therapist explains that this is an exercise in listening and attunement and how the playlist can be used. The playlist helps the client to explore, identify, and pay healthy attention to emotions and needs: comfort, sadness, anger, joy, pleasure, courage, strength, etc. Movement can be encouraged, both literally and figuratively. The effects of timing—that is, when the client listens to the music—can be explored. A playlist is also easy to share with others.

Additionally, the therapist explains that the exercise is about making choices: What do I like? What does/doesn't help me? For example, the client can listen to different arrangements of the same song.

AIM

- Connect with and recognize feelings, emotions, and needs.
- Strengthen autonomy.

Connection to healthy ego functions

- Healthy emotion regulation.
- Contact with one's own emotions/needs and those of others.
- Seeking enjoyment and fulfillment in a mature manner.

Materials

Cell phone, iPad, or PC, access to a music source (e.g., iTunes, Spotify, or YouTube), and speakers.

Group/pair/individual

- Group.
- Subgroups of two or three.
- Individual work in a group setting.
- Individually.

Further details

The playlist can be designed and used in many different ways. For example, it could be linked to the client's life story, or parts thereof, or it could be based on specific (adaptive) modes or musical elements. It can also be created interactively with the therapist.

An advantage of a playlist is that it can be modified over time, from minor change to deleting it entirely.

EVALUATION

- What emotions do you experience when listening to this music?
- What effect does this music have on you?
- When might you use this playlist?
- At what point might you need this playlist?

5.9 Rescripting

Description

Part 1

The client reflects on a moment when they felt very safe. They describe the moment, after which the therapist and the other participants play music to match this moment. The client decides who stands where, what they play, and on what instruments. They also choose where they themselves stand and whether to participate.

After the performance, the client is asked what they would like to change about the music to make it feel even safer. They can make adjustments, and then the music is played again and the client is again asked what they would change. This is deliberately asked as a leading question, to prompt clients who usually display socially desirable behavior to think critically. This is repeated until the client cannot think of anything else to change and is satisfied.

The client is asked to make a "mental recording and picture" of this moment and to pretend to put it in a breast pocket or similar. It can also be physically anchored by a photo, a small instrument, or something symbolic that the client can take with them.

Part 2

The client is asked to recall the last time they felt uncomfortable with their thoughts. Then, the client is asked to hold onto this feeling and try to erase the memory itself. Next, the client is asked to recall the first time they ever felt a similar way. This helps the client to choose a moment that was long ago but is still relevant.

Part 3

The client is asked to describe this moment. Then, the client is once again asked to depict this musically:

- What instruments are needed?
- Where does the client position themselves?
- Are other individuals involved in this memory? If so, where do they stand and what/how do they play?

Preferably, the client plays the part of themselves.

The client may turn the improvisation down (or off) at any time by "turning a volume knob" (making a pinching motion with their hand in the air and then twisting). If the client turns down the volume, the therapist asks if the client would like to share something about the experience.

Part 4

Next, the therapist asks what the child's need is. What could be offered to meet that need? Preference is given to adding an additional element rather than removing an existing element. For example, a Healthy Adult could be added, who is able to exert influence on the other instruments. It is important that the client gives instructions for this; to do so, they will have to take on the role of the Healthy Adult themselves and therefore become the agent who meets their own needs.

Then this situation is played out again. The addition may help the child's needs to be more easily identified and/or met.

In the debriefing, the therapist examines how the client experienced this part of the exercise. If it is considered an improvement/a more positive experience, they move on to the next part of the exercise. If not, the therapist invites the client to explore what (else) is needed.

Part 5

The client is asked to hold on to this memory. Again, they may take a mental picture or "record" the memory in some other way.

Finally, the outcome of Part 1—the safe situation—is repeated.

AIM

- Connect with the Vulnerable Child mode.
- Fulfill the basic needs of the Vulnerable Child.
- Strengthen the Healthy Adult.

Connection to healthy ego functions

- Personality integration and the formation of a self-image.
- Contact with one's own emotions/needs and those of others.

Materials

Something that can serve as an "anchor," perhaps something that can serve as a volume control, a (phone) camera or a Polaroid camera.

Group/pair/individual

- Individual work in a group setting.
- Individually.

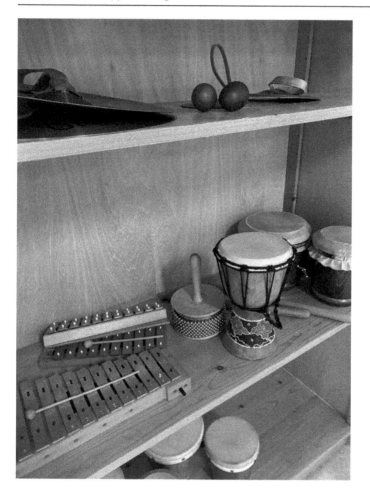

Further details

During Part 1, the therapist explains that the client can take this safe moment as an anchor for the rest of the session (and beyond). When stressed, the client can return to this moment, either using their imagination or by grasping the physical anchor. If this does not relieve the stress, the client can always pause the exercise and take a short break. If needed, the procedure outlined above can be restarted and performed again.

The goal is to ensure that any later moments of stress that the client experiences are manageable. As a guideline, the client should not experience so much stress that they panic or can no longer think clearly, nor experience so little stress that they are cut off from the memory or feelings. Part 1 could be developed in a separate session.

The added value of the volume button is that it gives the client some control over the unpleasant memory, and serves as a brake if the emotions become too intense.

In Part 4, the memory being rewritten should ideally be as close as possible to the original memory. Adding an element to provide for the child's need is likely to be more constructive than removing something and pretending it wasn't there in the first place, though the therapist and client can, of course, decide what suits the situation best.

EVALUATION

- What was the moment in which you felt very safe?
- What would you like to change about the music to make it feel even safer?
- Are you satisfied with the piece? If not, what would you like to change?
- When was the last time you felt uncomfortable?
- In your recollection, when was the first time you felt this way?
- How did you give visual and aural shape to the situation in the space?
- Where did you position yourself? Where did you place the others and have them play?
- What additional element could meet the child's need in this moment?
- What was it like to add this element?
- How did you experience this part? Is it an improvement? Is anything else needed?

5.10 Turn up the volume

Description

This exercise is about taking up space and experiencing boundaries. In preparation, the therapist leads a body-based warm-up, including breathing and voice exercises.

The therapist gives the following instructions: "Close your eyes and visualize a circle one meter wide around you. You're going to fill this circle with the volume of your voice. You can sing along with me. I'm going to make repeating sounds and you can copy them, though it doesn't have to be exactly the same tone; you can even come up with your own melody if you prefer. When I call out the number two, the circle expands to two meters and you fill up that larger circle with your voice. I'll keep going up to 10, so beyond the walls of this room. From 10, we'll go all the way back down to one meter."

"In this exercise you can get out of your comfort zone and try something new. You don't have to force it. Do monitor your own limits and stick with whatever feels good for you."

The therapist plays a simple chord sequence of no more than four bars on an accompanying instrument. For each chord, a tone is sung that is easy for the client to sing along with.

AIM

- Take up space.
- Acknowledge your boundaries.
- Connect to your strengths.

Connection to healthy ego functions

- Healthy emotion regulation.
- Contact with one's own emotions/needs and those of others.
- Seeking enjoyment and fulfillment in a mature manner.

Materials

An accompanying musical instrument for the therapist, such as a piano or guitar.

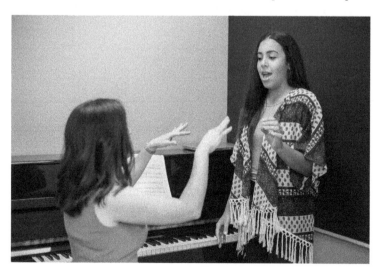

Group/pair/individual

- Group.
- Individually.

Further details

This exercise deals with the basic needs of self-expression, spontaneity, and play, as well as setting realistic limits and pushing boundaries. How far is the client prepared to go?

Coping behaviors, overcompensation, and/or avoidance can be identified and challenged. The exercise may also bring to the fore primary schemas, such as distrust or a sense of inferiority.

This exercise can also be offered using only voices, without an accompanying instrument. In practice, however, clients then often seem to be less daring and willing to take up space with their voice.

EVALUATION

- What went through your mind when I explained this exercise? (Link to schemas and modes.)
- Did these thoughts persist, or did they fade as we engaged in the exercise?
- What else happened to you while singing? What emotions did you experience?
- What bodily reactions did you feel?
- Did anything change when we started singing more loudly?
- What schemas or modes did you encounter while singing, and what did you try out with your Healthy Adult?
- At what number did you feel you had reached your own limit? What did you do then? Did you push your boundaries, or was it important for you to stay within them?
- What happened between you and the other person (groupmates or therapist)? Were you able to feel the connection? And your own strength?

5.11 Together alone

Description

Clients are asked to identify how they are feeling at the start of the session and then choose an instrument that matches that feeling.

The music therapist asks why they chose this instrument. If necessary, this is explored further, and participants can also question one another.

Then the therapist explains: one client is going to start, based on the therapist's rhythm. A key might be predetermined and the therapist leads with a melodic or harmonic instrument. When a client is "in" the game they call the name or nod to another who then also joins in. This participant then calls another name (or nods), and so on. The game can last 15–20 minutes.

The music therapist intervenes using musical (Bruscia) techniques (e.g., exaggerating/intensifying) to hold the participants' attention. The therapist may also ask participants to make eye contact with one another.

After the game, everyone is first asked to close their eyes and let the musical experience sink in, after which they are asked to speak or write about it.

AIM

- As an individual, connect with the group.
- Transition smoothly between participating in the group and practicing autonomy.

Connection to healthy ego functions

- Testing reality and assessing situations, conflicts, and relationships.
- Seeking enjoyment and fulfillment in a mature manner.

Materials

Chairs, pen and paper, a range of small instruments such as a woodblock, xylophone, samba balls, and flutes, as well as large instruments such as a guitar, piano, cello, and drum kit.

Group/pair/individual

- Group.

Further details

Participants may switch instruments, when appropriate, to reinforce the formation of their own self-image or personality.

It may be appropriate for participants not to join in at first and just listen to the music.

It is important to keep each participant involved throughout the game to maintain the musical interaction and to strengthen and develop their attention span and Healthy Adult mode.

EVALUATION

- At what point did you feel connected to others (Healthy Adult mode)?
- What made you feel connected? What did you do?
- What dysfunctional modes did you notice (Compliant Surrenderer, Avoidant, or Overcompensating mode) when you withdrew from and/ or "got into" the music?
- In these moments, what was your experience in terms of contact with other participants?
- How would you sum up the musical piece in three words?
- Did your instrument suit you and the piece as a whole?
- How would you describe the ways in which this instrument suits you?
- Is this different from at the beginning?

5.12 Who's singing?

Description

At the beginning of the session, the music therapist draws clients' attention to their bodies. Encourage them to relax and be in the here and now; this helps them engage with their feelings. Stomping, stretching, shaking, bending, walking, waving their arms: the clients are given space to discover which physical exercises feel good to them.

At the same time, they are invited to use their voice, to vocalize freely. The therapist can be a role model in this and participate if necessary. These can be "aah" sounds, "grr" sounds, or sounds that mimic complaining, for example. They can indicate or be a response to how the client feels at that moment. If the client says they feel nothing, the same exercise can be continued with variations. At which point does the sound begin to vibrate?

Observe which physical exercise does most justice to the client's voice. When does it sound most free? What feelings are present? Which schema is identifiable? Have the clients pause to reflect and identify what the feeling is telling them. Then modify the exercise based on this reflection, taking into account the Healthy Adult on the one hand (what does the client need?) and, on the other hand, the expression of emotions that fit different modes.

Accompany the client instrumentally, matching their pitch and dynamics and taking their lead. Do clients dare to rely on themselves? Only playing along with others may strengthen their lack of independence.

Clients can also sing and play an instrument simultaneously. Playing can reinforce singing and vice versa.

AIM

- Recognize and express dysfunctional and healthy schemas and modes.
- Learn to express the Vulnerable Child mode.

Connection to healthy ego functions

- Personality integration and the formation of a self-image.
- Contact with one's own emotions/needs and those of others.
- Developing a healthy internal dialogue.

Materials

A quiet, secluded, and open space where the client can move freely; a range of accompanying instruments such as a piano, guitar, and percussion instruments; chairs; drinking water (singing can result in a dry mouth).

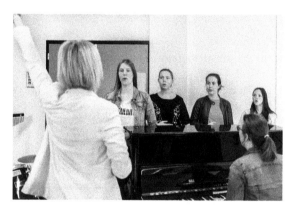

Group/pair/individual

- Subgroups of two or three.
- Individually.

Further details

When clients have no experience with free vocalization, attention must first be paid to breathing and connecting with one's own voice. This exercise is suitable for clients who already have a developed sense of self and an affinity for working with the voice, but who are emotionally inhibited.

It is important that the music therapist is freely able to use her own voice and recognize how schemas and modes manifest through it. This way, the therapist can recognize modes in the client and ask about them.

When the relevant emotions and needs have already been identified, the therapist can use this as material from the start of the exercise.

Experience shows that when feelings related to dysfunctional coping/parenting modes are expressed, the Vulnerable Child mode also almost always emerges.

If the language of schema therapy does not seem to resonate with the client, it may be effective to use words such as *silence, desire, hope, trust, letting go,* and *want.*

The therapist can support clients in processing their emotions by placing a hand on the client's back, holding hands, or working with eye contact.

If working in groups of two or three, participants can sing for each other. The listener then shares their own observations and helps the singer to explore what modes are at play. When singing together, a focus on the Happy Child is advisable.

EVALUATION

While working, the therapist asks the client questions, giving space for anything that the client needs to express.

*   How does this feel?
*   Where do you feel this in your body?
*   What would this feeling want to say to you?
*   Is the emotion or feeling recognizable to you?
*   Do you recognize this from your daily life?
*   What schema terms can you link to this?
*   When are/were there examples of avoidance, overcompensation, or submission?
*   When did you feel happy? When were you in your Happy Child mode? Did you create space for this?
*   What sounds fit with this? What made you feel inhibited?

5.13 Self-care

Description

The music therapist instructs clients to find a place in the room where they feel comfortable. They can also use a blanket and/or pillow to wrap themselves in something that feels warm and soft.

The therapist then leads a modified body scan, accompanied by soft, melodic piano music, to allow the participants to connect to their emotions. The clients do not speak, though they can sigh. Their eyes are closed. Have them tense and relax their feet, and repeat this for the pelvic area, shoulders, and forehead. Ask them to pay attention to their abdomen and take some deep breaths. When they are ready, they can make sounds that come naturally, such as "aah" or "ooh."

When the participants are "grounded," ask them to imagine a situation in which they felt vulnerable and used a dysfunctional coping mode, such as the Overcompensator, to deal with this. (Note that this is not an imagery rescripting exercise.)

Have the participants pay attention to what is happening to them both emotionally and physically. What did they feel in that moment? What was their need? Ask them to sing for this need, or vocalize freely, or sing the word "yes" in recognition of the Vulnerable Child. Monitor the participants closely and assist them as needed, playing the role of Healthy Adult.

Finally, have the participants turn down the volume until the singing fades out completely. Allow a moment for silent reflection, then ask participants to return their attention to the room. In pairs, they exchange experiences and take notes.

AIM

- Connect with emotions and underlying needs.
- Verbalize your own needs.
- Recognize your schema.

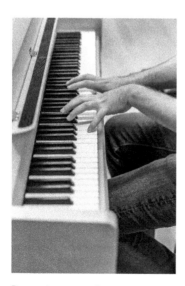

Recognize your schema.

Connection to healthy ego functions

- Contact with one's own emotions/needs and those of others.
- Developing a healthy internal dialogue.

Materials

Chairs, blankets/cushions, dim lighting to create atmosphere, piano (played by music therapist) or a music system to play piano music. Pen and paper.

Group/pair/individual

- Individual work in a group setting.
- Individually.

Further details

If the therapist finds it difficult to lead the exercise and play accompanying music simultaneously, piano music of the appropriate duration can be selected in advance and played through a sound system.

This exercise can also be done in pairs, though it is advised that each client initially works by themselves. When they are able to make connections with the child modes and/or identify feelings related to dysfunctional coping modes, they can work with their eyes open, and possibly sing to a fellow group member.

This exercise is not appropriate for clients with an underdeveloped sense of self, dissociative symptoms, or severe trauma.

EVALUATION

- What was it like to make a pleasant place for yourself?
- What did this place look like?
- Did you manage to relax and start making sounds?
- Could you recall a moment when you felt vulnerable?
- How did that feel? How did you feel in that moment?
- How did it feel to create a sound focused on fulfilling the needs of the Vulnerable Child?
- How did that feel in your body?

5.14 Happy Child music

Description

The therapist asks clients to choose a piece of music they think represents the Happy Child mode. This can be contemporary music or music they know from the past. If they find it difficult to identify music that makes them happy, encourage them to think of music that evokes a pleasant feeling.

Before listening to the music, the therapist explains, "Allow yourself to be carried away by the music and see what it does to you. Feel free to move or dance and sing along!" If needed, set an example by joining in, or standing up and moving along with the clients.

AIM

- Enhance the Happy Child mode.
- Relax and have fun.

Connection to healthy ego functions

- Healthy emotion regulation.
- Developing a healthy internal dialogue.
- Seeking enjoyment and fulfillment in a mature manner.

Materials

Instruments, sound system, mobile/tablet, possibly also CD player and CDs, enough space to move around.

Group/pair/individual

- Group.
- Subgroups of two or three.
- Individual work in a group setting.
- Individually.

Further details

The Happy Child mode can be stimulated at an early stage in therapy, even when many dysfunctional modes are still active. This helps the client to learn to create more space for enjoyment, positive feelings, and relaxation. It also helps to regulate stress and emotions.

In this exercise, the therapist demonstrates one way in which happiness can be expressed, and supports the client in practicing this.

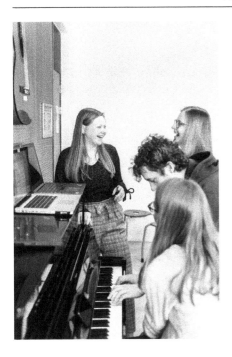

This can also take the form of a mini-intervention in a group setting, for example, to conclude the session or if a particular client needs extra support in fostering their Happy Child mode. In such cases, the group could also choose music for their fellow group member.

Alternatively, the clients can also play the music themselves.

EVALUATION

- How did you experience the music?
- Could you relax into the positive feeling?
- If so, what changed as a result?
- Could you try to activate this mode more often at home?

The following questions might be used if the client is finding it difficult to activate the Happy Child mode:

- Why, in your opinion, does this not work so well?
- Which mode plays a role in this or prevents you from relaxing?
- How could we put that mode/those modes aside to create space for your Happy Child mode?

5.15 Passing the beat

Description

The therapist asks clients to choose a rhythm instrument. They do not have to be able to play the instrument well; the important thing is that they join in.

Step 1

Everyone plays one beat on their instrument. That's it! The participants play their beat one after another, taking turns around the circle until the therapist stops the game.

Step 2

Step 2 is similar to Step 1 in that a beat is passed around the circle. But now an extra element is added: if someone beats their instrument twice in rapid succession, the direction reverses. (It can be helpful for the therapist to demonstrate this.) Anyone may change the direction at any time with two quick beats. The therapist starts and sets the direction, or instructs another player to start.

Step 3

After the therapist checks if everyone is able to keep up, another element is introduced: if someone beats their instrument three times in a row, the next player skips a turn.

The other two rules remain the same. So, participants have the option to keep the direction the same (one hit), change the direction (two hits), or skip the next person in line (three hits). Once this is clear to everyone, the therapist starts again and sets the direction, or instructs another player to start.

Step 4

After checking again whether the group is able to keep up, a final element is introduced. At this point, it can be useful to remind participants that although it's getting more complicated, it's just a game!

The fourth element is that when someone beats their instrument four times, the beat is passed back one player and then forward again. The therapist demonstrates how this works, and then starts again or instructs another player to do so.

Finally, the therapist brings the exercise to a close.

AIM

- Strengthen the Happy Child mode and encourage relaxation.
- Increase sense of belonging.

Connection to healthy ego functions

- Healthy emotion regulation.
- Contact with one's own emotions/needs and those of others.
- Seeking enjoyment and fulfillment in a mature manner.

Materials

Rhythm instruments such as drums (djembé, hand drum, bongo, conga) or boom whackers.

Group/pair/individual

- Group.

Further details

This exercise creates space for the Happy Child. The therapist assesses how the exercise is proceeding and how many steps the group can handle, ensuring a safe atmosphere.

EVALUATION

- Did you manage to access your Happy Child mode?
- If yes, what was this like? If not, what mode was active?
- What might the Healthy Adult do next time you take part in a similar exercise to create space for the Happy Child?
- How could you make more space for the Happy Child at home, too?

5.16 Musical modes dialogue

Description

In this exercise, the client practices restricting the space given to the parent mode and strengthening the Healthy Adult mode. The therapist emphasizes that what is important is not to play well, but to explore their feelings and modes.

The therapist asks, "Can you choose an instrument that fits your […] Parent mode? What fits in terms of sound or appearance?" If needed, help the client select an instrument. "Place this instrument somewhere in the room. Then choose an instrument to represent your Healthy Adult mode, and another for a child mode, and place these somewhere in the room too."

Once the client has done this, the therapist continues, "Can you try to make the sound of the [...] Parent mode? What does this voice sound like? Is it loud, harsh, fast, etc.?"

The client may need help in playing the sound of the chosen parent mode. After that, the therapist says, "Will you now stand/sit by the instrument of your child mode? I'll play the [...] Parent mode as you just did. How does it feel to hear this from the position of your younger self? Turn this feeling into a sound."

After this musical dialogue has taken place, the therapist asks, "How does your younger self feel when the [...] Parent mode goes on like that? What does this side of you need in this moment?" The client responds.

The therapist continues, "Would you like to try stopping the [...] Parent mode from your Healthy Adult, for example, by banging energetically on your instrument?"

If the client does not yet feel able to do this, the therapist gives an example. Again, the roles can be switched.

"How does the child feel when the [...] Parent mode is stopped?" The client responds.

"Shall we see what happens if a dialogue now arises between the Healthy Adult mode and your child mode?"

This is played out, again with the roles reversed if required.

AIM

- Do away with the parent mode.
- Make space for the feelings of the child mode.
- Strengthen the Healthy Adult.

Connection to healthy ego functions

- Personality integration and the formation of a self-image.
- Contact with one's own emotions/needs and those of others.
- Developing a healthy internal dialogue.

Materials

Any instruments can be used.

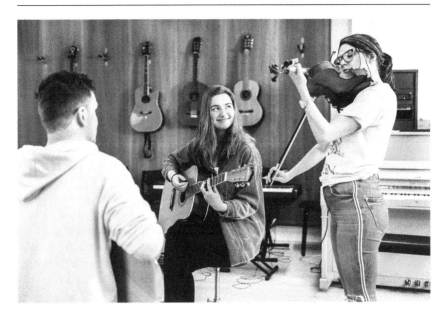

Group/pair/individual

- Individually.

Further details

The client should already understand what modes are and that they are parts of their personality. The musical modes dialogue can be used at various stages of therapy to explore and change modes.

EVALUATION

- What was it like to put a stop to the parent mode?
- Did this change anything for you?
- Could you imagine stopping the parent mode more often in your mind as well?
- Do you understand that this mode is not good for you and is not going to help you?

5.17 Drum battle

Description

The therapist explains, "We've talked about the importance of expressing the feelings of the Angry Child. Let's try this out with an exercise using drums. You don't have to worry about whether you can follow the rhythm or not. It's not about performing; the point is just for you to try something out and experience it. We'll do this together and help one another.

"I know how difficult it is for some of you to permit your feelings of anger. It might help to remember that anger also gives us strength and that you can also have fun!

"Now you can all choose a drum. We'll sit in two groups facing each other. Then we'll alternate playing our instruments in four beats per measure (4/4 time), which may consist of different rhythm variations. I will demonstrate.[...]

"Use your instrument to let us hear that you're angry or irritated. Be as loud as you like! If you're not feeling angry right now, let yourself be carried away by the sound and the playful dynamics. You can also recall a previous situation in which you did feel angry."

Then start the game, first with one group, then with the other. Keep an eye on all participants, and bring the game to a close when it is finished.

AIM

- Create space for the Angry Child and thus also the Happy Child.
- Regulate emotions on the basis of the Healthy Adult.

Connection to healthy ego functions

- Contact with one's own emotions/needs and those of others.
- Developing a healthy internal dialogue.
- Testing reality and assessing situations, conflicts, and relationships.

Materials

Drums that can be played with the hands.

Group/pair/individual

- Group.
- Individually.

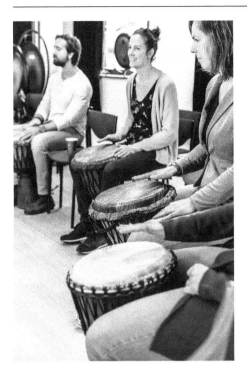

Further details

For participants with severe trauma, the sound of the drum-battle may be too much. The therapist may then make modifications, for example, by asking someone to stop and listen from a distance.

If a client has a strong protective mode and does not want to participate, the therapist can use empathic confrontation to encourage them to join in (e.g., suggest they watch once and then have a go).

EVALUATION

- How did it feel to drum loudly?
- Were you able to really feel your anger and/or irritation, and accept that this is okay, or even enjoyable?
- Did you experience any other modes?
- Do you have any other ideas for expressing anger and the Angry Child mode? (The therapist can also give examples here, such as singing along loudly during the game.)

5.18 From blues to swing

Description

This exercise is suitable when someone is feeling sad and alone. First, the therapist verifies their impression with the client: "You just said you feel sad and alone. Is this your Vulnerable Child mode? I know you find it difficult to let yourself be vulnerable."

Part 1

The therapist continues, "I think we can help you process this difficult feeling more easily so that you can better care for your Vulnerable Child's feelings. Is that all right with you? Can you choose a piece of music that fits what you are feeling right now?" (The client may need help with this.)

"You don't have to do much except listen. Try to open yourself up to the music and feel what it does to you. We'll do this together. If it becomes too much for you, just let me know. I'm here to help."

After listening to the music, discuss how it went.

Part 2

"I think it's brave that you showed your vulnerability through your choice of music. I'd like to show you what you can do to calm and/or comfort the Vulnerable Child. Are you okay with that?

For this, I want to ask you to choose music that suits your Happy Child mode or your Healthy Adult mode. It can be music that cheers you up, or that makes you feel calmer or more relaxed. Do you have an idea what this might be?"

Once again, after listening to the music, discuss how it went.

AIM

- Create space for the feelings of the Vulnerable Child.
- Learn to consciously change your state of mind.
- Strengthen the Healthy Adult mode.

Connection to healthy ego functions

- Healthy emotion regulation.
- Contact with one's own emotions/needs and those of others.
- Developing a healthy internal dialogue.

Materials

Instruments, sound system, possibly a mobile phone/tablet, CD player and CDs.

Group/pair/individual

- Individually.

Further details

If the client finds it difficult to engage with the language of schema therapy, the therapist may talk instead about, for example, creating space for difficult feelings and changing those feelings into more positive ones.

The exercise can also be performed using instruments instead of a piece of music.

EVALUATION

- How did it go?
- Were you able to accept that it's okay to make space for your Vulnerable Child?
- If not, why not?
- Did you find that ending with positive music helped to relax and/or reassure you again?
- Would you also like to try this at home?

5.19 Musical family sculpture

Description

The client is challenged to create a musical "sculpture" of their family. The therapist has the client choose an appropriate instrument for each family member, asking questions such as "Who is in this family? Are you looking for a big/small, high/low, loud/quiet, versatile/regulated instrument? Is there a family member for whom you can already think of an instrument?"

Emphasize that the client should select the instruments intuitively; their choices do not have to be well reasoned. Encourage the client to look around and try out different instruments.

When the client selects a certain instrument, they place it in a certain location in the room, for example, front and center or tucked away in a corner. When placing subsequent instruments, the client considers their position in relation to those already placed.

Once the client has placed an instrument in the space for all family members (including themselves), the family sculpture is complete and they can, if they wish, take a picture of the sculpture. The other group members are then asked to say what strikes them about the sculpture and what emotions it evokes for them. Before doing this, the therapist explains that everyone is welcome to give their impressions freely, and reminds the participants that only the client who created the sculpture really knows the family represented. The client can reflect on what they hear from fellow group members: "I do/don't recognize what you're saying," "this is new to me; it's something to think about," "that's not useful to me," "that doesn't seem right to me," and so on.

The therapist can make changes to the sculpture, such as moving the instruments representing the parents closer together. The client considers what emotions this triggers. Then, the therapist returns the sculpture to its original form.

The client can ask group members to take a seat at one of the instruments and play the role with which that instrument is associated. Group members may refuse to do so (e.g., if the assigned role is too stressful for them), but they are encouraged to participate as far as possible in order to help one another.

Then, the musical sculpture is brought to life through improvisation. Afterward, the client can ask how the participants experienced the exercise and their role in the sculpture. Any group members who did not participate can give voice to their experiences too.

Next, the client can occupy their own place in the sculpture, repeat the performance, and again ask for feedback and reactions from the other participants.

In consultation with the client, the therapist may decide to leave it here or to focus on a particular part of the sculpture, such as the interplay between the children.

AIM

- Gain insight into the influence of family relationships on your behavior.
- Develop independence and individuality within these relationships.

Connection to healthy ego functions

- Personality integration and the formation of a self-image.
- Healthy emotion regulation.
- Contact with one's own emotions/needs and those of others.
- Developing a healthy internal dialogue.
- Testing reality and assessing situations, conflicts, and relationships.
- Seeking enjoyment and fulfillment in a mature manner.

Materials

Various instruments, a keyboard as an easy-to-handle version of the piano, one or more double bass sound bars.

Group/pair/individual

- Group.
- Subgroups of two or three.
- Individual work in a group setting.
- Individually.

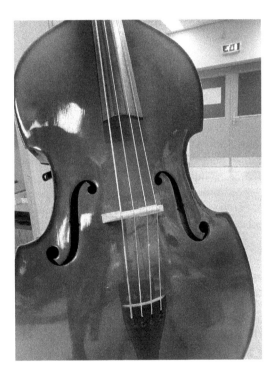

Further details

This exercise often arouses emotions even in those group members not participating directly. It is important that the therapist pays close attention to all participants.

Experience also shows that participants have a tendency to start giving advice to the client. The therapist should dissuade them in advance from doing so.

This exercise requires careful preparation on the part of the therapist. It is advisable to be well-informed of what the exercise entails and its effects (Verburgt, 2008).

EVALUATION

Evaluation is an integral part of the working process of this exercise.

If used within the context of schema therapy, a link should be made during the debriefing between the client's experience and their schemas and modes.

5.20 Musical modes sculpture

Description

Using musical instruments, one of the clients creates a sculpture portraying the relevant modes and the relationships between them.

With the help of the therapist, the client chooses an instrument that fits their Happy Child or Free Child mode, for example, and places this instrument in a certain location in the room (e.g., front and center or tucked away in a corner).

The client repeats this with another instrument for another mode, considering the distance from the first instrument. This is done for all relevant modes, creating a sculpture that provides insight into the importance of the various modes and their interrelationships.

Feedback

The other group members and the therapist share the thoughts and feelings that the sculpture evokes in them. The therapist explains that participants can say whatever they like, emphasizing that these are just subjective impressions. It's up to the client to consider whether or not the information is useful.

The therapist verifies with the client that it's okay to make changes, such as removing a certain instrument (mode) that stands between the Healthy Adult and the Happy Child. Ask the client what feelings and thoughts this change evokes.

The client chooses groupmates to represent a particular mode by playing the relevant instrument. Explain that they may refuse if necessary, but that it's important to try to participate if possible.

The sculpture is brought to life when the group members start improvising on their assigned instruments. The client directs when the playing begins and ends. Afterward, the client asks what this was like for the various group members.

The client can then choose to take their own place within the sculpture, working with the other participants to bring it to life.

Another option is to focus on a particular pair or trio within the sculpture, for example, by performing a dialogue between the Healthy Adult and the Happy Child.

At the end of the exercise, each participant is given the opportunity to share their experience: "What did you recognize in yourself, what touched you, inspired you?" The therapist reminds the participants that it is not their role to offer advice or value judgments.

AIM

- Recognize which modes are active in the present moment.
- Learn how to deal with your own inner dynamics as a Healthy Adult.

Connection to healthy ego functions

- Personality integration and the formation of a self-image.
- Contact with one's own emotions/needs and those of others.
- Developing a healthy internal dialogue.

Materials

Various instruments, a keyboard as an easy-to-handle version of the piano, one or more double bass sound bars.

Group/pair/individual

- Group.
- Individual work in a group setting.
- Individually.

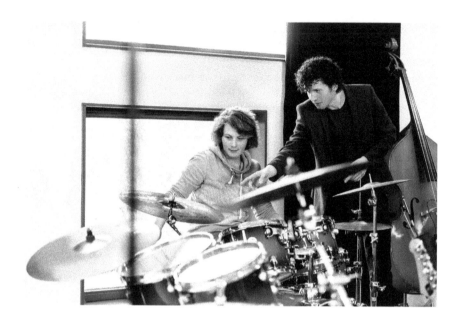

Further details

The exercise often arouses emotions even in those group members not participating directly. It is important that the therapist pays close attention to all participants.

Experience also shows that participants have a tendency to start giving advice to the client. The therapist should dissuade them in advance from doing so.

This exercise requires careful preparation on the part of the therapist. It is advisable to be well-informed of what the exercise entails and its effects (Verburgt, 2008).

EVALUATION

Evaluation is an integral part of the working process during this exercise.

If used in the context of schema therapy, a link should be made during the debriefing between the client's experience and their schemas and modes.

5.21 Beautiful and ugly

Description

Clients are divided into two equal groups. One group receives the following assignment: "Make as beautiful a piece of music as possible, lasting one to two minutes, with a beginning, a middle, and an end. You have 15 minutes to practice."

The other group leaves the room. Each member of this group, the "judges," decides what aspect they will pay attention to during the performance; for example, do the performers sound nice together, do they cooperate well, do they play with enthusiasm?

Then the piece of music is performed. The judges each focus on their chosen aspect, grade it from 1 to 10, and together reach an overall/final evaluation.

Next, the roles are reversed, but with one difference: this time, the task is to create a piece of music that sounds as ugly as possible. The players start practicing, and the judges leave the room and decide which aspect each will focus on; for example, do the instruments fit together badly, is the structure unclear, is the performance lackluster?

The piece is played, and the judges make their assessment.

AIM

- Connect with the Healthy Adult and the Happy Child.
- Recognize behavioral patterns in yourself and others.

Connection to healthy ego functions

- Developing a healthy internal dialogue.
- Seeking enjoyment and fulfillment in a mature manner.

Materials

Free choice.

Group/pair/individual

- Group.

Further details

Although participants are expected to follow the rules of the assignment, this exercise allows for spontaneity and fun, combining the Healthy Adult with the spontaneity of the Happy Child. The High Standards and Failure schemas are also discussed.

Participants often find it difficult to evaluate each other or feel stressed when being assessed. The therapist can link this directly to their personal schemas.

It is advisable to have two therapists lead this exercise, one to guide the players and the other to guide the judges.

In terms of cooperation, different patterns may be observable in the two groups. Sometimes, a group member will immediately take control and leave little space for others to contribute; others may remain passive/detached. Again, the therapist can relate this to the relevant schemas and modes.

EVALUATION

- What was it like to try to perform a very beautiful/ugly piece together?
- What was it like for you to be assessed and to give an assessment?
- Were you able to be spontaneous?
- Did you manage to stick to the assignment?
- Which part was more fun/easier to do—making beautiful or ugly music?

5.22 The sound portrait

Description

The therapist explains the exercise and asks for a volunteer to take center stage. This client temporarily leaves the room while the group gets to work preparing a sound portrait.

First, the group creates an inventory of the client's traits and behaviors. The therapist records these on a flip chart.

Then the group is asked what they would like to give this person to help them further develop and strengthen their Healthy Adult. This is written in a separate column.

Next, the group brainstorms how all this can be performed: on what instruments, in what style, and in what order, and so on.

The group also reflects on the division of its own roles: the therapist asks each player to choose a trait, instrument, or playing style from which they can learn something in the context of their own treatment goals.

The client is called back into the room and the group performs its composition. The client is asked to first just listen and only later, during the debriefing, to read what has been written on the flip chart.

AIM

- Collaborate
- Connect with others
- Increase healthy self-expression.

Connection to healthy ego functions

- Personality integration and the formation of a self-image.
- Healthy emotion regulation.
- Testing reality and assessing situations, conflicts, and relationships.

Materials

Various instruments, a blackboard, or flip chart

Group/pair/individual

- Group.

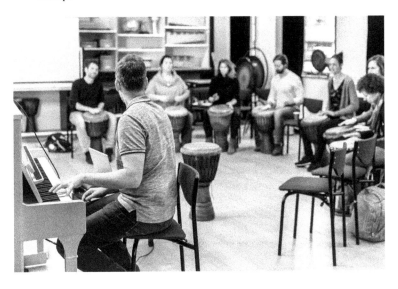

Further details

A precondition for this exercise is that the group feels safe working together and displays no exclusionary or destructive processes. It is important that most group members already know each other well.

When introducing the exercise, the therapist explains that it can at first be quite complicated and stressful, but that participants are almost always very satisfied afterward and the therapist will, of course, provide active support.

The link with schema therapy can also be outlined, though this may be unnecessary as it is often already clear to the participants how musical elements such as tempo, harmony, volume, timbre, and rhythm are connected to the manifestation of modes and schemas.

Most clients want to take a picture of what has been written about them afterward. They may also ask if they can make an audio recording of the piece. It is important that there is no filming and that everyone involved gives their consent.

If needed, the therapist can provide input for the design and execution of the sound portrait. It is also advisable for the therapist to be one of the performers, so that they can stimulate structure and coherence.

Sometimes, a group chooses to invite the client for whom the music is being made into the performance (usually the final part).

EVALUATION

First, the listener is asked to respond and share their observations. Once the initial emotion has sunk in, they are asked to reflect on the music and on what the group might have meant by it.

- How was it for you?
- What did you hear/notice?
- How did this feel to you?
- What do you think the group wanted you to hear?

The group is asked to offer any required explanations, followed by further discussion.

To conclude, the therapist also asks the performers what it was like for them and whether they learned anything while shaping their part of the performance.

5.23 Listen with your body

Description

This exercise is about linking an auditory stimulus—music track chosen by the therapist—to an emotional or bodily response.

The therapist starts the exercise with a brief body scan to bring the client into a state of bodily awareness. Then the therapist explains, "We are now going to listen to this music together. You may close your eyes or look at a calm spot in front of you. While listening, pay attention to your body and what you observe in it: your breathing, any muscle tension, whether you are warm or cold, any pain, pressure in your chest, and so on. Maybe something will change when you begin listening to the music. Anything you feel is okay, including emotional block-ages, or if you have no reaction at all. If it becomes too much for you, let me know and I will stop the exercise. Afterward, we will have a moment of silence so you can also experience how that feels in your body."

For clients with dissociative symptoms or a strong Distant Protector mode, add the following:

"I will also stop the exercise if I see signs that you're distracted or no longer present. If you feel yourself getting distracted, let me know so we can monitor this together."

AIM

- Become aware of your own bodily reactions and emotions.
- Become aware of and expand your window of tolerance.
- Become aware of triggers and modes that are evoked.

Connection to healthy ego functions

- Healthy emotion regulation.
- Contact with one's own emotions/needs and those of others.
- Testing reality and assessing situations, conflicts, and relationships.

Materials

Speaker, music system, and music tracks.

Group/pair/individual

- Individual work in a group setting.
- Individually.

Further details

This exercise is suitable for people who find it difficult to overcome a chronic coping mode, such as the Perfectionist Overcontroller or the Distant Protector. Such clients have little or no connection to and constantly avoid acknowledging their bodily sensations. Others may have a constant sense of insecurity due to underlying trauma. Clients may be dealing with a stalled grieving process or a lack of epistemic confidence. Some may get along well with their therapist and fall into a kind of pseudo-process where they use schema language and reduce certain coping modes, but their Healthy Adult does not develop. Others may be unable to reflect on their different modes due to fear or anxiety.

In this exercise, clients can learn that a stimulus can cause a reaction in their body, that their body does not always feel the same, and that they can exercise control over this process. They practice the skills that they will later use to recognize modes.

When choosing the music, the therapist considers how clients are likely to respond. The therapist carefully monitors their reactions when listening and reports these back afterward; for example, a shrug, a smile, or a bouncing leg.

In the case of an underlying trauma, the auditory stimuli may trigger a trauma reaction such as dissociation. In this case, additional interventions may be necessary to help the client stay in touch with their own bodily reactions and remain within their window of tolerance. Have the client keep their eyes open and direct their focus toward breathing or the positioning of their body weight and contact with the chair.

Alternatively, have them walk around the room barefoot, possibly over different materials, focusing on the contact of their feet with the ground while listening at the same time. This can foster a sense of being in the here and now. Other sensory stimuli, such as a balance cushion or stress balls, can also be helpful.

During the evaluation, speak slowly and softly, tuning into the client's language and repeating their words. Ask open-ended, body-based questions, and use experiential language rather than schema language so as not to disrupt the connection to sensations. You may, however, signpost the modes, and perhaps discuss them with the client at a later time. What is important is that the client begins to feel comfortable while exploring. Exaggerate differences such as good/not good, pleasant/unpleasant, to encourage greater awareness of emotion in the body. Psychoeducation about bodily reactions that the client doesn't understand can be offered, and critical thoughts can be linked to punitive modes.

EVALUATION

- Which area caught your attention the most: your body, your feelings, or your thoughts? Where else did your focus go? To the lyrics or music? Or did your mind wander?
- When were you more in touch with your body: while listening, during the moment of silence, or during the body scan?
- What bodily sensations did you observe and when? Are they still present now? Put your hand on the spot where you feel something.

- Try to describe the bodily sensations in as much detail as possible. Can you describe them through associations? Let's focus on those, such as the image of a stone in the stomach or a closed throat.
- What emotions did you observe while listening? Do these match your body's reaction?
- I thought I saw that your body reacted with [...] (bodily reaction) when [...] (musical observation) happened in the music. Does that resonate with you?
- Can you view your reactions without judgment, or do you also feel critical of them?
- Could you choose one word that is coming to you right now? This could be a sensation in your body, a thought, an emotion, or an association. It could also be a need or desire.

5.24 Each to their own experience

Description

In this exercise, participants listen to three musical excerpts without lyrics. These can be classical music, but need not be. What is important is that the pieces differ in terms of timbre, rhythm, and composition.

On the floor, lay out postcards showing different landscapes: a meadow with flowers, a barren desert, a volcano, a raging sea, a calm sea, a road wreathed in fog, and so on.

While listening to each piece of music, the participants mentally select one or more cards. The cards are left where they are so multiple clients can choose the same one.

Then everyone shares which card(s) they chose and how it fits with the music.

AIM

- Recognize your own perception (hearing, seeing, feeling).
- Recognize differences in experience between yourself and others.

Connection to healthy ego functions

- Personality integration and the formation of a self-image.
- Contact with one's own emotions/needs and those of others.
- Developing a healthy internal dialogue.

Materials

Sound system, stack of postcards with different landscapes.

Group/pair/individual

• Group.

EVALUATION

• What did you feel while listening to this music?
• Can you explain this using the postcards you selected?
• Can you say something about points of similarity or difference between yourself and the other participants?

Further details

One option is to ask group members about everyone's preferred music for certain moods. You can create a playlist and then listen to it together.

5.25 Exploring boundaries with djembés and egg shakers

Description

The group and therapist form a circle. Each group member has a djembé or conga. One person sets a rhythm that the others follow.

The therapist has four egg shakers and, once the rhythm is underway, throws them one at a time to a group member.

The group member who receives an egg shaker can decide what to do with it: hold onto it and play with it, pass it to another group member, or ignore it.

Meanwhile, the group maintains the rhythm on their djembé or conga. A game ensues with multiple egg shakers flying through the air, some group members having one, another suddenly having three.

After some time, the therapist stops the game and there is an interim evaluation where the focus is on observing what happened to each individual.

Then, each participant is challenged to come up with a different strategy than the one they were using so far. For example, if someone collected all the egg shakers and put them on the floor next to them, this time they are asked to pass the shakers on to other participants. Someone with the tendency to get rid of the egg shaker immediately can be asked to do something with it before passing it on.

AIM

- Experience in a playful manner where your personal boundaries lie.
- Experience the Happy Child/Free Child.

Connection to healthy ego functions

- Personality integration and the formation of a self-image.
- Contact with one's own emotions/needs and those of others.
- Seeking enjoyment and fulfillment in a mature manner.

Materials

Djembés and/or congas for all group members and the therapist, and at least four egg shakers.

Group/pair/individual

- Group.

Further details

This exercise allows participants to experience how much they can handle and how they deal with it. Healthy people have some sense of how much they can have on their plate at any one time. In this exercise, participants can experience through play how it feels to allow themselves to relax so the djembé game can continue.

For some people, such as those with complex trauma, this exercise can be too chaotic and therefore triggering. The therapist can give someone the option of not participating but instead playing the role of observer.

EVALUATION

Interim evaluation:

- What happened when an egg shaker came at you?
- What were you thinking? What did you feel? What did you instinctively want to do? and What did you actually do with it?
- Did you manage to maintain the djembé rhythm?
- How many egg shakers could you hold while maintaining the rhythm?

- Do you recognize the strategy you employed here from other situations?
- Which strategy will you practice next?

Evaluation after the second round:

- What was it like to employ a different strategy?
- How did it feel to pass on the egg shakers when initially you held onto them?
- How could you translate this to other situations?
- Did you feel a boundary or not? How did others perceive it?
- Do you recognize this from other situations?

5.26 Invitation to spontaneity and playfulness

Description

The participants begin by sitting in a circle, each with a different rhythm instrument. Cards showing different commands—such as slower, faster, louder, softer—are laid out on the floor.

As soon as someone wants to change something about the game, they take a card and show it to the others. Everyone has to do what is written on the card.

The exercise builds up from here, with the therapist continually adding cards: everyone takes a different instrument, swaps instruments, performs a solo, performs a duet, everybody uses wind instruments, makes a sound without their instrument, sings along, makes animal noises, and so on.

There is also a stack of blank cards; any idea from a group member is welcome.

If a client is shown the card "solo," they have to perform something alone, but can quickly grab a new card if they find doing so too stressful.

Everyone must take at least three cards during the exercise.

AIM

- Express wants and needs.
- Dare and permit yourself to be playful.
- Practice leadership.

Connection to healthy ego functions

- Healthy emotion regulation.
- Contact with one's own emotions/needs and those of others.
- Seeking enjoyment and fulfillment in a mature manner.

Materials

A range of instruments, a stack of cards with various tasks (see Section 5.26.1 "Description").

Group/pair/individual

• Group.

Further details

Choosing cards allows a person to take control.

EVALUATION

• How many cards did you take?
• What was it like to have to do what the card said?
• What did you do if you found a task too difficult (e.g., "solo")?
• What would you have liked to do?
• Which card did you like?
• Did you try anything that was new to you?

5.27 Sound of connection

Description

In this exercise, clients practice recognizing and receiving support from their environment.

Each group member takes three sound bars from the various xylophones and metallophones. They can choose from the bass, tenor, alto, and soprano sounds. All sound bars are tuned to an A-minor chord.

Participants put the sound bars in a circle and sit beside them on the floor. The group member with the bass sound bars starts playing a basic rhythm and, one by one, everyone joins in. Once a common cadence is established, the tempo and dynamics are varied in a wave motion until the piece flows smoothly and participants are in tune with one another.

Group members then take turns leaving the circle to play a melody on the piano while the group continues to play the basic chords on the sound bars. The soloist can practice exploring emotions on the piano, with a focus on being allowed to make mistakes, while the group continues to provide the safe foundation for the soloist to fall back on.

The soloist should feel that the connection between themselves and their environment remains even when they "isolate" themselves temporarily. They are reminded by the group's continued playing that they are not alone.

AIM

- Increase awareness of your surrounding environment.
- Take up space.
- Express yourself.
- Accept support and recognize sources of help.

Connection to healthy ego functions

- Personality integration and the formation of a self-image.
- Healthy emotion regulation.
- Contact with one's own emotions/needs and those of others.
- Developing a healthy internal dialogue.
- Testing reality and assessing situations, conflicts, and relationships.
- Seeking enjoyment and fulfillment in a mature manner.

Materials

Metallophones; xylophones in bass, tenor, alto, and soprano sound; a piano.

Group/pair/individual

- Group.
- Subgroups of two or three.
- Individual work in a group setting.
- Individually.

Further details

In this exercise, the client gradually comes to recognize that they can achieve harmony together with a group while also being an individual with their own story. The exercise therefore addresses both connection with others and awareness of one's own autonomy.

EVALUATION

- What is it like to be part of an exercise in which the whole group uses the same sounds?
- How does it feel to play your own melody (story) while the group plays on?

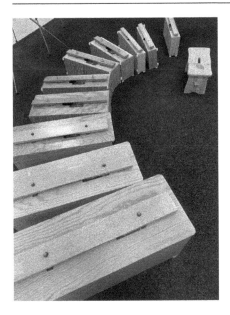

5.28 Let us hear what you feel!

Description

The group forms a circle. In the center is a pile of cards, each with a different emotion written on it.

The group is asked to think about which instruments they think fit the different emotions. In turn, each individual is asked how they think the emotion should sound. For example, one group member might consider "angry" to be best represented by an explosive drum sound, while another would choose three psalters (stringed instruments from the harp or zither family) that can be played with a bow.

The client places different group members by the instruments they feel represent the designated emotion and gives instructions on how it should sound: what rhythm, what build-up and/or fade-out. The emotion is then "performed" while the other group members listen and give feedback on what they hear. The individual plays along while conducting.

Every individual has one turn.

AIM

- Express emotions.
- Jointly give shape to emotions.

Connection to healthy ego functions

- Personality integration and the formation of a self-image.
- Healthy emotion regulation.
- Contact with one's own emotions/needs and those of others.

Materials

A range of instruments.

Group/pair/individual

- Group.
- Subgroups of two or three.

Further details

This exercise can also focus on the current emotions of the group members. This makes it more personal, while still allowing the group to explore how each member would musically portray particular feelings. This exercise is suitable for advanced groups.

EVALUATION

- How does it feel to give sound to your inner feelings?
- Are there similarities and differences with how other group members experience and display the same emotion?
- What do you need when you experience this emotion?
- What do you tend to do when you feel this?
- What is your underlying need with this emotion?

5.29 Voice it!

Description

The therapist announces an exercise involving the use of voice.

Step 1

Ask group members to stand in a circle and think of a word that does not have strong emotional connotations and that rolls off the tongue nicely, preferably with two or three syllables. Make suggestions if needed. Then ask the group to take turns saying this word (going clockwise around the circle) in a neutral manner.

Step 2

Next, the group chooses a particular emotion or mood. Everyone says the word again, but this time in a way that represents the chosen emotion or mood. Variations of the basic emotions can also be chosen.

The therapist helps the group brainstorm as needed, suggests areas that have not yet been practiced, and pauses the exercise after a few rounds so that a new word can be chosen.

Step 3

Finally, the therapist suggests practicing with the sentence: "No, I don't want that," or with a phrase that indicates what someone does want. The clients can also suggest phrases to use.

AIM

- Express yourself in a healthy manner.
- Have fun.
- Increase assertiveness and autonomy.

Connection to healthy ego functions

- Personality integration and the formation of a self-image.
- Healthy emotion regulation.
- Testing reality and assessing situations, conflicts, and relationships.

Materials

None.

Group/pair/individual

- Group.
- Subgroups of two or three.
- Individual work in a group setting.
- Individually.

Further details

The therapist takes an active stance, participating and providing verbal and non-verbal encouragement and affirmation.

Often, the beginning of the exercise involves a lot of fun and free play. When the phrase "No, I don't want that" is introduced, the atmosphere changes and many controlling thoughts arise in clients, such as the Punitive Parent, who forbids the setting of boundaries. It is important that the therapist and fellow group members encourage one another to continue to express themselves freely and connect with others, as they did earlier in the exercise.

EVALUATION

- What was it like to use your voice in these ways?
- How can you apply this exercise in your everyday life?
- What did you do well in this exercise?

5.30 Djembé

Description

The therapist asks all group members to take a djembé and sit in a circle. The therapist demonstrates the different djembé strokes (slap, tenor, and bass) and has the group practice them. Then the therapist explains that this exercise will consist of several steps.

Step 1

First, teach the participants an opening rhythm. The entire group learns it together, though later it will be played individually.

Step 2

Teach a rhythm that the entire group will continuously repeat after the opening rhythm.

Practice the sequence of Steps 1 and 2 several times. When this runs smoothly, move to Step 3.

Step 3

Teach the group a third rhythm that they will play over the second rhythm later in the exercise.

Step 4

Now assign the players a role and put Steps 1, 2, and 3 together.

Step 5

Finally, teach the group a closing rhythm that is also played by one person.

AIM

- Increase autonomy.
- Increase connection.
- Have fun and engage in play.

Connection to healthy ego functions

- Seeking enjoyment and fulfillment in a mature manner.

Materials

One djembe per participant.

Group/pair/individual

- Group.
- Subgroups of two or three.
- Individual work in a group setting.
- Individually.

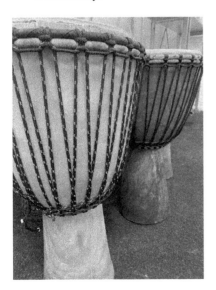

Further details

For a variation on this exercise, add free improvisation or (African) singing, for example.

EVALUATION

- What happened to your attention and focus, for example, were they directed more toward your own part or to the other participants?
- Do you recognize this from your daily life?
- What helped you to collaborate as well as focus on yourself?
- What did you notice physically while playing? Where in your body did you notice this?
- What emotions arose while playing? What did you feel?

5.31 Feeling nothing

Description

The therapist asks the client (as homework) to look for music about which they do not have strong feelings.

Based on the contact with the client and/or the setting, consider setting specific parameters that help with perception, including both physical (e.g., breathing rhythm) and mental sensations (e.g., positive thoughts).

During the next session, the client/group and therapist listen to the music together, discussing the search process and making observations. This feedback can help the client move toward recognizing, generalizing, and connecting to emotions.

This exercise may later be extended to include music that evokes different emotions in the client at different times.

AIM

- Explore and recognize emotions.

Connection to healthy ego functions

- Personality integration and the formation of a self-image.
- Healthy emotion regulation.
- Develop a healthy internal dialogue.

Materials

Spotify or another streaming service, such as YouTube.

Group/pair/individual

- Group.
- Subgroups of two or three.
- Individual work in a group setting.
- Individually.

Further details

This exercise raises the client's awareness that feelings and schemas are always present and active. People sometimes repress their emotions, feel highly anxious, or are overly analytical. The exercise helps people recognize that feelings can also be something very ordinary, like smiling or frowning, getting goosebumps, or feeling a small thrill.

The client is encouraged to really observe and perceive their feelings.

EVALUATION

The evaluation is entirely focused on client feedback.

- How did you search for this music?
- How did the assignment affect you?
- What surprised you?
- What did you actually already know?
- Do you recognize a pattern?
- Do you recognize these emotions from other situations?

References

Bruscia, K. (1987) *Improvisational Models of Music Therapy*. Charles C. Thomas, Springfield.

Verburgt, J. (2008). Werken met muzikale gezinssculpturen [Working with family sculptures]. *PSYC*, *10*:158–162. https://doi.org/10.1007/BF03077557

Verburgt, J. (2010). *Muziek en schema - Schema en muziek. Wat kunnen muziektherapie en schematherapie voor elkaar betekenen? [Music and schema – Schema and music: Music therapy related to schema therapy]*. HAN University of Applied Sciences.

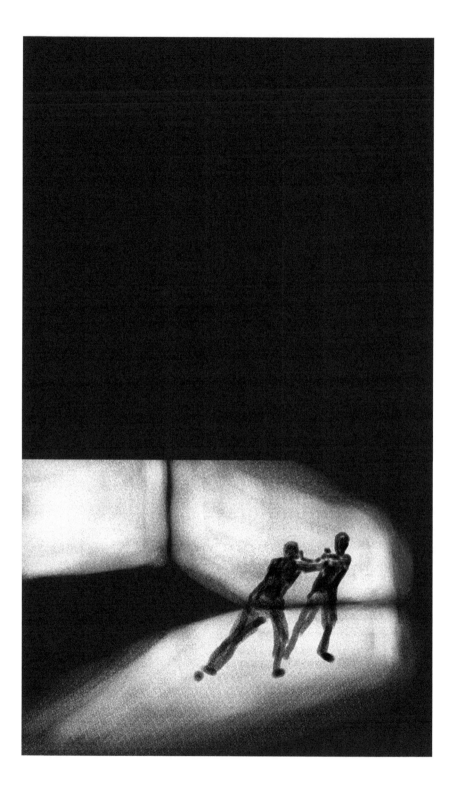

Chapter 6

Body-based therapy working methods

Summary

Body-based or psychomotor therapy focuses on psychological complaints and problems that manifest themselves in part through movement and body perception. Body-based therapy uses movement activities and body-oriented techniques. Movement activities include exercise situations from sports and physical education, while body-oriented techniques involve concentrating on the experience and perception of one's own body, for example, relaxation exercises, breathing exercises, sensory awareness, and bioenergetics. Within therapy, various interventions such as relaxation methods and impulse regulation methods may be used, with the goal of strengthening coping skills in dealing with emotions, cognitions, and behaviors. Specific attention is given to negative body appreciation and self-regulation, empathy and intimacy. Practice-oriented, experiential, and discovery-oriented work can be done to address the client's (help) needs.

DOI: 10.4324/9781003456988-6

6.1 Letting an elastic band be shot

Description

The therapist indicates that this working method is about tension regulation.

The client holds the end of an elastic band in front of his abdomen with both hands. On the other end of the elastic band is a group member or the therapist in the role of accommodator.

Part 1

The client makes the accommodator walk backward step by step so that the elastic band becomes taut. After each step, a moment of rest is taken so that the client can observe how the body reacts to the increasing tension of the elastic band. The therapist makes the client register what is changing in his body and what this means:

"What do you feel happening in your body? Where in your body do you feel something change? How would you describe the experienced feeling?"

The therapist has the client add quality characteristics to the experienced feeling (hard, tense, stinging, moving, turning, solid). This helps to become more connected to his body signals (*felt sense*). The therapist mirrors and names body signals that the client does not perceive. The therapist asks about emotions, thoughts, and can name modes, while the elastic band is tense.

The therapist provides psychoeducation about anxiety reactions.

The therapist encourages the client to increase or decrease the distance to make him aware of the change in his body.

Part 2

The client now searches for the distance from which he wants the elastic band to shoot off. In doing so, he allows himself to be guided by his body reactions. The therapist explains that the client will not hurt himself if he is in connection with his bodily sensations. The client finally instructs the group member to let go of the elastic band so that it will shoot back to him. Monitoring body reactions is the conclusion, as usual.

AIM

- Healthy tension regulation.
- Being in touch with needs through noticing body signals.
- Recognizing modes in the body.

Connection to healthy ego functions

- Personality integration and the formation of a self-image.
- Healthy emotion regulation.
- Contact with one's own emotions/needs and those of others.
- Testing reality and assessing situations, conflicts, and relationships.

Materials

An elastic magic cord (red and white elastic) several meters long.

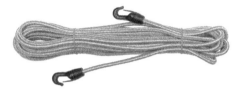

Group/pair/individual

- Individually in the group.
- Individually.

Further details

The therapist explicitly monitors safety in this working method. Do not use this working method with clients if you doubt that they can keep to the agreement to let go of the magic cord only if they give their permission. Intervene as soon as you see that the client is not properly attuned to his own body and is about to hurt himself. The therapist is always the last to give permission to release the cord.

Accommodators must also be able to take responsibility for their own body reactions and anxiety. Clients accustomed to being in tension-filled situations are willing to go too far in tolerating tension (accommodating from the schemas of self-sacrifice or submission).

Modes seen with regularity in this working method:

- The Detached Protector: The client has difficulty signaling his bodily sensations.
- The Self-aggrandizer/Demanding Parent: The client wants to show others how far he can go.
- The Punishing Parent: The client feels the tendency to hurt himself; the tendency to let the cord shoot off from too great a distance.
- The Detached Self-Soother: Tension can also be used to distract from other emotions.
- The Impulsive Child/insufficient self-control: Link to risky behaviors such as *thrill seeking* or drug use.

- The Vulnerable Child: The client feels fear or loneliness. Schemas such as mistrust/abuse may become activated.
- The Healthy Adult learns to trust his body responses and experiences being in control of increasing and decreasing tension.

This working method can be followed up with rescripting.

EVALUATION

- What did you experience during this exercise?
- Which mode became active?
- How did you feel?
- Hold this feeling and bring your attention back into your past. What memories come up? (affect bridge)
- Does this tension remind you of anything?
- What role does the elastic cord take on/what significance does the elastic cord take on?
- What role does the group member on the other side of the elastic cord take on?

In this way, a link is made between the client's activated mode or schema and his history.

6.2 Ball shower

Description

This working method involves the basic need: spontaneity and play.

"There is one big ball in the middle of the room and we all have small balls that you can throw against the big ball. Two sections are marked on the floor. There are two teams, and we all try to get the big ball across the other side's line.

You may retrieve small balls from the field, but do not throw them until you are back in your own section. Are the rules clear? 3, 2, 1, start!"

If the ball gets behind the line, have the ball quickly put back in the middle and distribute the small balls equally and count down again. After about ten rounds, ask participants if they have any requests regarding breaks, field adjustments, rules, or teams.

AIM

- Being able to enjoy movement and play.
- Recognizing inhibitions.

Connection to healthy ego functions

- Healthy internal dialogue.
- Seeking enjoyment and fulfillment in a mature manner.

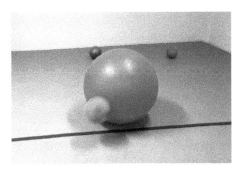

Materials

A yoga ball, the same number of balls (preferably foam balls) as there are participants. More or less is also possible. Lines on the floor to mark sections.

Group/pair/individual

- Group.
- Individually.

Further details

This activity focuses on the ability to enjoy movement and play. The client can recognize in this if he feels inhibited in anything and can focus his attention primarily on fun and fanaticism within the activity, rather than on winning/losing or succeeding/failing.

The therapist's attitude is inviting. He shows pleasure in movement by joining in, cheering, complimenting, and by showing that everyone misses the ball now and then and that this is not a problem. This game can also be played one on one.

Interventions

- In the beginning do not focus on winning/losing but on the game itself, if the group likes it, a competition element can be attached. For example, the team that has ten points first is the winner. Then revenge.
- Change groups if there is a clear difference.

- More or fewer small balls.
- Make space bigger or smaller.
- For a small space: one point if the yoga ball hits the wall.

EVALUATION

- Did you have fun playing the game? Why/why not?
- Did you feel inhibited in anything? If so, in what area?
- What is the difference in your mood now compared to before the game? (Possibly link to green/yellow/orange/red of body thermometer.)
- In what way did you act as a Healthy Adult here?
- Was there a moment/situation where it didn't work out to act/think as a Healthy Adult? How do you think this came about? How can you link this exercise to the basic need "spontaneity and play" (Domain 5: Excessive vigilance and inhibition)?
- Were you triggered into something (modes) and how did you deal with it?
- Have you experienced space for the Happy/Free Child?

6.3 Body chart with modes

Description

Create a life-size body drawing filled in with how you experience the various modes "in person." What shapes, colors, symbols, energy do you use to shape your modi world?

AIM

- Understanding which modes are active.
- Physical awareness of modes.
- Understanding modi dynamics from a Healthy Adult perspective.

Connection to healthy ego functions

- Personality integration and the formation of a self-image.
- Contact with one's own emotions/needs and those of others.
- Healthy internal dialogue.

Materials

Drawing paper for each participant (large format, 1 × 2 m), chalk, pencil, marker, etc.

Group/pair/individual

- Subgroups/twos or threes.
- Individually in the group.
- Individually.

Further details

Experience has shown that some people experience a great barrier with this working method. It may help to work in pairs, for example, to help outline the body on paper. Doing a body exercise beforehand can help lead to inspiration. The objective is that the client gains insight and overview of what modes are at play from the experience in the body.

In visual art therapy, this working method is also done more often, focusing on artistic self-expression and the symbolization of different modes in the body. In that case, it is desirable to use more diverse materials, for example, different paints or inks, and to work in a more image-filling way.

EVALUATION

- What was it like to have your own body outlined?
- Can you present your own drawing?
- What would you like to say about it?
- Where in your body have you shaped different modes?

6.4 Creator

Description

The therapist indicates that this working method focuses on safety, on making choices, and on making your own wishes known.

The therapist and clients select three objects and place them in the center of the room; these may be anything in this room. A brief reflection follows on how easy or difficult this task was and what thoughts come to the client's mind.

"The idea is that we are going to make a game together with the materials we have chosen. How shall we begin?"

As an idea develops, the game can be implemented and possibly modified along the way to make it more fun or challenging.

The client can offer his own ideas and indicate when he disagrees with the other person.

AIM

- Being able to make choices that lead to action.
- Expressing one's own wishes and opinions.
- Collaboration.

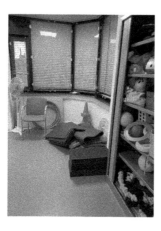

Connection to healthy ego functions

- Contact with one's own emotions/needs and those of others.

Materials

Three objects for each participant (e.g., hard/soft balls, field hockey sticks, pawns, chairs, balloons, hoops, rackets, stopwatch).

Group/pair/individual

- Subgroups/twos or threes.
- Individually.

Further details

The therapist's attitude is stimulating, reliable, inviting to trust and be satisfied with one's own ideas.

The initiative may lie with the client, but do not make the client feel he has to do it alone. Give compliments or offer ideas if the client gets stuck.

Interventions here may be to agree that the therapist should suggest more ideas and the client should assertively indicate when he disagrees and come up with counterproposals. The therapist contributes to making the game fun and encouraging the client to move in a relaxed way and have fun.

This working method is best implemented in a small group.

EVALUATION

- Are you satisfied with our game? Why/why not?
- What went easily in shaping the game?
- What did you find challenging in shaping the game?
- How was the division of roles between us? Do you recognize this from other situations at home or at study/work?
- In what way did you act as a Healthy Adult here?
- Was there a moment when you failed to act/think as a Healthy Adult? How would that come about?
- How can you link this exercise to the basic need "secure attachment" (Domain 1: Disconnection and rejection)?
- Were you triggered into something (modes) and how did you deal with this?

6.5 The Healthy Adult anchored

Description

We are going to look for the Healthy Adult in your body.

Optionally, as a start, a mindfulness exercise can be done to get in touch with one's own body.

You imagine what signals you can feel in your body that have to do with the Healthy Adult. Think of foundation, balance, strength, energy, breathing space, compassion, wise voice, certain thoughts.

Is there a particular spot in your body where you can connect the Healthy Adult with a particular posture or movement?

AIM

- Recognizing the Healthy Adult side through body signals.
- Mindfully connecting with oneself.

Connection to healthy ego functions

- Personality integration and the formation of a self-image.
- Contact with one's own emotions/needs and those of others.
- Healthy internal dialogue.

Materials

None. Quiet therapy room.

Group/individual/pair

- Group.
- Individually in the group.
- Individually.

Further details

Knowledge of schedules and modes is important. If this is still difficult, the initial focus can be on getting to know the Healthy Adult, for example, by doing activities. When in session or in daily life does one "meet" the Healthy Adult side? Ask for thoughts and descriptions of the Healthy Adult.

EVALUATION

- How did it go?
- Where in your body could you feel the Healthy Adult?
- What signals/sensations did you observe?
- What other words can you associate with it? And what situation?
- Did something new emerge in relation to the Healthy Adult?
- Is there an appropriate sentence/message from the Healthy Adult to remember?

6.6 The Lighthouse

Description

Starting exercise with the goal of getting more into the Healthy Adult side and from here an easier connection with your goals, to where you want to get to.

"Stand in a posture that is appropriate for you for your Healthy Adult side. Close your eyes for a moment or direct your gaze in front of you, if you prefer that. Focus your attention on your breathing; gently breathe in and out.

Are your shoulders hunched up? Are they tense or relaxed? Focus your attention on your face, on your forehead, eyebrows, eyes, nose, jaws, and mouth. And if you want to change anything because it is more appropriate for you in the Healthy Adult mode, you may do so.

If you had closed your eyes, now open them."

A pawn has been placed on one side of the room. The therapist and client(s) stand on the other side of the room. The pawn on the other side is meant to be a kind of lighthouse, symbolizing something that is important to you, something you would like to achieve, where you want to go. You can think of a value, or one of your goals that you have set up for this therapy.

For example, "I would like more social contacts." Imagine you are in a boat on your way to the lighthouse, which is where you want to go, to more social contacts. You are well on course, but then a strong gust of wind comes from the right, taking you off course. What could that gust of wind be, what causes you to take no action in daily life to expand social contacts?

Brainstorm about this with the group.

"When you are just getting back on course, strong waves come and make you change direction again. What else keeps you from staying on track to where you want to go?

This is how we get started. Who wants to start? Do you want to be the first worker?"

When it is clear what the lighthouse stands for, stock is taken of what modes are holding the client back from taking steps.

The Vulnerable Child who says, "I can't do it at all."

Parenting modes that say, "You'll never succeed at this, you can't do this at all, there are other much more important things you need to pay attention to, you'll let me down if you're going to do this," and so on.

Guardians who say, "Just go with us, you'll feel a lot better. Why go to all that trouble? Let it go. Stick to the familiar."

Physical complaints, for example, headaches, fatigue, joint pain.

Practical issues, for example, no/insufficient money, no/insufficient time, not mastering certain skills.

Family and friends/acquaintances who are not supportive.

The worker is asked how far he is currently from his target.

"The maximum distance in the room is 100%. You cannot stand further away from your target. Where are you now? You may already have taken steps and are halfway there."

Group members and co-therapists are used as "obstacles" and stand between the client and the pawn. They carry materials symbolizing the obstacle in question.

Example: Group member 1 holds a pad and repeats several parent messages, while using the pad to impede the worker from walking further or he tries to push him in another direction. Group member 2 tries to entice the worker to resume his old coping. For example, come sit on the couch, snuggle under a blanket watching TV, you feel much more like that, don't you? Group member 3 hands the worker two weights to hold. These symbolize physical discomfort: "You have a tough time as it is." Group member 4 makes a loop of a long rubber band, which he puts around the worker. He pulls the worker away from the pawn, away from his goal with obstacles previously mentioned by the worker.

It is up to the worker to relate to the obstacles and experience the extent to which he manages to resist and stay on course or regain his course.

A group member or the therapist can stand next to the pawn and help the client by naming what the pawn stands for or asking the client, "Where were you going again?" This can be very helpful when the obstacles are too strong and the client is struggling.

AIM

- Increasing one's own motivation to take steps toward personal goals.
- Increasing realism; What obstacles must I relate to as I begin to take steps toward my goal?

Connection to healthy ego functions

- Healthy internal dialogue.
- Testing reality and assessing situations, conflicts, and relationships.

Materials

Various sports and games equipment, a large pawn, punching pad or boxing gloves, rope or long elastic (possibly hand or fitting mirror).

Group/pair/individual

- Group.
- Subgroups/twos or threes.
- Individually in the group.

Further details

The pawn/lighthouse can be replaced with another object that symbolizes what the client wants to get to.

When there is negative body valuation and this is a barrier to taking or not taking steps toward the goal, a hand or fitting mirror can be used. A group peer can repeat negative self-talk from the client and ask him to look in the mirror.

EVALUATION

- At which obstacle did you experience the most difficulty?
- Is it the same in everyday life?
- At which obstacle did you notice that you were doing well?
- Has your motivation to take steps toward your goal changed? Increased, decreased, stayed the same?
- If increased: Can you think of a first step now for today/this week?
- Next time, will you let us know how this went?

6.7 This makes me happy

Description

"We are going to do a short Happy Child exercise as an introduction."

"We are going to stand in a circle and throw a ball to each other. Each time you throw the ball to someone, name something (object/situation) that makes you happy. So, 'I get happy from....' It can be something small or large."

"Gradually, that's how you hear from everyone what makes him happy."

"Next, when you throw the ball to someone, you will name that person's object/situation: 'You are made happy by ....'"

"This is about making contact with the objects/situations in your life that make you happy and that you begin to feel it too, also because of the affirmation you receive from others."

AIM

- Becoming aware of what makes you feel happy.
- Play and collaboration.

Connection to healthy ego functions

- Contact with one's own emotions/needs and those of others.
- Testing reality and assessing situations, conflicts, and relationships.

Materials

Lightweight ball in cheerful color(s) that is easy to throw.

Group/pair/individual

- Group.

Further details

Variations on this exercise can be introduced, for example, mentioning cases/situations related to one's own childhood: "When I was little, I liked to..." (positive play experiences) or related to coping behavior: "When I come home very tired, I'm going to enjoy..." (daring to share maladaptive behavior).

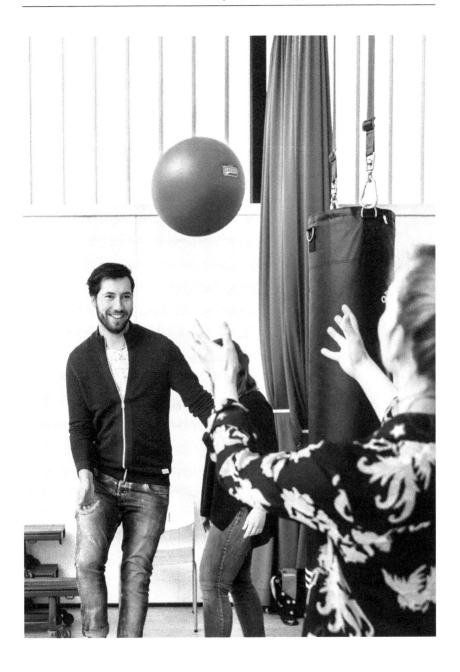

EVALUATION

- Was it easy to come up with something?
- Could you connect with your choice of something that makes you happy?
- What happened to your feelings? Did they change? Did they get stronger?
- What was it like getting affirmation from others about what makes you happy?
- Did that change the feeling?

6.8 Rolling in a mat

Description

"In this working method, you can explore the experience of being rolled into a mat. Here you are in control: you give directions on how the group is going to roll you in. This is done step by step and you keep in touch with your body and your Healthy Adult. If you want to get out, you can tell us and we will roll you right back. In a while, you will feel for yourself how far you want to go and whether you want to get out of the mat on your own, or whether it is just nice to stay in it for a while. We cannot predict what you will feel; for some people this task is about loss of control, for others it leads to a pleasant feeling. Lie down on the mat. Your head stays off the mat. Choose a group member who keeps contact with you by your head. Feel what it is like to lie here. Tell us what you perceive. When you are ready, instruct the group to roll you in a bit. And do you want that a quarter turn or all the way to your belly?"

The therapist maintains eye contact and explores body reactions. If there is too much coping, the therapist does an empathetic confrontation. If the client cannot stay in his Healthy Adult, he is rolled out of the mat and it is discussed that he is then going into too much coping.

"What do you feel? Stay with that feeling and associate. What do you think about? What role does the mat take on? What role do your groupmates take on? Do you know these feelings from the past? Hold on to that feeling and direct your attention to the past (affect bridge)."

The next step in an unpleasant experience linking to a scheme is to follow the steps of imagination and guide a rescripting in which the client is liberated by his own strength (deploying the Healthy Adult) and ends the entrapment.

The next step in a pleasant experience is to have the client share the pleasant memory or perhaps express the lack of a similar cherishing. Have him choose a person in the role of a Good Parent/Ideal Parent and role-play a positive scene.

AIM

- Connecting with the needs of the Vulnerable Child.
- Exploring emotions evoked by entrapment versus cherishing.

Connection to healthy ego functions

- Contact with one's own emotions/needs and those of others.
- Testing reality and assessing situations, conflicts, and relationships.

Materials

A roll-in heavy mat or heavy blanket (size about 3 × 3 m).

Group/pair/individual

- Group.
- Individually in the group.

Further details

In this exercise, the client gets in touch with the experience of letting go of control and surrendering. For many, this means getting in touch with the Vulnerable Child mode and it is linked to the schemas of self-sacrifice or submission (mode: Compliant Surrenderer), as well as the schemas of distrust or abuse. Abandonment or emotional deficit may play a role. The therapist explains that being able to surrender is also a characteristic of the Healthy Adult and that surrender can also go hand in hand with having control.

This working method is appropriate for clients with some level of emotion regulation and who want to look for/explore a fear. The group should be safe and familiar.

This exercise is deliberately offered material based. The meaning is given only from the evoked experience. It may be experienced very differently from what you think you see. The rationale that something that is very frightening can also feel very safe and cherishing is important as well as emphasizing that the control lies with the protagonist.

While explaining the exercise, some clients may already get scared. Therefore, the therapist asks for the reactions of group members before starting. He makes it clear that this exercise is voluntary and a lot of therapeutic things can happen even from the side. The therapist exudes confidence in the good outcome and validates the fear.

EVALUATION

Because of the intensity of the experience, the evaluation takes place specifically in the next session. The open question then asked is, "What does this exercise mean for your life when you look back at your trauma or the lack that has led to your schemas?"

The therapist emphasizes the fact that if things were different now, the client would be able to mobilize his Healthy Adult power or allow nurturing. "Your body is capable of this.""

For group members, the sharing of experiences, associations, schemas, and modes takes place after the exercise. The protagonist is allowed to let the experience sink in and does not have to share verbally directly.

6.9 Obliging people can bear much

Description

"You recognize the coping mode Compliant Surrenderer (also called Adjuster or Pleaser), you are primarily focused on what is good for others and less or not at all on what is good for you.

"You indicate that you do not have time or do not make time to dwell on yourself, to dwell on what you need, on the needs of your Vulnerable Child.

"On your needs as a Healthy Adult. Apparently there are other things that are more important or that you make more important.

"Let us dwell on what demands your attention on an average weekday. What keeps you so busy?

"Would you like to come and stand? For everything you name, I give you an object from the materials cabinet. The idea is that you hold it. You are not allowed to put the objects down, you keep holding everything, or clasp it under your arm, or as far as I am concerned you can put it on your head, as long as you don't put it down.

"Which day do we take? For example, yesterday.

"Okay, what time did you get up yesterday? What was the first thing you started doing?

I went downstairs to make breakfast for my husband and children.
I woke them up.
I prepared sandwiches for the lunch boxes.
I stripped the beds.
I put the bed clothes in the washing machine.
I called my mother-in-law, she is not so well.
I called the dentist to make an appointment for my daughter.
And so on."

After each activity/task described by the client, he is given an object by the therapist. Consider different materials, such as balls, hoops, pawns, blocks, sticks, tennis rackets, weights, and yoga mats. The therapist varies the weight and size of the object. When the client talks about an activity/task, it is often audible and/or visible whether it was a big or small strain on him.

"Here you have a heavy ball, it sounds as if calling your mother-in-law was quite a strain on you." For making the dentist appointment, a light bag of seeds may be more appropriate.

In between, the therapist asks if the client has already done something for himself on this day, or he asks if there was something that was pleasant or of value to the client himself (directly or indirectly). We may decide that an object can be removed or replaced by another object.

We continue in this way until the client has named his activities for the whole day (until bedtime) or until the client can no longer hold objects indicating this or drops objects.

In between, the therapist stops the client to consider the amount of materials he is holding and how this is experienced. "Can you carry it all well or is it heavy, does your body feel okay under the ballast you are carrying or is something starting to bother you?"

If there is a mirror in the room, you can ask the client to take a look in the mirror to see what it looks like. "Does this more or less picture what you do in a day? And does this include anything in terms of relaxation? Cup of tea, inga walk, reading a book, something like that?"

The therapist asks the client if it is okay for him to take a picture with the client's phone, so that the client can see what it looks like and to remind himself to ask the Healthy Adult: Is this how I want it? Is this right for me?

AIM

- Understanding patterns that prevent the Healthy Adult side from being strengthened.
- Increasing insight by experiencing (seeing and feeling).
- Onset of behavior change: Understanding what one can do to take better care of oneself.
- Taking care of one's own needs.

Connection to healthy ego functions

- Personality integration and the formation of a self-image.
- Contact with one's own emotions/needs and those of others.
- Healthy internal dialogue.

Materials

Many different sports and play materials: Different shapes and sizes of balls, hoops, pawns, blocks, sticks, tennis rackets, weights, yoga mats, and so on.

Group/pair/individual

- Group.
- Subgroups/twos or threes.
- Individually in the group.
- Individually.

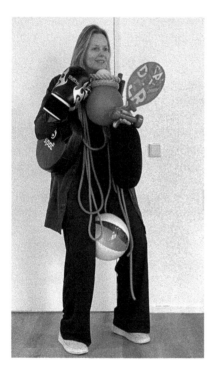

Further details

Through this working method, the client gains insight into coping modes, how powerfully they are often present and cause the client to not take good care of himself.

In terms of therapeutic attitude, the therapist may choose to be supportive and to encourage the client to take good care of himself, to indicate boundaries.

The therapist may also be a bit more confrontational, provocative, and encourage the client to persevere, to endure discomfort. The therapist can give tips on how the client can ensure that the materials do not fall out of his hands, even when the therapist sees that this causes physical discomfort. This is to encourage the client to indicate his own limit. When he does this, fully validate it.

When you choose to make the discomfort palpable from a therapeutic point of view, you can indicate materials that are difficult to hold because they are large and/or heavy, such as a large physio ball or a chair.

If working in a group and several group members recognize the Compliant Surrenderer mode, this working method can be performed simultaneously. For example, the three clients who recognize this stand up, the other group members hand out the materials.

EVALUATION

- We have got a picture of what your day looks like. Pretty impressive how many balls you keep in the air. What's that like for you?
- Almost everything was focused on others; there was hardly anything you did just for yourself. You hardly seemed to dwell on your own needs during the day. Do you recognize that?
- Which mode is mostly active during the day? Which protector mode? Which parent mode?
- Did you notice them during the working method?
- Would you like to keep it this way or would you like it to be different? Would you as a Healthy Adult like to keep it this way or is it important that something changes in this?
- Can you look at the picture every morning for the next week, holding all that stuff and ask yourself, "Do I want to do it this way today or do I make different choices?" I'd love to hear next time how this went.

6.10 Yes and no

Description

"In this working method, we will play with opposing interests, being able to feel your power and express yourself.

"Stand opposite each other as a pair with a few meters between you.

"You bounce one ball at each other. When bouncing, one says 'yes' and the other says 'no.' The harder you bounce, the louder you say 'yes' or 'no.' The softer you bounce, the softer you say 'yes' or 'no'. Play with your voice. Agree on who says what.

"Alternate between 'yes' and 'no.'"

The therapist makes the clients observe differences in themselves (including in the use of force and volume) with both words and keeps inviting the clients to play with the use of voice and bouncing hard.

When working individually, the therapist can be an example of how it can be done. In a group, you can do this working method with pairs where experiences are shared all the time. If possible, you can also switch partners and do it again. Are there differences with whom you do it?

Finally, choose the word that suits you best. It can be the same word as the other person's.

AIM

- Self-expression, expressing oneself both physically and verbally.
- Connecting with the Healthy Adult side.
- Understanding schemas/(coping) modes and needs.
- Gaining corrective experiences.

Connection to healthy ego functions

- Personality integration and the formation of a self-image.
- Contact with one's own emotions/needs and those of others.
- Seeking enjoyment and fulfillment in a mature manner.

Materials

One (properly) bouncing ball per pair.

Group/pair/individual

- Subgroups of pairs.
- Individually.

Further details

In this working method, clients can practice nuanced appropriate emotional expression, both physical and verbal. It can be a playful way in which much interaction takes place, but where clients can also express themselves in contact with someone else from the Healthy Adult side.

Clients can gain insight into schemas/(coping) modes and needs by paying attention to how they do the exercise. They can gain corrective experiences from the Healthy Adult and validate this through the experience.

Frequently, a client throws the ball first and speaks/calls only afterward. The therapist then invites him to say/call "yes" and "no" while bouncing the ball. The therapist also asks after the perceived difference.

Sometimes it is difficult for a somewhat inhibited client to do this exercise. You can then first practice imitating each other by bouncing the ball in equal volume and equal force. This can also be done in opposite ways: one hard and the other softly. Then the therapist can invite the client to play with it.

This working method can give the client great energy and pleasure from the Healthy Adult or from the Happy Child, but there are also clients who may find it intimidating and end up in coping modes. The therapist then gives attention to both experiences.

EVALUATION

- What is it like to vary your voice and power while bouncing the ball?
- What do you like in this and what is difficult?
- Do you respond to the other person or do you always do it your own way, or does it alternate?
- Which suits you best, "yes" or "no"? Did you expect that? Do you recognize yourself in what you are most comfortable with? Is that new?
- What is it like for you to do something opposite to what the other person does? What is it like for the other person to do something opposite to what you do? How do you respond to this?
- Does it evoke memories, recognition?
- What modes/schemas do you encounter?
- What do you need to get into the Healthy Adult/Happy Child mode?

6.11 Children's party

Description

"We are going to work with children's games. These are old games reminiscent of the first game you play as a very small child with your caregiver, such as peekaboo, catch me if you can, Annamaria Cuckoo, duck, duck, goose, goose, play tag, and hide-and-seek.

We will explore different games and see if you can connect with the Happy Child or if there are barriers. In any case, try to open yourself up to the experience of playing with others."

AIM

- Experiencing the Happy Child.
- Examining barriers in experiencing fun in play.

Connection to healthy ego functions

- Healthy emotion regulation.

Materials

Large room. Tag or hide-and-seek can be played outside.

Group/pair/individual

- Group.

Further details

Sometimes encouragement is needed, but in a group there are always people who spontaneously suggest these forms of play. The therapist always accepts other ideas from the group, if appropriate.

Sometimes, grief comes up because one missed this experience in the past. Sometimes, another mode comes up, such as the Punishing Parent.

EVALUATION

- What happened to you in your game?
- Did you have contact with others?
- How did the Happy Child mode feel to you (emotion, energy, laughter, etc.)?
- Did other things come up?
- Did you feel any obstacles?

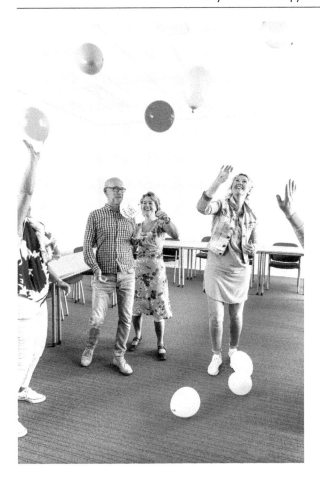

6.12 Hitting a bat with restriction

Description

"It can be nice to use all the strength you have, but this includes restrictions."

Place a mat on the floor. Holding the ball, the therapist stands on one side of the mat and the client with the bat on the other side, facing each other. The client has the bat above his head and stands with feet slightly apart. The therapist throws the ball with an arc, the client hits the ball on the mat with the bat with all his strength.

The ball must land on the mat, this is the restriction. Any ball hit outside the mat must then land on the mat with a control hit before the client is allowed to hit again as hard as possible.

During the working method, the therapist repeats the instructions: aim at the mat, watch your way of striking. The therapist protects himself.

After five hits, the therapist asks, "How much force did you use? 100% is maximum." The therapist tries to find out what inhibits the client when he does not make 100%. Then the therapist and client together look for a way to try and reach 100%.

AIM

- Understanding one's own pattern in using or not using force.
- Experiencing restriction.
- Understanding schemas/(coping) modes.
- Experiencing and experimenting with self-empowerment from the Healthy Adult side.

Connection to healthy ego functions

- Personality integration and the formation of a self-image.
- Healthy emotion regulation.
- Seeking enjoyment and fulfillment in a mature manner.

Materials

One (small) thick mat, one baseball bat, one light ball the size of a hand or soccer ball. For groups, use several balls.

Group/pair/individual

- Individually in the group.
- Individually.

Further details

In this working method, the client is invited to experience in a safe environment what it is like to use his strength 100%. By dwelling on what happens in the working method, the client can also gain insight into what inhibits him from using force or what restriction by the mat and the situation does to him. One can experience that appropriate restriction can be helpful in using force, especially when inhibition or boundlessness is involved. What is evoked often has to do with schemas/(coping) modes. From the Healthy Adult the client can experiment with force and discover what is needed to do so.

The therapist encourages and validates the force used by the client. The client may experience hitting as a release of anger. Explore together what is experienced and what it means to use force.

The restriction allows an inhibited client room to experiment with force. It gives direction and safety to an uninhibited client. The therapist is mindful that the client may be "too quick" to say he is using his strength 100%.

This working method can be done in a group. Everyone then takes turns hitting, say, ten times. In this case, use several balls. Group members collect the balls that have been hit.

Seeing group members during the exercise can evoke much. Group members may feel encouraged to try it themselves but may also feel fear using (all of) their own strength or become anxious at seeing the force used by someone else.

Take time to place the working method in the present and get a clear picture of the underlying story.

EVALUATION

- What is it like to use (all your) strength?
- What percentage of your strength did you use?
- What schema(s) and (coping) modes do you recognize?
- How can you use all/more of the Healthy Adult strength?
- What is it like to see others doing this exercise? What does it evoke in you?
- Which part of what has been evoked belongs to your past? How is this for you in the present?

6.13 Walking across an inverted bench

Description

"An inverted gymnastics bench with the balance beam facing up is in the room.

"The idea is to walk with full attention from one side to the other the way you always walk, and be aware of and focus on what can be observed while walking. This is a metaphor of life.

"Walk from one side of the beam to the other to get used to it.

"Walk across the bench one more time, mindfully, step by step, and observe what body signals and thoughts you encounter along the way. How do you deal with them?

"Walk across the bench and stop the moment you feel imbalance (cannot 'walk in an ordinary way'). Start walking again when you are balanced. If necessary, step off the beam for a moment, then step back on and continue walking.

"We are going to do this quite a few times."

AIM

- Focus on and awareness of body signals, thoughts, and movement.
- Becoming aware of schemas/(coping) modes.
- Acting from the Healthy Adult side.

Connection to healthy ego functions

- Personality integration and the formation of a self-image.
- Contact with one's own emotions/needs and those of others.
- Healthy internal dialogue.

Materials

Balance beam under gymnastics bench.

Group/pair/individual

- Group.
- Subgroups/twos or threes.
- Individually in the group.

Further details

This working method involves making the client aware of what he perceives (body signals, thoughts, and how he moves) and paying attention to it, dwelling on it rather than passing it by. From this awareness, the exercise continues. Here, the therapist asks the client to connect to daily life, where schemas/(coping) modes may come into view. By doing the exercise several times, the client can learn to tap into their own Healthy Adult side in order to achieve corrective experiences and make the transfer to daily life.

Sometimes, a client walks quickly across the bench with a purpose (end of bench) and insufficiently observes what happens along the way. The therapist then asks the client to slow down or stop and pay attention to what he encounters along the way. Only then does the client move on.

Clients may feel looked at in a group, are afraid to fail (e.g., the Punishing Parent is triggered). The therapist then appeals to the Healthy Adult by indicating that the client can ask for some help.

Clients are often amazed that there is so much to experience along the way. They frequently remark that they find much more peace in walking and are actually more balanced as a result.

The therapist then tries to make a transfer to life outside of therapy.

EVALUATION

- After the first time: What did you encounter along the way, such as body signals and thoughts, and how did you deal with them?
- How do you put your feet on the bench? Do you walk in the same way you walk on the floor?
- What is it like to stop for a moment at imbalance and only then continue?
- Do you recognize the way you walk across this bench compared to how you experience life?
- If so, in what way?
- Do you recognize schemas/(coping) modes in how you did the working method?
- How do you recognize these?
- How can you walk across the bench from the Healthy Adult side?

6.14 My Healthy Adult Attitude

Description

"Examine how you are sitting in your chair right now. Try not to change anything for the moment. Observe yourself: Are you sitting straight, slightly slumped, does your back make contact with the backrest, are your shoulders pulled up, have you relaxed them, how are your feet positioned, where do they make contact with the surface? Look at your legs: What is the position of your legs, lower legs in relation to your upper legs, how do you hold your arms, your hands, what do you notice in terms of muscle tension? What do you notice about your facial expressions? What do you notice about your breathing? And so on.

"Which mode is active right now? Your Healthy Adult side, one of your guardians, one of your parent modes, your Vulnerable Child mode?

"In case you don't know this very well, try magnifying your posture a little, it may give you more information."

In the group there is an exchange of what mode was noticed, clients show what posture fits with this, and something might be said about what is noticed about body signals (inside) in this. The therapist invites group members to react to each other. They will recognize certain aspects of an attitude from earlier moments in the therapy.

"Now you may 'shake loose' your limbs in a circle or walking around the room, 'shake out,' stretch, spin around, stamp, jump."

This as mode regulation; physically releasing the old mode. The above directions can stimulate the Free Child mode.

"Next, we will look for an attitude which fits the Healthy Adult side or which can help encourage it. For those who have noticed the Healthy Adult side in themselves during a previous exercise, the attitude may be the same, but it is also quite possible that you will notice differences.

"What can you do physically (posture, facial expressions, muscle tension/ relaxation, breathing, etc.) to more fully engage your Healthy Adult side? You can sit down or stand, whatever is comfortable for you and best suited to activating your Healthy Adult side at this moment.

"First, turn your attention to your breathing. Follow your inhalation and exhalation, feel the movement of your breath. If it feels okay to you, try extending your exhalation a little. Move your attention to your face. What do you notice about your forehead, eyebrows, eyes, around your nose, lips, jaws, tongue? If you want to change something, for example, if you have noticed tension and would prefer to release it a little more, do so. Find out to what extent it works. Go with your attention to your shoulders, neck, and back. Go with your attention to your hands. And so on.

"If I have skipped a body part or muscle in which it does feel important to change something, feel free to go ahead.

"What feels to you like a Healthy Adult attitude or one in which you easily activate your Healthy Adult side? Explore this; try a few things."

AIM

- Mode regulation to Healthy Adult using body awareness and bodily changes.
- Exploring the Healthy Adult.
- Giving and receiving feedback.
- Recognizing modes.

Connection to healthy ego functions

- Healthy emotion regulation.

Materials

Chairs or seating blocks, cushions.

Group/pair/individual

- Group.
- Subgroups/twos or threes.
- Individually.

Further details

It is important to consider that the Healthy Adult is not necessarily active when you have a calm and relaxed posture. For example, the Healthy Adult can also be angry. Then, something very different is happening in the body and the posture is probably different from the posture you found appropriate for the Healthy Adult side in the working method.

The working method works well for some as mode regulation. Others may be better off going for a walk or a bike ride to do so.

Group peers and the therapist provide feedback on the client's postural and movement image to better recognize the modes.

In this working method, the focus is on posture. Giving attention to the way you move, to walking through the room may be a nice extension.

Another variation is working in pairs. Then the client walks up to the other twice: the first time in a Protector mode, the second time in the Healthy Adult posture. The question to the other person is: What did you see? And which do you think is the Protector side and which is the Healthy Adult side?

EVALUATION

- What do you take away from today?
- How can you make sure you consciously engage your body as a mode regulator?
- What concrete exercise can you think of for yourself to do next week?

6.15 Exploring my space

Description

"Explore in three exercises which literal space suits you.

1. Stand in the room and place a rope tightly around your closed feet.
2. Bound the largest possible space that can be made in the room with ropes; you can also use the walls as boundaries.
3. Bound the most appropriate space in the room for you with ropes."

In the first exercise, the therapist emphasizes the feet together and the rope tight around them.

In the second exercise, the client is invited to really use the maximum space, in which the therapist and materials cannot leave the space and the ropes are around that maximum space.

The therapist invites the client to take time to stand still and always asks about body signals, thoughts, and impulses or actions. A connection can also be made to schemas/(coping) modes.

At the end of the exercises, the client cleans up his own space.

AIM

- Becoming aware of body signals, thoughts, and impulses on the theme of "personal space."
- Becoming aware of autonomy and boundaries.
- Exploring what needs there are from the Healthy Adult.
- Understanding one's own patterns regarding personal space.

Connection to healthy ego functions

- Personality integration and the formation of a self-image.
- Contact with one's own emotions/needs and those of others.
- Seeking enjoyment and fulfillment in a mature manner.

Materials

Various short and long ropes.

Group/pair/individual

- Individually.

Further details

The client explores, recognizes, and acknowledges body signals, thoughts, and impulses that can be observed in various spaces. The client is invited to make connections to situations outside therapy for autonomy and boundaries.

In this way, the client becomes aware of his own space and what this does to his own experience. The client can explore from the Healthy Adult where needs lie, discovering by experience what the most appropriate space is and what is important in it. Transfer to outside therapy is sought.

Exercise 1 often involves negative experiences, but it can also be experienced as pleasant. Exercise 2 involves experiences such as it's too big, I come to nothing. Exercise 3 is all about the Healthy Adult: I can move and am able to go to someone myself, but also keep more distance.

Clients often also create a "door" because others are also welcome. The therapist then emphasizes their own space where no one can enter.

The therapist respects boundaries and therefore does not enter the client's own space, even if the client would like him to.

The therapist also makes the client dwell on figurative space, such as in conversation.

EVALUATION

- 1. What do you perceive in your body? What thoughts arise and what action/impulse does it evoke? Do you recognize this situation/signals from other moments in your life? If so, how, where, when?
- 2. Ditto.
- Do you recognize schemas and modes of yourself in these two previous working methods so far?
- 3. What is important to create an appropriate space for you from the Healthy Adult? What do you perceive in your body? What thoughts and what action/impulse?
- Do you recognize situations in your life where there is an appropriate space?
- If so, how, where, when?

6.16 Modes with material

Description

The therapist explains that the purpose of this working method is to become more aware of and in touch with a particular mode. It can be used with all the different modes, including the Healthy Adult and Happy Child modes.

"Choose an object from the materials available in the body-based therapy room that symbolizes a particular mode for you. Anything goes, from very small to very large, light or heavy. Hold it, look at it, move through the space with it, make contact with it." The client tells about his choice and what happened. The mode is thus introduced to the group.

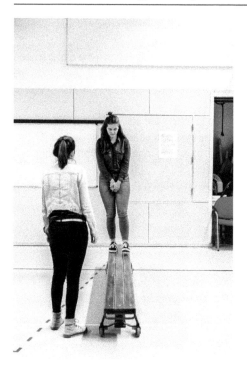

AIM

- Becoming aware of and in touch with a particular mode.
- Self-expression.

Connection to healthy ego functions

- Personality integration and the formation of a self-image.
- Healthy emotion regulation.
- Getting in touch with one's own feelings and needs.

Materials

All sorts of things, including "unusual" objects that are in use in the body-based therapy room. Diversity in size, weight, shape, color, hard/soft, and so on.

Group/pair/individual

- Group.
- Subgroups/twos or threes.

Further details

For some clients, it may be a problem to work with symbolism when they think too literally. The therapist then first engages in conversation, focusing on how a mode may feel to the client. In this, leads can be sought in the way of experience.

EVALUATION

- What did the symbol and moving with it teach you?
- Were there any new insights or recognition with your experience with this mode?
- How can you take this into your life? What are good reminders to hold on to this?

6.17 Fussbudget

Description

This activity is about expressing one's own feelings and needs within healthy frameworks.

"We have one basketball for the two of us, with which we are going to throw over to each other with one bounce on the floor. Try to do this symmetrically, with both legs side by side, applying equal force with both arms. You can also try to bounce the ball toward the ceiling."

With the encouragement to do it as hard as possible, this may be about expressing anger through force.

The therapist indicates: "inhale with the ball overhead, exhale when throwing the ball. If this works for the client as an emotional release, keep repeating this several times without going directly into conversation."

After this variation, a switch may be made to an intervention where explosive power makes room for relaxed and precise movement. To do this, lay down a hoop.

"There is one hoop between us. Again we throw the ball over to each other with one bounce, but the intention is for the ball to bounce into the hoop."

When this feels under control, "In how many hoops do you think we can bounce the ball?" The therapist can then invite the clients to do the same with two hoops, that is, two bounces. Ditto for three and four hoops.

Try everything to check if expectations come true.

AIM

- Expressing anger within frameworks.
- Getting in touch with one's own needs and boundaries.
- Indicating boundaries.
- Tolerating discomfort or relativizing when failing to meet one's own performance goals.

Connection to healthy ego functions

- Healthy emotion regulation.
- Contact with one's own emotions/needs and those of others.

Materials

One basketball per pair, three to four hoops. Preferably a room with a high ceiling (up to 4 m). If the ceiling is low, a softly inflated (basketball) ball might be used so that more force can be applied without the ceiling being restrictive.

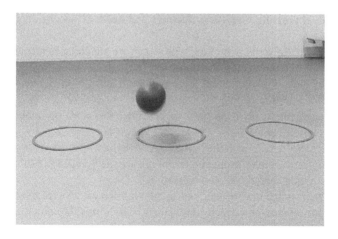

Group/pair/individual

- Subgroups/twos or threes.
- Individually.

Further details

Within the working method, the therapist encourages taking up space, making choices, and gives room for emotions. In the "force" part, the therapist also participates actively and seriously himself. In the "precision" part, he emphasizes playfulness more.

The challenge for the client is to also endure discomfort or to be able to put it into perspective when he fails to meet his own performance goals.

EVALUATION

- On release: What did you like most about this exercise (e.g., applying force, the sound)?
- What muscles did you feel working while throwing the ball? Where is your breathing?
- What difference did you notice between the "force" and "precision" variation?
- How did we manage to bounce the ball over via 1/2/3/4 hoops? Do you recognize this strategy of yours in other situations?
- In what way did you act as a Healthy Adult here?
- Was there a moment when you failed to act/think as a Healthy Adult? How would that come about?
- How can this exercise be linked to the basic need "freedom" (Domain 4: Orientation toward others)?
- Were you triggered into something (a mode) and how did you deal with this?
- Have you experienced space for the Free Child?

6.18 Sparring together

Description

This working method addresses the basic need for autonomy and is about connecting with the other person while giving and receiving force.

"We hold a stick horizontally between us with both hands. Then, one of us starts pushing and the other one pushes back, but in such a way that we go in the direction of the pusher. So counterforce may be given, but the pushed person will not work the pusher backward. The pushed one can also verbally indicate how much force the other one can give."

The starting point is a wall or a line on the ground, the end point is a wall or a line across the room, about 10 meters away.

Next, the roles are switched, agreeing when breathing and muscles have recovered sufficiently for another round.

AIM

- Trusting each other.
- Recognizing and acknowledging boundaries.
- Understanding one's own patterns (thoughts, feelings, behaviors).
- Becoming aware of body sensations during contact with the other person.

Connection to healthy ego functions

- Healthy emotion regulation.
- Testing reality and assessing situations, conflicts, and relationships.

Materials

One stick (1 m long) per pair. Room (approximately 2 × 10 m) without obstacles.

Group/pair/individual

- Subgroups/twos or threes.
- Individually.

Further details

In this working method, the client learns to trust the other person, which becomes visible by reaching the other side while sparring with force/pushing within each other's boundaries. During the exercise, the client observes what thoughts arise in him and focuses his attention on his body sensations while maintaining contact with the other person.

The therapist encourages from trust and challenges the client to use his own strength.

The therapist is alert to the fact that being pushed away may be perceived as uncomfortable and provides a safe and playful mindset in which both parties maintain a sense of control.

The therapist emphasizes that it is not a competition.

In a group, one can switch sparring partners; this may be someone physically similar (in terms of gender, strength, weight, height) or, on the contrary, someone physically completely different.

The therapist can agree to provide more variation in force which may cause balance disturbances (e.g., by tilting a stick or suddenly increasing force). This can encourage feeling and indicate boundaries.

EVALUATION

- How did you feel about being the pusher?
- How did you feel about being pushed?
- Did you feel that we stayed in touch with each other?
- What do you notice about your body during this exercise? Do you recover at rest?
- What expectations did you have after the instruction of the activity? Were they met?
- In what way did you act as a Healthy Adult here?
- Was there a time when you failed to act/think as a Healthy Adult? How would that come about?
- How can this exercise be linked to the basic need "autonomy" (Domain 2: Impaired autonomy and impaired functioning)?
- Were you triggered into something (modes) and how did you deal with it?

6.19 Tower of Hanoi

Description

This is a puzzle assignment called "the tower of Hanoi." (See also YouTube—Tower of Hanoi 4 Disc Solution in the Fewest Moves.)

There are three mats next to each other, and on one of the mats there is a tower made of four materials from large to small.

The goal is to move the entire tower from the first mat to the third mat. The rules are as follows:

1. Only one of the materials may be moved at a time.
2. Only the top piece of the tower may be moved.
3. Materials can be placed on an empty mat or on a larger piece. Never large on small.

AIM

- Recognizing emotions.
- Practicing self-control strategies.
- Translating rules into correct action, or asking for clarification.

Connection to healthy ego functions

- Personality integration and the formation of a self-image.
- Healthy emotion regulation.
- Healthy internal dialogue.

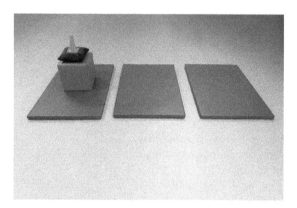

Materials

Three mats or sections and four materials of varying sizes that can be stacked (e.g., pouf, cushion, pylon, tennis ball).

Group/pair/individual

- Individually.

Further details

This working method addresses the client's problem-solving ability to adequately deal with success or failure and associated thoughts, feelings, and behaviors.

The client also learns to recognize signals associated with various emotions that are addressed during the activity and can practice strategies to maintain self-control when stuck in the task (tolerating, acting rather than thinking, asking for tips, standing back, breathing calmly, slowing down).

The client is challenged to translate the enumeration of rules into correct action or ask for clarification.

The therapist emphasizes experimentation (not right/wrong, "just try something"), is patient, gives feedback on emotion regulation. The therapist is strict on adhering to the rules, and asks, for example, during breaking them if the client can list the rules again so that he can see for himself what goes wrong and fix it himself.

Possible additional interventions include:

- deploying more materials; each additional piece doubles the minimum resolution time;
- deploying fewer materials (minimum of three) for a guaranteed successful experience;
- performing with a group which requires consultation.

EVALUATION

- If successful: How does it feel? How did you do it? Are you open to more challenges?
- If failed: How does that feel? What are you inclined to do? Are you open to tips?
- How do you look back on the way you regulated your emotions? Do you recognize that in yourself?
- Have you considered... (asking for help, taking a break, etc.)? Why/why not?
- In what way did you act as a Healthy Adult here?
- Was there a moment when it was not possible to act/think as a Healthy Adult? How was this?
- How can this exercise be linked to the basic need "realistic boundaries" (Domain 3: Weakened boundaries)?
- Were you triggered into something (a specific mode) and how did you deal with it?

6.20 Varying circle sizes

Description

The group stands in a circle facing inward with a gap of about 1 m in between. In turn, each person (the protagonist) can experiment with three self-selected circle diameters and explore what it evokes (body sensations, thoughts, feelings, memories, and so on).

The protagonist can make the diameter as large or as small as possible or something in between. Finally, he sets the circle at the distance most comfortable for him and considers what this means.

The protagonist indicates non-verbally what the intention is, and group members follow. For example: he takes three steps backward and the group imitates. After each change, take time to reflect on it. The protagonist is the first to indicate what has been experienced, then the group members.

AIM

- Dwell on body signals (and thoughts, actions) becoming aware of their meaning.
- Awareness of the influence of place, distance, and proximity to the other person.
- Strengthening self-direction (autonomy).

Connection to healthy ego functions

- Personality integration and the formation of a self-image.
- Contact with one's own emotions/needs and those of others.

Materials

None.

Group/pair/individual

- Group.
- Individually in the group.

Further details

In this working method, the client practices dwelling on body signals (and thoughts, actions) and becomes aware of their meaning. The client may experience the body as a source of information (barometer). In this way, the client becomes aware of the influence of place, distance, and closeness in relation to the other person and from here can better understand himself and recognize schemes/modes. The client practices self-direction (autonomy) in a group and might have a corrective new experience from the Healthy Adult.

In a large group, the therapist can invite some clients to be the protagonist. The protagonist may be specifically invited to experiment from the Healthy Adult.

The therapist invites the protagonist to take more time when things are going fast, looking at what schedules/modes are at play. After each distance change, the protagonist's experience is reviewed; it is still fresh then. At the end of the turn, the protagonist is in a better position to compare. The therapist gives group members the opportunity to share experiences after the protagonist.

The therapist gives the protagonist validation for doing the working method, including the situation in which the protagonist has entered into a new experience from the Healthy Adult.

This working method can evoke fear in a client. Being allowed to watch it once can be helpful. The therapist pauses to consider what this client is experiencing and tries to appeal to the Healthy Adult.

The circle format often contributes to group formation (Perquin, 1987).

EVALUATION

- What was it like to practice autonomy?
- What did you experience in your body and what thoughts came up? Does it have any particular meaning?
- Do you recognize schedules/modes in this working method? How did you deal with them from the Healthy Adult perspective?
- What aspects of the Healthy Adult emerged in this working method?

Questions to group members:

- What was it like to be steered?
- See further evaluation questions above.

6.21 Wobble course

Description

The wobble course is made as follows: The gymnastics bench is hung in the rings. A gymnastics box is placed in front of this as a step. At the end, a thick mat is placed under the bench.

The idea now is to walk across the wobble bench from one side to the other.

If there is no gymnastics equipment, the alternative is to make a course out of chairs or blocks, with one person having to get to the other side through this course without touching the floor. The course is set up in such a way that there is a balance between feasibility and challenge. The next step is to see who wants to start.

Once it is known who wants to start, the working method begins by paying attention to the client's feelings. It is examined at what level the client starts. Here, it is important that the client dares to ask for attention and care for what he is feeling.

AIM

- Emotion regulation, noticing rising tension and taking actions from the Healthy Adult (making adjustments, asking for help, and experiencing support).

- Knowing what coping occurs when tension mounts.
- Rescripting past experiences.

Connection to healthy ego functions

- Healthy emotion regulation.
- Contact with one's own emotions/needs and those of others.
- Healthy internal dialogue.

Materials

Gymnasium, rings, gymnastics box, thick mat, hoops, chairs, or blocks. Sufficient space to make a course.

Group/pair/individual

- Individually in the group.

Further details

The therapist makes sure it stays safe. He mirrors and limits modes when someone is out of touch with his own body signals.

Some clients experience a lot of anxiety in this exercise. If so, as a therapist, make space to meet the underlying need for safety. This can be done by making the course easier or by using support figures. For example, a wobble course can be modified to a more stable course by using hoops lying on the ground.

The therapist pays attention to feeling, but also seeks a balance between talking and acting. Too much talking can be distracting and stagnating.

Through asking about the connection of the experience in the present with the past, an affect bridge can be made to an early experience and the need from that experience can be met (rescripting). Needs that can be satisfied include the need for safety, connection, autonomy, and boundaries.

The group members then come into the role of Ideal Parent. They make the client feel how he wants to be supported. The therapist also asks the group members in the role of Ideal Parent to name the need while walking across the bench. Examples of such phrases might be "You don't have to do it alone; We support you; or We provide stability."

The modes regularly seen in this working method:

- The Self-aggrandizer shows there is no fear, does not dwell on his own body, and is focused on showing achievement. May want to hang the wobble bench higher and higher.

- The Detached Protector is not in touch with body signals, has difficulty perceiving mounting tension, and gives many cognition-based responses.
- The Demanding Parent ignores mounting tension in his body, crosses the bench or course with great anxiety, turns down offers of help or of making things easier, or feels that the exercise has then failed.
- The Vulnerable Child feels very anxious, dependent, or inferior, fears things will go wrong or fail. Emotions are easily felt.
- The Healthy Adult is able to perceive increasing tension in the body. Can take actions to decrease or increase this tension, and in this way takes care of the need for safety, connection, and autonomy.

EVALUATION

- Can you feel how your body is responding?
- What would your body need right now? Does it need something to relax?
- From what mode are you walking across the bench now? What makes you notice this?
- Do you recognize this wobbly, unstable feeling?
- Where in life have you felt this?
- What did you want then? What were your needs?
- How can we meet them now?
- What can we (therapist/group members) do for you now to shape that?
- How does that feel?

6.22 Changing trees

Description

This game can be played both indoors and outdoors. Outdoors, it can actually be done with a group of trees several meters (5–10 m) apart.

In the hall, this game can be played with hoops placed on the ground as markers. As many trees/hoops are used as there are participants, minus one.

All but one participant can stand near a tree/hoop. Everyone standing near a tree can try to switch trees/hoops. You seek contact with a group member and together choose a time to switch. Once you leave your tree/hoop, you are not allowed to return to the spot you came from. The participant who was not near a tree or hoop then tries to get to the abandoned tree/hoop faster to take that spot.

Do this for several rounds and use an evaluation moment to try out new behaviors in the next round. Consider: Daring to step into the game more, daring to stand in the middle, being allowed to fail.

AIM

- Taking risks, choosing and taking action.
- Connecting with the other person.
- Allowing failure; not allowing the critical voice to prevail.

Connection to healthy ego functions

- Contact with one's own emotions/needs and those of others.
- Healthy internal dialogue.
- Seeking enjoyment and fulfillment in a mature manner.

Materials

Hoops.

Group/pair/individual

- Group.

Further details

The therapist takes the clients' condition into account and, if necessary, allows time for breaks.

EVALUATION

- Where was your attention during the activity?
- What did you experience/notice about yourself?
- What thoughts did you have about yourself and the other person?
- In what way did you participate?
- Were you able to stay with yourself and your own choices or did the other person influence your choices as well?

6.23 Live Bowling

Description

Two sides play against each other. As in real bowling, each team has two turns to knock over ten cones. It is not played with a ball, but with a participant on a cart. One participant sits on a cart. A team member stands behind it and pushes his teammate with (a little) speed toward the cones further down the hall. Behind the cones there is a thick mat.

The participant on the cart allows himself to ride toward the cones, his arms and legs staying inboard.

AIM

- Experiencing tension, being able to release fear.
- Giving space to enthusiasm, fun, and spontaneity.

Connection to healthy ego functions

- Personality integration and the formation of a self-image.
- Testing reality and assessing situations, conflicts, and relationships.
- Seeking enjoyment and fulfillment in a mature manner.

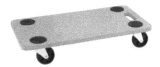

Materials

Ten cones, cart with flexible wheels, thick mat.

Group/pair/individual

- Group.
- Subgroups/twos or threes.

Further details

Participants must be able to sit on a small cart.

EVALUATION

- What did you experience?
- Was there room to express your feelings? Why/why not?

- Where was your attention during the working method?
- Did you manage to have fun in the game?
- Did you choose to sit on the cart yourself or not? (What role did everyone have in the game?)

6.24 Ping-pong plop

Description

This working method involves landing a table tennis ball in a cup.

Initially, this game is played in pairs. Each pair has a cardboard coffee cup with a little water in it. The idea is for the ping-pong ball to land in the cup after bouncing twice on different types of surfaces. The water is meant to make the ball stop bouncing as soon as it is in the cup.

The pair determines which two surfaces are used and whether the ball bounces from top to bottom or vice versa.

AIM

- Collaboration: Consulting, coordination, testing, and adapting.
- Being absorbed in a challenge.
- Experiencing the Happy Child.

Connection to healthy ego functions

- Personality integration and the formation of a self-image.
- Healthy emotion regulation.
- Contact with one's own emotions/needs and those of others.

Materials

Coffee cup or other type of container or jar, table tennis ball, different types of surfaces.

Group/pair/individual

- Subgroups/twos or threes.
- Individually.

Further details

In this working method, the clients learn to become absorbed in a challenge that they know can be done, despite the fact that the chance of failure is greater than of success, but success creates excitement and experience. The idea is that this experience is allowed to prevail.

The game starts in pairs but can very well be expanded to the whole group. Instruction could then be to roll the ping-pong ball via a "marble track" into a cup. in this case, the participants must roll the ping-pong ball from a certain spot in the room along the track into the cup. By working together, they must try to arrive at a construction.

EVALUATION

- What did you experience?
- What determined your thoughts and feelings?
- How did you deal with (negative) thoughts and feelings?
- Were you able to experience pleasure? What caused this?
- How did you deal with yourself, your ideas in relation to the other person?

6.25 Rolling is also fooling around

Description

You play this activity alone or in a (sub)group.

Lay a hoop on the ground at a distance of your choosing (about 4 or 5 meters). The person whose turn it is has three soft tennis balls in his hand and tries in one turn to roll three balls into the hoop one after another.

AIM

- Awareness of thoughts about performance.
- Becoming aware of modes that are triggered.
- Understanding that play is more important than results.

Connection to healthy ego functions

- Personality integration and the formation of a self-image.
- Healthy emotion regulation.
- Healthy internal dialogue.

Materials

Three soft tennis balls, a hoop.

Group/pair/individual

- Subgroups/twos or threes.
- Individually in the group.
- Individually.

Further details

This working method aims deliberately high. It is up to the clients to decide what to do with this aim. Do they go along with it? Can they distance themselves from the aim? Can they playfully deal with what is presented? They can become aware of thoughts arising from the outcome of the performance that will influence the continuation of the working method.

A variation on this form of work is to try to bounce the ball into a hoop three times in a row while playing tennis against the wall. Playing tennis against the wall is not interrupted after a bounce in the hoop but remains dynamic.

EVALUATION

- What did you experience in the working method?
- Were certain modes triggered?
- How did you deal with (negative) thoughts?
- The working method requires a certain performance. What choice(s) did you make in this?
- What have you been guided by?
- How do you look back on that now?

6.26 Counting ten in the jungle

Description

The therapist explains that the mode of the Free Happy Child will be central to the working method. "Free children are absorbed in the moment; they do one thing at a time and feel the pleasure that play brings. In the working method, you can experience being absorbed in the moment. Participating in what we are doing. And possibly experiencing pleasure as well. The excitement of being seen or not seen. The surprise when you do not see anyone but know they are there.

"Undergo, experience, and play. Later, you might be able to look back at moments when you momentarily forget your worries. That you are in the now.

"The game being played is a form of hide-and-seek. The seeker has a fixed area, such as a corner of the room, available to 'search'/see if he sees group members.

"Many different hiding places are created in the remaining parts of the room.

"The seeker stands in the corner of the room facing the wall and says, 'counting 10 in the jungle.' Then, the seeker counts backward from 10 to 0. Having arrived at 0, he turns around and looks to see if he sees group members hidden. If so, he says who he sees sitting where. If it is correct, that person is found. If not, everyone stays put.

"If the seeker sees no one (anymore), he turns his face to the wall again and says, 'counting 9 in the jungle.' Then the seeker counts from 9 to 0. In the meantime, the group members come out from behind/out of their hiding spots, tap the wall near the searcher, say their names, and hide again. Arriving at 0, the seeker turns around and looks to see if he sees group members while staying in the section marked off in the corner.

The above process repeats from counting 9 to 8 in the jungle, to 7, and so on until everyone has been found."

AIM

- Being able to be absorbed in the moment.
- Allowing fun, spontaneity, and optimism.
- Different emotions can coexist.

Connection to healthy ego functions

- Personality integration and the formation of a self-image.
- Contact with one's own emotions/needs and those of others.
- Seeking enjoyment and fulfillment in a mature manner.

Materials

The idea is that hiding places can be created in the room. Think of tables, chairs, rugs, cloths, curtains, cart for mats, table tennis table, and so on.

Group/pair/individual

- Group.

Further details

Participants must be physically able to hide behind something, get up quickly, run a short distance, and then hide again. For the seeker, the effort intensity is lower.

EVALUATION

- Where was your attention during the activity?
- What feelings did you notice in yourself during the activity?
- Did you have any judgments about yourself?
- What were they?
- What did you do with the judgments?
- Did you experience pleasure?
- At what moments?
- How did you notice this about yourself?

6.27 Seeing the Healthy Adult

Description

"We will practice seeing the Healthy Adult and expressing the messages from this side to yourself. We will do this in front of the mirror."

Step 1

"You can stand in front of the mirror and take a look at yourself."

Step 2

"What thoughts do you notice when you see yourself?"

Have the client reflect on what it evokes, what modes the client recognizes in this (often the Critical Parent or the Demanding Parent). The therapist pays attention to body language, posture, movement, whether or not the client looks at himself.

Step 3

"What feeling does it evoke? Is there fear or sadness (Vulnerable Child)? Do you also feel it in your body? Where do you feel it?" As a therapist, you allow space for this feeling. The client can then step away from the mirror.

Step 4

The client is now asked to think of Healthy Adult messages he would like to express to the Vulnerable Child. This is about acknowledging difficulty: "I can see that it's affecting you/that you are sad," as well as about positive messages: "You are good just the way you are, you have beautiful eyes, you are allowed to be there."

Step 5

The client writes these messages on Post-its (each message on a new Post-it).

Step 6

The client starts looking again, saying the Healthy Adult messages aloud one at a time. Then, the client sticks the Post-its on the mirror.

AIM

- Strengthening the Healthy Adult.
- Practicing Healthy Adult messages; coming up with them and expressing them to oneself.

Connection to healthy ego functions

- Healthy emotion regulation.
- Contact with one's own emotions/needs and those of others.

Materials

Mirror, preferably a full length one.

Group/pair/individual

- Individually in the group.
- Individually.

Further details

The therapist encourages, and acknowledges that it is difficult but also stresses the importance of practice.

As a therapist, you reinforce expressing Healthy Adult messages. You ask to repeat them and practice with them. Every small step counts and the therapist emphasizes its importance. The therapist validates the client by acknowledging that the working method may have been exciting but that the client has practiced well. It is important that the client continues to practice this at home so that his Healthy Adult continues to grow.

EVALUATION

During the working method:

- What thoughts do you notice when you see yourself?
- What feelings does it evoke? Do you also feel it in your body? Where do you feel it?
- What Healthy Adult messages would you like to express to the Vulnerable Child?

Afterward:

- Did you manage to come up with supportive and positive messages?
- What was it like to express these to yourself?
- How can you continue to practice this concretely at home?

6.28 The floor is lava

Description

The group is given the task of getting from spot A to B without their feet touching the floor. To do this, the participants have a limited number of materials at their disposal.

Step 1

The group is asked to come to one side of the room. "You are instructed as a group to get to the other side together without touching the floor. The floor is full of lava, so you cannot stand on it. To get to the other side, you can use the materials that are here."

Step 2

The group gets to work. As therapist, you observe the behavior, both verbal and non-verbal. How is the cooperation? Does everyone dare to have input or express his feelings?

Step 3

Evaluation: "What was it like? What did it evoke? What modes did you recognize?"

Step 4

"Now we are going to do this again but this time very deliberately from the Healthy Adult mode. In what way would he carry out the assignment?" Each client may have a different focus, for example, take the lead or wait and see, express feelings, not go first or last.

AIM

- Playing and needing to be inventive.
- Recognizing which modes become active.
- Practicing with the Healthy Adult side.

Connection to healthy ego functions

- Contact with one's own emotions/needs and those of others.

Materials

Various materials, such as seating blocks, chairs, cubes, cushions, and mats.

Group/pair/individual

- Group.

Further details

It is important to be able to work from safety. Should distance and proximity be difficult, the group can make a bridge that participants can walk around and over.

EVALUATION

- How did you experience this exercise?
- What mode was invoked?
- How did you recognize this?
- Was your Healthy Adult active?
- What was it like doing this from the Healthy Adult?

6.29 Overcoming parent mode with the Healthy Adult

Description

Step 1

Demanding Parent or Punishing Parent mode

Consider your Demanding Parent or Punishing Parent. Perhaps it will help you to dwell on a situation where you felt very vulnerable and the Demanding Parent or Punishing Parent mode was present. What does that mode say? What is this mode like?

Step 2

Portraying the Demanding Parent or Punishing Parent mode with materials

The next step is to symbolize the Demanding Parent or Punishing Parent with materials. This can be done with any material present in the room (or in the storage room). The material should symbolize the parent mode. Think about the size of the material, color, shape, etc.

The clients look for objects that symbolize the parent modes. If necessary, you may help the clients with this (e.g., is it big or small, do you have a particular color in mind?). For some, it is one object, for others a whole pile.

Step 3

Reflecting on what the parent mode evokes for the Vulnerable Child

Stand for a moment very consciously in front of the Demanding Parent or Punishing Parent mode and feel what it evokes in you (Vulnerable Child) (e.g., small, alone, anxious). Do you feel the same in your body?

Step 4

Try to get to the feeling of injustice/anger (injustice of the parent mode toward the young Vulnerable Child: "This is no way to treat a child")

As a therapist, you can help a little with this, especially if clients find it difficult to feel this anger/injustice. You might name what it evokes in yourself when you see the parent mode like this.

Step 5

Preparing to deploy anger toward the Parent mode and dismissing it

You discuss with the client beforehand what he would like to do; you may give some examples. The next step is that you also deploy these feelings of anger/injustice toward the parent mode. How to do this is up to you

- What do you want/are you going to say? (stop, get out, I'm done with you)
- What emotion do you want to express? (anger)

- What attitude goes with this? (stop sign, angry facial expression, turning away)
- What movement goes with this? (pushing away/throwing away, pushing over the parent mode)

Step 6

Actually implementing and sending away/pushing away the parent mode (possibly with group members)

"Okay, now we're also going to do what we have just prepared ... go ahead." (You as therapist encourage the client to express his anger.)

Step 7

Applause (by fellow clients and therapist). As therapist, you re-validate the expression of anger; you validate that this may be expressed.

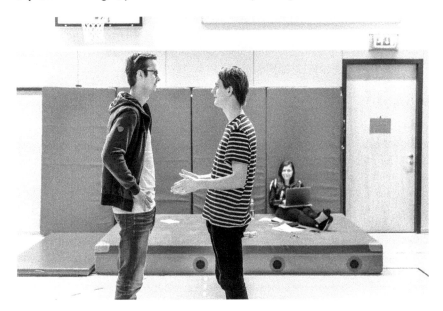

AIM

- Practicing dismissing the Demanding Parent or Punishing Parent mode.
- Using anger constructively (Healthy Adult and Angry Child mode).
- Corrective experience.

Connection to healthy ego functions

- Healthy emotion regulation.
- Contact with one's own emotions/needs and those of others.

Materials

Various materials, different shapes and sizes so that a client can build his own parent modes, also in a size that suits the client.

Group/pair/individual

- Individually in the group.

Further details

Variant 1

In the early stages, clients may collectively construct a Demanding Parent or Punishing Parent mode. Although they can recognize and name this mode in others, they may struggle to recognize it in themselves.

Variant 2

Clients often do not initially feel anger toward the parent mode. In this case, the therapist can use the group to express this anger from the Healthy Adult and assist the client to express it. Or possibly as a therapist or group, express the anger against the parent mode.

Variant 3

Later in the treatment, two clients can stand next to the symbolic parent mode and demonstrate resistance by digging in their heels (e.g., offering resistance in the materials, answering back). Then check in the group, "Would you really cool it or leave?" The exercise concludes when the client has succeeded in creating the change.

See also the exercise with anger overcoming the parent mode, in Reubsaet (2018).

EVALUATION

- What was it like to express your anger/feelings of injustice toward the parent mode?
- What was it like to be able to do this both physically and verbally (pushing materials over, throwing them away, shouting stop, etc.)?
- What did you experience in this?

6.30 Parenting modes pilloried

Description

"We will do an exercise in which we will work with the parent modes and express dissatisfaction/anger toward the parent modes."

Step 1

Write on Post-its some parent mode messages that are recognizable to you.

Step 2

Stick these messages on the newspapers hanging on the line here.

Step 3

We will go through the messages. You can take turns reading a Post-it aloud. Dwell consciously for a moment on the Punishing Parent mode and feel what it evokes in you (Vulnerable Child) (e.g., small, alone, anxious). Do you also feel it in your body? Where do you feel it?

Step 4

Also try to get at the feeling of injustice/anger (injustice of the parent mode toward the young Vulnerable Child: "This is no way to treat a child"). If you find this difficult, imagine this is being said to a group member.

Step 5

We will engage this feeling of anger toward the parent mode by throwing bags of seeds against the parent messages.

Step 6

Actually performing and throwing the bags of seeds toward the messages of one's parent mode (possibly together with group members).

Step 7

Applause (by group members or therapist). Affirmation of anger, validation that this may be expressed.

AIM

- Practicing expressing anger toward the parent mode.
- Using anger constructively (Healthy Adult and Angry Child mode).

Connection to healthy ego functions

- Healthy emotion regulation.
- Contact with one's own emotions/needs and those of others.

Materials

Post-its in various colors, a taut line (such as a magic cord/rope, between two walls or two poles) with newspapers to cover the line, seeds, possibly pawns or hoops to determine the throwing distance.

Group/pair/individual

- Group.

Further details

There may be the risk of clients regarding this working method as a game and somewhat losing the link with the Parent modi messages. So, as therapist it is good to keep pointing this out. Deliberately asking to touch the Post-its.

EVALUATION

- What was it like to express your anger/feelings of injustice toward the parent modes?
- What was it like to be able to do this both physically and verbally (throwing bags of seeds, effect of newspapers falling off the line)?
- What did you experience in your body in the process?

References

Perquin, L. (1987). *Exercises in Pesso-psychotherapy.*

Reubsaet, R.J. (2018). *Schematherapy: Working with phases in clinical practice.* Bohn Stafleu van Loghum (p. 122). http://doi.org/10.1007/978–90-368–2115-5

YouTube – Tower of Hanoi 4 disc solution in the fewest moves. https://youtube/mDA4YclG3uE. Practice it yourself: Google 'Tower of Hanoi online'.

Chapter 7

Evidence for treatment of personality disorders in arts and body-based therapies

Suzanne Haeyen

Summary

This chapter reviews the current scientific evidence for arts or body-based therapies for personality disorders. This concerns an intensive literature review conducted as part of the revised national multidisciplinary guideline (MDR) for the
treatment of personality disorders (2022). The purpose of this guideline revision
was to update and expand the 2008 guideline to include a number of specific
areas of focus, including adolescents and the elderly, antisocial personality disorder, recovery, and patient perspective. In addition to focusing on symptomatic
recovery, the mental health system is increasingly focusing on functional recovery, social recovery, and personal recovery.

The MDR Personality Disorders was developed according to the methodology
of evidence-based guideline development (EBRO) (Burgers & Van Everdingen,
2004; Van Everdingen et al., 2004) by the MDR Personality Disorders working
group, commissioned by the Dutch Psychiatric Association, methodologically
and organizationally supported by the Trimbos Institute.

This present chapter describes conclusions and recommendations for the use
of arts and body-based therapies. A number of people provided feedback during
the writing process. Thanks for this to Ellen Willemsen, Theo Ingenhoven, Piet
Post, Rosi Reubsaet, and Paul Ulrich.

In this chapter, the focus is not specifically on schema therapy in combination
with arts and body-based therapies, but on arts and body-based therapies in a
broad sense. However, the combination with schema therapy will be discussed.

7.1 Introduction

This chapter and the formulated guideline deal with personality disorders as
defined in the DSM-5 (American Psychiatric Association, 2013).

We know of three main groups of personality disorders.

DOI: 10.4324/9781003456988-7

- Cluster A - Strange and eccentric behavior. People with this disorder often lead reclusive lives. Included are the paranoid,schizoid and schizotypal personality disorders;
- Cluster B - Emotional and unpredictable behavior.People with this disorder actually draw attention to themselves. This includes the antisocial, borderline, theatrical and narcissistic personality disorders;and
- Cluster C: Highly anxious and insecure behavior. This includes the avoidant, dependent, and compulsive personality disorders (NVvP, 2021).

A personality disorder is a common psychiatric disorder. People diagnosed with a personality disorder are present at a wide variety of places and times in care. The estimated prevalence of personality disorders as found in studies among the general population ranges from 4 to 15% (Coid et al., 2006; Torgersen et al., 2001; Torgersen, 2014). Differences in the prevalences found may be partly explained by differences in methods and criteria used (Trull et al., 2010). Cluster C personality disorders are the most common, followed by Cluster B and Cluster A personality disorders (Torgersen, 2014). Personality disorders are approximately equally common in men and women (MDR Personality Disorders Revision Working Group, 2022).

In the mental health system, personality disorders are much more frequent. Nearly half of people in the care of the mental health system meet the criteria for a personality disorder, often in addition to one or more symptom disorders (Zimmerman et al., 2008; Friborg et al., 2013, 2014). Among patients in addiction care, the prevalences of personality disorders range from 34 to 72% (Bowden-Jones et al., 2004; Köck & Walter, 2018; Parmar & Kaloiya, 2018). Among people in forensic care, an estimated 36–40% of patients meet the criteria for a personality disorder, and among probationers around 70% (DJI, 2012, 2018).

Personality disorders usually manifest in adolescence or early adulthood. Contrary to popular belief, personality disorders can be reliably diagnosed even before the age of 18. This is of great importance in order to provide appropriate treatment at an early stage (Hutsebaut & Hessels, 2017, Working Group Revised MDR Personality Disorders, 2022).

Arts and body-based therapies are often part of psychotherapeutic or social psychiatric treatment for people with personality disorders. Arts and body-based therapies are offered individually as well as in groups, customized or modular. Arts and body-based therapies are usually part of a treatment program within an outpatient clinic, day clinic, or clinic. In multidisciplinary programs, arts and body-based therapies are usually embedded in a consistent and common therapeutic framework, such as dialectical behavior therapy (DBT), schema-focused therapy (ST), and mentalization-based treatment (MBT), psychodynamic psychotherapy, or in general or generic psychotherapy treatments such as *acceptance and commitment therapy* (ACT) or, for example, *guideline-informed treatment for personality disorders* (GIT-PD). Arts and body-based therapies can also be part of psychotherapeutic treatment with freelance working psychologists and psychotherapists in the context of interdisciplinary collaboration/professional networks.

Arts and body-based therapists, like all other health care disciplines, face the question of evidence for their interventions. What evidence is available for interventions, and how do you determine what is good evidence?

At the national level, multidisciplinary guidelines are developed for the treatment of people in a particular diagnostic category. Such guidelines are often developed by an umbrella institute such as NICE (National Institute for Health and Care Excellence, 2021) or the Federation of Medical Specialists in collaboration with the Trimbos Institute (https://richtlijnendatabase.nl/). Similarly, there is a guideline for the multidisciplinary treatment of personality disorders. A guideline focuses on what is the best care for patients with a personality disorder according to current standards. The guideline covers a whole range of topics, such as the patient and family perspective in treatment, diagnosis and indication, psychotherapeutic interventions, nursing care, and arts and body-based therapies, as well as crisis intervention, pharmacotherapy, cost-effectiveness, and organization of care. A guideline is intended for all healthcare providers involved in the care of patients with personality disorders.

Evidence-based medicine (EBM) refers to the application of the best available research to clinical care, which requires the integration of evidence with clinical expertise and patient values (Evidence-based Medicine Working Group, 1992; Strauss et al., 2011). The object of EBM is to support the patient by contextualizing the evidence with their preferences, concerns, and expectations. This results in a process of shared decision-making in which the patient's values, circumstances, and setting determine the best care. The widespread use of EBM in many healthcare disciplines (e.g., nursing, psychology, arts and body-based therapies, medicine) reflects its broad impact. EBM plays a prominent role in policymaking; research data inform decision-making as a statement of legitimacy (Malterud et al., 2016).

7.2 Arts and body-based therapies in the treatment of personality disorders

The starting question for arriving at the text on arts and body-based therapies in the multidisciplinary guideline was as follows:

What is the effect of arts and body-based therapies as a treatment for personality disorders?

In answering this question, we distinguish between the various arts and body-based therapies if possible.

Definition and purpose of the intervention

Arts therapies (ATs) and body-based therapies include visual art therapy, drama therapy, dance therapy, music therapy, and psychomotor therapy (PMT). Play therapy is also included in the professional group of arts and body-based therapies, but is not considered in this guideline because this form of arts and body-based therapy is not used and has not been studied in personality disorders. Arts and body-based therapies have an experiential, action-oriented, and creative quality and make methodical and goal-oriented use of various working methods, materials, instruments, and attributes, for example, with a lot or little structure. Feelings, thoughts, and behavioral patterns that emerge through design, play, physical, sensory sensation, or movement offer points of departure for awareness and (self) reflection. This occurs through observation and through contact with others about this, impulse and emotion regulation, addressing patterns in feeling, thinking, acting, and practicing new roles and skills (AATA, 2024; Akwa GGz, 2019; BAAT, 2024; FVB, 2024; National Steering Committee on Multidisciplinary Guideline Development in the Mental Health Care, 2008/2022).

7.3 Method: Systematic review by GRADE

7.3.1 What is GRADE?

GRADE (Grading of Recommendations, Assessment, Development, and Evaluations) is a transparent framework for developing and presenting evidence summaries. It also provides a systematic approach in which clinical and practical recommendations can be made (Guyatt et al., 2008a, 2008b , Guyatt et al., 2011a, 2011b, 2011c). GRADE is the most widely used tool for evaluating the quality of evidence and for making recommendations. First, authors determine what the clinical question is and for which population this question is relevant (Guyatt et al., 2011b). A systematic review then includes the best estimate of the effect size of each outcome (e.g., the difference in emotion regulation) (Guyatt et al., 2011a). The authors assess the quality of the evidence for each outcome measure. The quality of the evidence often varies between outcomes (Balshem et al., 2011). A GRADE quality assessment can be applied to a *body of evidence* of different outcomes, usually taking the lowest quality of evidence for outcome measures for decision-making (Guyatt et al., 2013).

GRADE format

The guideline texts answering the starting questions have been prepared according to an established structure based on the GRADE methodology. The starting question for each form of therapy is, "Is treatment X recommended for condition Y?" This question is introduced for each form of therapy with a brief introduction describing the nature of the treatment and its presumed mechanism, supported by literature references. Following this introduction is the summary of the scientific rationale consisting of the discussion of the reviewed research. This leads to a set of conclusions consistent with the starting question. This is followed by the transition from conclusions to recommendations, which was previously called "other considerations." Because the GRADE methodology was used, the procedure was slightly different than in previous guidelines. Four significant factors have been taken into account (Post, 2020):

1. The trade-off between the beneficial and adverse effects of treatment.
2. The degree of certainty about the effect estimates found (uncertain for low-quality evidence, fairly certain for high-quality evidence).
3. The degree of certainty about patients' values and preferences (ideally based on systematically collected information but otherwise at the working group's estimation).
4. The strain that the recommendation of treatment has on available resources.

Assessing evidence

Depending on the factors mentioned, treatment may or may not be recommended. A distinction is made between strong and weak recommendations. With a strong recommendation, treatment X is recommended for all patients with Y. With a weak recommendation, for example, it depends on the preferences of the patient in question. It is important in this section to explicitly state on what basis a treatment is or is not recommended and also why that recommendation should be weak or strong. This is actually the essence of GRADE (striving to explicitly and transparently describe choices). In this guideline working group, a strong recommendation was chosen if the benefits outweigh the harms for almost all patients.

GRADE has four levels of evidence—also known as "certainty in evidence" or "quality of evidence": very low, low, medium, and high (Table 7.1). Evidence from randomized controlled trials (RCTs) starts at high quality and observational data starts at low quality (due to confounding factors). Certainty of evidence is increased or decreased for several reasons, as described below (BMJ, 2021).

GRADE is subjective

There is always a certain amount of subjectivity in any decision. GRADE therefore provides a reproducible and transparent framework for assessing certainty of evidence (Mustafa et al., 2013). Evidence becomes more uncertain with any risk of bias, imprecision, inconsistency, indirectness, and publication bias. The option exists to adjust the level of certainty somewhat up or down. GRADE is

Table 7.1 GRADE uncertainty assessments

Certainty	Meaning	Preferred formulation
STRONG FOR	The benefits outweigh the harms for almost all patients. All or nearly all informed patients are likely to choose this option. *The authors have a lot of confidence that the true effect is similar to the estimated effect.*	We recommend [intervention]
MILD FOR	The advantages outweigh the disadvantages for a majority of patients, but not for all. The majority of informed patients are likely to choose this option. *The authors believe that the true effect is probably close to the estimated effect.*	Consider [intervention], discuss pros and cons
MILD AGAINST	The disadvantages outweigh the benefits for a majority of patients, but not all. The majority of informed patients are unlikely to choose this option. *The true effect might be markedly different from the estimated effect.*	Be cautious about [intervention], discuss pros and cons
STRONG AGAINST	The disadvantages outweigh the benefits for almost all patients. All or nearly all informed patients are unlikely to choose this option. *The true effect is probably markedly different from the estimated effect.*	We do not recommend [intervention]

used to assess the *body of evidence* at the outcome level rather than the study level. The risk of bias can be determined using available tools (Guyatt et al., 2011c). The certainty of a *body of evidence* is highest when there are multiple studies that show consistent outcomes. Evidence is most certain when studies directly compare interventions in the given target population and when the most important outcomes for decision-making are reported. Certainty can be rated down if the patients studied are different from those for whom the recommendation applies. More information on GRADE can be found in the GRADE guideline series (such as Guyatt et al., 2011).

A guideline text not only includes the result of a systematic literature review but also includes, for a large part, the patient and family perspective in relation to treatment, diagnosis and needs assessment, psychotherapeutic interventions, nursing care, and arts and body-based therapies, crisis intervention, pharmacotherapy, cost effectiveness, and the organization of care. A guideline presents the state-of-the-art evidence as well as all other relevant aspects that should be taken into account in making clinical choices in treatment.

Table 7.2 PICO for search (Patient group, Interventions, Control, Outcomes)

P	People with a DSM classification for a personality disorder
I	One of the arts and body-based therapies interventions listed below: · Visual art therapy · Drama therapy/psychodrama · Dance/movement therapy · Music therapy · Psychomotor therapy (PMT)
C	· Standard treatment or Treatment as usual (TAU). · Waiting list condition or no treatment · Comparison with one or more other treatment(s)*
O	Crucial: · Quality of life · Positive mental/psychic health Important: · Emotional functioning · Suffering and dysfunction · Symptomatic recovery · Social recovery · Failure (surrogate for adverse events)

*No conclusions can be drawn from this comparison that concern effectiveness of *individual* treatment

Search strategy/review protocol

To answer the above starting question, a search was conducted in September 2019 for systematic reviews, meta-analyses, and randomized controlled trials on the treatment of personality disorders within Medline, Embase, PsycInfo, and the Cochrane database of Systematic Reviews (Table 7.2 and 7.3). The search strategy used can be requested from the editor. An additional search was also conducted in June 2020 with search terms focused on arts and body-based therapies.

Process of conclusions and recommendations

The guideline working group discussed each step of the described process. The conclusions and recommendations as formulated in this chapter represent the outcome of this discussion and relate to the opinion of the working group.

Table 7.3 Relevant outcome measures

Outcome measure protocol	Outcome measure study
Quality of life/positive mental/ psychic health	· Well-being and psychological flexibility
Emotional functioning	· General psychological functioning (emotional functioning subscale) · Emotional states of mind (modes)
Symptomatic recovery	· General psychological complaints (social functioning, emotional functioning, social role)
Social recovery	· Subscale social functioning

7.4 Results

Scientific foundation

Included and excluded studies

The first broad search yielded 1874 results, from which 27 articles were selected for full-text viewing. The additional search yielded 23 articles. The majority of all articles found ($n = 38$) were excluded because the study did not exclusively involve patients with personality disorders and this group was not analyzed separately. In addition, it appeared that several studies lacked a control group or had no effect data available for some other reason ($n = 8$). Also, no clinically relevant outcome was reported ($n = 1$). Finally, one RCT and two pilot studies of participants in RCTs on arts and body-based therapies were included to answer the baseline question (Table 7.4). The search strategy and selection procedure are described in the review protocol.

In a recent RCT (Haeyen et al., 2018a, 2018b) on the effect of **(visual) art therapy,** 57 patients with cluster B/C personality disorder were examined. The patients were randomized between a group with a weekly session of imagery therapy (90 minutes, 10 weeks) and a waiting list group. After a five-week follow-up, the primary outcome of improved psychological flexibility (decrease in experiential avoidance, more acceptance of unpleasant inner experiences) was measured using the Acceptance and Action Questionnaire-II. Effect sizes were calculated with the change in Cohen's d, which indicates the effect over time. The AAQ-II-total showed a small effect ($\Delta d = 0.11$, d posttest -0.44 [-0.97, 08] 95% CI), while large effects were found on mental functioning measured with the Outcome Questionnaire 45 (OQ45—total score/decrease symptoms: $\Delta d = -1.67$, d posttest -1.24 [-1.81, -0.68] 95% CI). The experimental group showed a decrease in personality disorder pathology, specifically in the degree of presence of maladaptive schema modes measured with the Schema Mode Inventory (SMI). There was a decrease in impulsivity *($\Delta d = -1.66$, d* posttest -088 [-1.42, -0.33] 95% CI), detachment *($\Delta d =- 1.31$, d* posttest -1.04 [-1.59,

Table 7.4 Characteristics of the included studies

Study	n	Country	Duration of therapy	Follow-up measurement	Mean age (SD)	Female (%)	Measured outcomes
Haeyen (2018 a, 2018b)	57	Netherlands	10 weeks (group sessions)	5 weeks	37.48 (SD = 10.45)	7025%	Psychological flexibility General psychological functioning (social/ emotional and in measure social role) Emotional modes
Van den Broek (2011)	10	Netherlands	4 individual sessions — (out of 3 months of treatment)		40.7 (SD = 7.4)	0	Emotional modes; healthy modes
Keulen -de Vos (2017)	9	Netherlands	5 individual sessions —		38.2 (SD = 7.6)	0	Emotional modes: vulnerability

Source: Haeyen et al. (2018a, 2018b).

–0.48] 95% CI), vulnerability $\Delta d = -1.24$, d posttest –0.64 [–1.18, –0.11] 95% CI), and punitive behavior ($\Delta d = -1.29$, d posttest –0.88 [–1.43, –0.34) 95% CI). Scores on the adaptive schema modes such as experiencing pleasant feelings, spontaneity (Happy Child mode) ($\Delta d = 1.55$, d posttest 1.19 [0.63, 1.75] 95% CI), and self-regulation (Healthy Adult) ($\Delta d = 1.60$, d posttest 1.38 [0.80, 1.96] 95%CI) showed an increase. Art therapy not only reduced personality disorder pathology and maladaptive modes but also helped patients develop adaptive positive modes, indicating better positive mental/psychic health and self-regulation.

In a second study reporting on the same RCT (Haeyen et al., 2018b), additional data were also analyzed to examine whether art therapy was effective on increases in mental/psychic well-being (positive mental health) or decreases in psychological symptoms (mental illness), or both. Five questionnaires (AAQ-II, Dutch Mental Health Continuum-Short Form [MHCSF], Mindful Attention Awareness Scale [MAAS], SMI-II adaptive and maladaptive scales, and two subscales of the OQ45) were divided into two domains: positive mental health and mental illness to compare the results on these two domains of effect. The effect of art therapy on indicators of positive mental health ranged between $\Delta d = 0.52$ on the MHC-SF (social well-being), F(2, 30) = 28.05, $p < 0.01$, and $\Delta d = 1.46$ on the AAQ-II, F(2, 30) = 60.00, $p < 0.01$. The results also showed large effect sizes for outcome measures for mental illness ($\Delta d = -0.82$ on the OQ45 Interpersonal Relationships scale, F = [2, 30] = 27.83, $p < 0.01$ and $\Delta d = -1.32$ for the SMI maladaptive modes, F[2, 30] = 109.85, $p < -0.32$). The mean effect on indicators of positive mental health was $\Delta d = 1.06$ and on indicators of mental illness $\Delta d = -1.09$. Art therapy was found to be not only a generic intervention to improve well-being and quality of life, but also a specific therapy to reduce specific symptoms of mental illness (Table 7.5).

Van den Broek et al. (2011)

A pilot RCT (Van den Broek et al., 2011) investigated the effectiveness of **visual art, drama, and body-based or psychomotor therapy** in evoking different emotional schema modes in forensic patients. This involved ten male patients with Cluster B personality disorders randomly assigned in a clinical trial of schema-focused therapy (SFT) versus "normal" forensic treatment (treatment as usual; TAU). The effects of vocational therapy versus verbal psychotherapy and of SFT versus TAU on emotional modes were examined. Patients showed significantly more healthy emotional modes in arts and body-based therapies ($d = 0.80$) than in verbal psychotherapy ($T = 7.00$; $p < 0.05$). Visual art, drama and body-based/psychomotor therapy and SFT were thus found to have the potential to evoke healthy emotional expressions in forensic patients with personality disorders (Table 7.5).

Keulen-de Vos et al. (2017)

Another pilot study investigated the evocation of emotions through **drama therapy** in male offenders with Cluster B personality disorder (Keulen-de Vos et al., 2017). Nine male patients in a forensic psychiatric clinic followed a protocol of five drama therapy sessions. Emotions were tested with the Mode Observation Scale (MOS), before and after each session. The participants showed significantly more emotional vulnerability in all experimental intervention sessions. After Session 2, the Vulnerable Child mode was seen more often ($M = 1.88$, $SE = 0.28$) compared to baseline scores ($M = 1.0$, $SE = 0.007$, $t[7] = -3.13$, $p = 0.017$, $d = 1.18$). This also appeared to be the case in Session 3 ($M = 2.06$, $SE = 0.30$ after the session compared to $M = 1.09$, $SE = 0.06$ before the session, $t[7] = 3.26$, $p = 0.014$, $d = 1.23$). In contrast, patients did not show more anger after the session focused on anger ($M = 1.17$, $SE = 0.12$) compared to before the session ($M = 1.00$, $SE = 0.008$, $t[8] = 1.41$, $p = 0.19$, $d = 0.50$). The results show that drama therapy has potential in evoking emotional vulnerability in forensic patients with Cluster B personality disorder (Table 7.5). However, there are limitations to this study: it does not discuss what is done with the emotions after they are evoked in drama therapy. The purpose of evoking emotional vulnerability in forensic clients remains somewhat unclear.

Conclusions

From evidence to recommendations

QUALITY OF EVIDENCE

The scientific evidence is formed by only one RCT and two pilot RCTs, which can be explained by the still limited research culture in this field.

- The effect sizes of the change in outcomes in the RCT of Haeyen and colleagues (2018a, 2018b) indicate a substantial improvement in the experimental group after the intervention. The imprecision due to the limited size of the study ($n = 57$) is contradicted by an adequate *sample size calculation*. The dropout analysis shows that there was no bias due to dropout. Due to some methodological limitations (allocation blinding), we are cautious about the robustness of the scientific evidence.
- The pilot RCTs by Van den Broek and colleagues (2011) and Keulen-de Vos and colleagues (2017) are very small in size ($n = 10$ and $n = 9$, respectively). This greatly limits the quality of evidence.

Table 7.5 Conclusions

⊕⊕○○ *Outcome measure: Improvement in psychological flexibility, positive mental health, and self-regulation*
There is evidence that visual art therapy has a beneficial effect on patients with personality disorder.#
Haeyen, 2018a/b

#downgraded for risk of bias and for imprecision

⊕⊕○○ *Outcome measure: Reduction in personality pathology and maladaptive functioning (reduction in vulnerability)*
There is evidence that visual art therapy has a beneficial effect on patients with personality disorder.#.
Haeyen, 2018a/b

#downgraded *for risk of bias and for* imprecision

⊕○○○ *Outcome measure: Evoking emotions*
It is uncertain, but there are indications that patients with Cluster B personality disorder show more emotional vulnerability in drama therapy.#
Van den Broek, 2011, Keulen-de Vos, 2017

#downgraded for imprecision (2x) and for risk of bias

OTHER EVIDENCE FOR THE EFFECT OF ARTS AND BODY-BASED THERAPIES IN PERSONALITY DISORDERS

There are also other indications that arts and body-based therapies are effective in the treatment of personality disorders. These indications can be found in the relevant studies that were excluded for the scientific evidence in this chapter. Given the limited availability of scientific evidence, they are nevertheless relevant to mention here. They are presented with mainly qualitative descriptions because they serve a different goal than the studies included for scientific substantiation. These include, for example, RCTs in which not the entire population but part of the group studied had a personality disorder, studies with a *pre-post design* or qualitative research. The group of people with a personality disorder was not analyzed separately in these studies, and therefore these studies were excluded as scientific evidence for the guideline. To give an impression of the most clinically relevant studies, they are briefly summarized descriptively below. These studies are potentially relevant because a substantial proportion of the group studied were diagnosed with a personality disorder. The final recommendations should be seen as an outcome of the complete process and as a guideline for daily practice in the treatment of PD patients.

Art therapy

- Karterud and Pedersen (2004) examined the effect of the components of a group-based, short-term day treatment program for personality disorders in 319 patients. Of the patients, 86% had a personality disorder, mostly avoidant personality disorder or borderline personality disorder. The treatment effect was evaluated with the question: How much did you benefit from the following groups during treatment? The benefit of the art therapy was scored significantly higher ($p < 0.001$) than that of all other groups. This score was contrasted with outcomes on the Global Assessment of Functioning (GAF) and the Group Style Instrument (GSI), among others. The art therapy group's score correlated significantly ($p = 0.005$) with the "overall benefit" of the program. Multiple regression analysis also indicated a stronger effect in the art therapy group. The authors mention that patients with personality disorder highly valued art therapy, particularly because of the "as if situation" (Fonagy et al., 2002), which provides a safe method of exploring, expressing, and assigning meaning (mentalizing) to the experiential world through self-objects in the form of artworks.
- In an RCT by Green and colleagues (1987), half of 28 chronic psychiatric *outpatients*, including patients with personality disorder, were randomly assigned to a supportive art therapy group supplementary to TAU, and half received TAU. The results of this study indicate that the patients in the experimental group improved in social functioning, in their attitudes toward themselves, and in their self-confidence.

Drama therapy

- Kipper and Ritchie (2003) conducted a meta-analysis based on 25 experimental studies of psychodrama techniques such as role reversal, doubling, and role-playing with various target groups including patients with personality disorders. Outcome measures of diminishing stress and avoidance, self-esteem, conflict management, reality check, empathy, and positive self-image are mentioned. They concluded that these techniques contribute positively to the development of empathy, getting in touch with one's own world of experience, and being able to see situations in perspective (e.g., distancing).
- In an experimental multiple baseline single-case design ($n = 8$), it was shown that overall, psychological, and social well-being changed positively after participation in the Dramatherapy Self-Esteem Module in women with personality disorder in an outpatient setting. These results indicate the

effectiveness of the DSM and drama therapy and provide directions for follow-up research on the transdiagnostic value of this module (Bodde, 2020).

- Popolo and colleagues (2018) focused on metacognitive interpersonal therapy (MIT) in which role-playing techniques (drama techniques) are used in an intervention for patients with personality disorders ($n = 17$) to gain awareness of their patterns and drives when interacting with others. In this study, medium to large magnitude changes from pre- to post-treatment on emotion dysregulation, well-being, alexithymia, and metacognition were found. It was stated that in group psychotherapy, experiential techniques are useful to practice experiences in a controlled and safe environment and to actually feel these experiences in the body (Dimaggio et al., 2020).

Music therapy

- Schmidt (2002) examined the effects of two months of group music therapy (twice weekly, 90 minutes) in 34 patients with borderline personality disorder (BPD) and 29 patients with "general neurotic/psychosomatic problems" (54% of total number had a diagnosis of BPD). The main descriptive results showed that patients with BPD were satisfied with music therapy after the study, reported better self-perception, felt more able to engage in new contacts, and felt calmer and more relaxed.
- Gold and colleagues (2009, 2013, 2014) showed that music therapy was an effective adjunct in patients with low motivation ($n = 144$, of whom only six had a BPD).
- Research by Gebhardt and colleagues (2014) showed that patients with personality disorders ($n = 34$, 18.8% of $n = 610$) more often applied music to reduce negative thoughts and achieve relaxation than "healthy" subjects.
- Van Alphen and colleagues (2019) investigated in an RCT the effects of musical attention control training (MACT; n = 35) for psychiatric patients with psychotic features, among whom some also had a comorbid personality disorder ($n = 7$). MACT was found to be effective in promoting attention skills.
- A small pilot study ($n = 10$) found that group music therapy in patients with mild intellectual disability (IQ 70-85) with *features* of Cluster B personality disorder was effective in improving emotion regulation and reducing avoidant and passive coping (De Witte, 2014).

Dance and movement therapy

- In a non-randomized parallel trial, Leirvåg and colleagues (2010) compared the treatment effects of psychodynamic group therapy (PGT) and body awareness group therapy (BAGT) as outpatient day treatment for female patients with severe personality disorders ($n = 50$). The patients who followed BAGT showed significantly higher scores in general and interpersonal functioning. They reported greater satisfaction with therapy and the group climate over time.

- A body awareness intervention (basic body awareness therapy; BAT) was investigated in an RCT by Gyllensten and colleagues (2003). This involved psychiatric patients ($n = 77$, of whom only seven [18%] had a personality disorder). BAT showed improvements in psychiatric symptoms, attitudes toward the body and exercise, self-efficacy, sleep, and physical coping.
- The effect of short-term dance and movement therapy on depressive and anxiety symptoms in patients with personality disorder ($n = 20$) was investigated in a pre-post design by Punkanen and colleagues (2014). Measurements before and after therapy sessions showed a significant decrease in depressive symptoms and improved recognition of one's own feelings.
- A systematic review focused on dance movement therapy (DMT) in personality disorders yielded an inclusion of four articles with expert opinions (Kleinlooh et al., 2021). Six overarching themes were found for DMT interventions for personality disorders. self-regulation, interpersonal relationships, integration of self, processing experiences, cognition and expression, and symbolization in movement/dance.
- Results of a meta-analysis based on 33 studies ($n = 1078$) by Koch and colleagues (2014) among patients with a diversity of psychiatric problems suggested that DMT and dance are effective for increasing quality of life and reducing clinical symptoms such as depression and anxiety. Positive effects were also found on increases in subjective well-being, positive mood, affect, and body image.

Body-based/psychomotor therapy

- A pilot study by Zwets and colleagues (2016) examined the effect of psychomotor therapy (PMT) as an adjunct to aggression replacement therapy (ART) in the treatment of aggressive behavior. Most patients in this study ($n = 37$) had a personality disorder (antisocial, narcissistic, and not otherwise specified). Clinically significant improvements were observed on aggressive behavior, social behavior, and self-reported anger, but there were no significant differences in treatment effects on these primary outcomes. A small improvement was found in secondary outcomes such as body awareness during anger and coping behaviors in the experimental group with PMT, compared with the control group.
- A study by Hutchinson and colleagues (1999), a quasi-experimental design with 37 psychiatric patients, 33% of whom had a personality disorder, showed that increasing physical fitness through a structured exercise program (15–20 weeks) can have a beneficial effect on mood, psychological

well-being, self-image, and self-esteem, and leads to reductions in depression, anxiety, and stress.

- Research by Knapen and colleagues (2003a/b, $n = 119$) provided evidence for increases in physical fitness and improvements in self-esteem in psychiatric patients, including those with personality disorders when targeted body-based therapy is applied.

- Comparative, non-randomized research with pre- and post-measurement showed that group therapy focused on body awareness using experiential techniques is more effective than psychodynamic group therapy in reducing problematic functioning in severe personality disorders (Leirvåg et al., 2010).

- A review article by Sanderlin (2001) described a number of studies on the treatment of excessive anger and aggression dysregulation in populations with antisocial personality disorder. These include prisoners, juvenile offenders, and hospitalized adolescents with impulse control problems. Four RCTs showed that aggression regulation training, sometimes combined with relaxation training and social skills training (two RCTs, n could not be ascertained), leads to a significant improvement in aggression regulation. The combination of cognitive therapy and relaxation training was reported to be most effective.

- An elaboration of PMT in personality disorders can be found in Drewes and colleagues (2019). A multicenter RCT is underway to study the effectiveness of schema therapy for older people with personality disorder enriched with PMT arrangements (Van Dijk et al., 2018, 2019).

- Various relaxation methods are used within PMT, such as functional relaxation (Krietsch-Mederer, 1988), progressive relaxation (Jacobson, 1929; Bernstein & Borkovec, 1977), Schulz autogenic training (Lehembre, 2003), and breathing training (Bolhuis & Reynders, 1983; Brooks, 1974). A pilot RCT in borderline personality disorder provided evidence of an effective contribution of mindfulness exercises, which are also used in PMT, but did not take place within that framework in this study (Soler et al., 2016). These methods could be useful for learning to control tension levels and regulate emotions in patients with personality disorders. Several modules have also been developed in practice for aggression and impulse regulation that incorporate PMT working methods (e.g., Kuin, 2005; Roethof & Van der Meijden-van der Kolk, 2000). There is often very little contact on the part of these patients with their own body awareness on account of chronic overstrain and for the patients themselves, increasing tension is not adequately observable. A pilot study with time series design in a mixed group of personality disorders/eating disorders showed that a PMT module "aggression regulation" has a rapid effect on coping with anger in patients who excessively internalize their anger (Boerhout & Van der Weele, 2007).

Contribution to observation, setting treatment indications, and goals

In practice, arts and body-based therapists make an often-valued contribution to observation, for the purpose of diagnosis and setting treatment indications, and goals. Observations by arts and body-based therapists, among others, can be of great importance in confirming a diagnosis of personality disorder and further establishing care needs (Akwa GGz, 2017). To this end, they have also developed some instruments.

- For example, **art therapists** can use the Diagnostic Drawing Series (DDS). This test, developed in the United States, is based on the DSM-5 and uses an objective structural analysis of three drawings (Cohen et al., 1998). The DDS thus contributes to diagnostics. The drawings are scored for structural features. The test must be administered by an art therapist trained in it. Mills (1989) studied a group of 32 patients with borderline personality disorder. The drawings were scored blindly on forty visual characteristics and compared with other diagnostic groups. This revealed a profile with a statistically significant indication of borderline personality disorder drawings with common features. In the tree drawing: disintegration and much use of space (67–99%); in the third drawing (question of feeling): containment, color mixing (not in the first or the second) and abstraction. The survey is large-scale in design and leaves little room for subjective interpretation. The instrument is described in a manual (Mills, 1993). There is a clearly defined control group. The DDS has high inter-rater reliability; of the items, 84.2% were scored accordingly (Cohen's kappa 0.57) (Mills, 1994; Fowler & Ardon, 2002). The DDS offers treatment indications because the test provides a profile of the patient in terms of coping with different appeals (coping with structure, with appeals to expression and with task, motivation, willingness or ability to reflect, content of experience and need to express oneself about it).
- **Drama therapists** sometimes use the Six Part Story Method (6PSM). The 6PSM is a projective technique in which the patient creates a fictional story according to structured instructions from the therapist. Research by Dent-Brown (1999) and Dent-Brown and Wang (2004) shows that the level of pessimism and failure in a patient's story represents the severity of the writer's borderline personality disorder. It is argued that 6PSM is especially important as a form of qualitative feedback to the patient.

Arts and body-based therapies combined with schema therapy

In the practice of treating personality disorders, it can be seen that arts and body-based therapies fit well with the combination of schema therapy and positive psychology (Muste et al., 2010; Claassen & Pol, 2015). Studies use and endorse the combination of arts and body-based therapies and schema therapy (e.g., Van der Broek et al., 2011; Haeyen, 2018). In a qualitative analysis by Brautigam (2013) into the evaluation of a multidisciplinary clinical schema therapy treatment of clients with complex personality problems, arts and body-based therapies emerges as a venue for experiencing positive emotions and practicing adaptive skills (Healthy Adult). The following quote from this study is about this practice with adaptive skills:

> "Yet I have also had a lot of trouble with this, the fear of doing it wrong, of saying the wrong thing, I have experienced that this is not so easy, that you have to let go of control precisely in improvising, and that I too can do that."
>   Alice, about drama therapy

In a year-long study of multidisciplinary clinical schema therapy (including three different arts and body-based therapies) with positive psychological interventions, in clients with complex personality disorders, the mean score of well-being was 1.34 (SD = .67), on a scale of 5, at the start of treatment. A very low score relative to the Dutch population and also lower than the norm group of personality disorders. At follow-up (six months after treatment), these clients scored an average of 2.33 (SD = 1.12). This is still below average relative to the Dutch population, but above average relative to the norm group of personality disorders. A large effect size emerged from this (Franken et al., 2019; Phagoe, 2018; Phagoe et al, 2022; Schaap et al., 2016).

General instructions and indications

In conclusion, the other relevant studies show that arts and body-based therapies can be used, and are often used, for (emotional) contact with difficult-to-reach aspects of the patient's world of experience in order to work on goals such as emotion, stress and tension regulation, identity/self-image, self-expression, mood/anxiety, relaxation, changing patterns and social functioning. Body-based therapy is often offered as an option to improve physical fitness, body image, relaxation or the treatment of aggression and impulse regulation problems. The use of arts and body-based therapies for patients with personality disorder is recommended because they value arts and body-based therapies and experience them as effective (see also *Patient Perspectives*). The above-described effects of arts and body-based therapies also emerge within the various panel discussions held among arts and body-based therapists (Kehr, 2020; Manders, 2020).

Specifically for adolescents and the elderly, despite the fact that there are hardly any studies on the effectiveness of arts and body-based therapies in adolescents or the elderly with personality pathology, in clinical practice one sees added value in the integration of arts and body-based therapies in a multidisciplinary treatment. Therefore, there are no reasons to assume that the recommendations as formulated for adults would not also be applicable to adolescents and the elderly.

It should also be noted that a large number of studies on multidisciplinary treatment programs include one or more forms of arts and body-based therapies. These programs are found to be effective, but here the influence on the found effect of the different treatment components has not been studied separately. For example, Styla (2014) described positive results of treatment programs for personality disorders, among others, in which psychodrama was part of the treatment offered. Van Dijk and colleagues (2019) describe the effect of a group-based schema therapy program enriched with PMT for the elderly. Many more examples could be cited (Bateman & Fonagy, 2009; Laurenssen et al., 2018).

Balance between desired and undesired effects

- There are no known undesirable effects or negative side effects of vocational therapy. It is necessary to mention, however, that certain conditions have to be met like in any psychotherapeutic intervention, such as safety, so that feedback can be processed in a regulated way (e.g., Meekums, 1999). A well-trained arts and psychomotor therapist is aware of the importance of this and will handle this as needed.

Patient perspective

- The majority of patients with personality disorder report that they rate arts and body-based therapies highly and perceive them as effective (among others; Karterud & Pedersen, 2004; Solli et al., 2013). The importance of this is recognized in multidiciplinary collaboration and in independent practice. Arts and body-based therapies are potentially motivating and contribute positively to treatment readiness.
- In a longitudinal study by Haeyen and colleagues (2020) among 528 patients with personality disorder who received art therapy in their treatment focused on personality disorders, these patients reported increasing and reasonable benefit from art therapy at repeated measurement times, particularly in the

areas of emotional and social functioning. The five highest scored goals, as identified by them, highest scored goals were:

1. Expression of emotions.
2. Improved (more stable/positive) self-image.
3. Making your own choices/autonomy.
4. Recognition, understanding, and change of personal patterns of feelings, behaviors, and thoughts.
5. Coping with one's own limitations and/or vulnerability.

The extent of perceived benefit was related to factors such as a judgment-free attitude of the therapist, feeling taken seriously, and experiencing sufficient freedom for expression in addition to sufficient structure offered. Age, gender, and diagnosis did not predict the extent of perceived benefit. It was argued that art therapy provides equal benefit to a broad target group, and thus can be used broadly. Experienced benefit and its increase over time were significantly ($\Delta R^2 = 0.03$, $p < .05$) related to the extent to which patients perceived that they could give meaning to feelings in their artwork.

*   It is usually different for each individual which art or body-based therapy is most indicated. This also depends on the patient's ability/willingness to open up to it, their affinity with the relevant form of art and body-based therapy, and the perceived possibilities within the therapy form in question, rather than on specific diagnostic or personal characteristics. It is therefore important to give shape to this in consultation with the patient so that they can also take and experience control in this.

Side effects perspective

*   Caregivers feel it is important that the (day) clinical use of arts and body-based therapies are preferable to forms of day care/activities in order to effectively use treatment time, so that personal therapeutic goals can be worked on in a focused manner (Kehr, 2020; Manders, 2020).

Professional perspective

*   Arts and body-based therapies are often part of psychotherapeutic or social psychiatric treatment (Akwa GGz, 2017). Day clinical psychotherapy must be conducted by a multidisciplinary team, consisting of at least a (clinical) psychologist and/or psychotherapist, a psychiatrist, sociotherapist(s), and arts and body-based therapist(s). Part-time programs and full-time programs that do not work from the principles of (day) clinical psychotherapy also often include arts and body-based therapies. Arts and body-based therapies are also very well possible in an independent setting within the

framework of interdisciplinary collaboration/professional networks. Thus, arts and body-based therapies are often part of a larger treatment program. This makes it difficult to isolate the specific effect in research (Bateman & Fonagy, 2004). Nevertheless, its value is widely recognized by professionals specializing in the treatment of personality disorders, both nationally (Ingenhoven et al., 2018) and internationally (Bateman & Fonagy, 1999).

- The combination of arts and body-based therapies with state-of-the-art psychotherapeutic treatment methods serves as a fruitful combination in practice, according to clinical experience (Akwa GGz, 2019; Haeyen, 2018; Haeyen, 2020). Due to their experiential and mentalizing-promoting nature, arts and body-based therapies are often boosters or perpetuators of psychotherapy in this interplay (Akwa GGz, 2017).
- It is important that arts and body-based therapies are carried out by a qualified arts and body-based therapist with certified training for this purpose (Akwa GGz, 2017, 2019).
- Arts and body-based therapists offer group therapy which they shape independently without the presence of a co-therapist, as is the case in many (psycho)therapies. This entails extra responsibility in handling the therapy situation. It also requires good team collaboration with attention to safety, regular consultation, and inter-/supervision (Akwa GGz, 2019).
- Ensuring optimal compliance can be facilitated by regularly evaluating the course of therapy with the patient(s) (Haeyen, 2018).

Resources

- Compared to the cost of specialty psychotherapies, arts and body-based therapies have a modest impact on the resource budget. Moreover, arts and body-based therapies are relatively often offered in group settings.

Organization of care

- Many effectively proven day treatment programs include forms of arts and body-based therapies, individually and/or in groups (Bateman & Fonagy, 1999; Karterud & Urnes, 2004; Wilberg et al., 1998). As a result, arts and body-based therapies are available in practice.
- Some psychotherapeutic treatment methods, such as schema therapy and emotion regulation training, also use experiential treatment techniques. This is closely aligned with arts and body-based therapies, and therefore psychotherapists often work directly with an arts and body-based therapist. Experts from different disciplines believe that arts and body-based therapies can be integrated into, and are a good complement to, for example, dialectical behavioral therapy, schema therapy, and mentalization based therapy. This view is expressed in several panels of experts (Kehr, 2020; Manders,

2020) and is also evident in descriptive literature (e.g., Haeyen, 2018, 2020; Thunnissen & Muste, 2002).

Social perspective

- The use of arts and body-based therapies early in treatment can contribute to treatment readiness and patient motivation, optimal patient rapport (personalized care), and efficient treatment progression.

7.5 Recommendations for practice

The combination of the conclusions based on the scientific evidence and all other considerations led to the formulation of the following recommendations:

- It is recommended that a treatment program for patients with personality disorder include arts and body-based therapies in its programme.
- As part of treatment, offering art therapy or another form of arts and psychomotor therapies should be considered, independent of age, sex, or specific diagnostic characteristics. It is recommended to educate patients about the various arts and psychomotor therapies and to include patient preferences in the process of together deciding on the indication for arts and psychomotor therapies. It is recommended to integrate psychotherapeutic verbal and arts and body-based therapies methods within an ambulant, part-time, day-clinical, or polyclinical treatment in order to best suit patients with different affinities, abilities, and learning styles.
- It is worth considering the use of arts and body-based therapies for the purpose of (emotionally) getting in touch with hard-to-reach aspects of patients' experiences.
- It is recommended to have arts and body-based therapies contribute to the diagnostic process, to problem analysis through observation, and to establishing treatment indication and treatment goals.

7.6 In conclusion

A guideline is never finished. The field evolves, new insights emerge, research data becomes available. At the same time, a guideline is an anchor point: here we are now, this we know, and from here we can proceed. Hopefully, the guideline will create room for designs other than RCTs that are better suited to practice or more feasible to conduct. Research on arts and body-based therapies is developing rapidly. From the overview provided here, follow-up steps can be taken, and new studies conducted.

References

AATA [American Art Therapy Association]. (2021). About art therapy? Accessed January 15, from https://arttherapy.org/about-art-therapy/

Akwa GGz. (2017). Persoonlijkheidsstoornissen: Zorgstandaard [Personality disorders: Care levelstandard]. GGz Standaarden. https://www.ggzstandaarden.nl/zorgstandaarden/persoonlijkheidsstoornissen/introductie

Akwa GGz. (2019). Vaktherapie: Generieke module [Arts therapies: Generic module]. GGz Standaarden. https://www.ggzstandaarden.nl/generieke-modules/vaktherapie/inleiding

Alphen, R. van, Stams, G.J.J.M., & Hakvoort, L. (2019). Musical attention control training for psychotic psychiatric patients: An experimental pilot study in a forensic psychiatric hospital. *Frontiers in Neuroscience, 13*. https://doi.org/doi.org/10.3389/fnins.2019.00570

American Psychiatric Association. (2013). *Diagnostic and statistical manual of mental health disorders* (5th ed[N1] .).

BAAT [British Association of Art Therapists]. (2024). *What is art therapy?* Accessed January 1815, from www.baat.org/About-Art-Therapy

Balshem, H., Helfand, M., Schunemann, H.J., Oxman, A.D., Kunz, R., & Brozek, J., et al. (2011). GRADE guidelines: 3. Rating the quality of evidence. *Journal of Clinical Epidemiology, 64*(4):401–406.

Bateman, A., & Fonagy, P. (1999). Effectiveness of partial hospitalization in the treatment of borderline personality disorder: A randomized controlled trial. *American Journal of Psychotherapy, 156*:1563–1569.

Bateman, A., & Fonagy, P. (2004). Mentalization-based treatment of BPD. *Journal of Personality Disorders, 18*:36–51. https://doi.org/10.1521/pedi.18.1.36.32772

Bateman, A., & Fonagy, P. (2009). Randomized controlled trial of outpatient mentalization-based treatment versus structured clinical management for borderline personality disorder. *American Journal of Psychiatry, 166*(12):1355–1364. https://doi.org/10.1176/appi.ajp.2009.09040539

Bernstein, D.A., & Borkovec, T.D. (1977). *Leren ontspannen: Handleiding voor de therapeutische beroepen [Learning to relax. Manual for the therapeutic professions]*. Dekker & Van der Vegt.

BMJ Best Practice. (2021). What is GRADE? Accessed from https://bestpractice.bmj.com/info/us/toolkit/learn-ebm/what-is-grade/

Bodde, R.E.A. (2020). The effect of the dramatherapy self-esteem module on well-being in people with personality disorders [Master thesis]. University of Twente. Accessed from https://essay.utwente.nl/81065/2/Bodde_MA_BMS.pdf

Boerhout, C., & Weele, K. van der (2007). Psychomotorische therapie en agressieregulatie: Een pilotonderzoek [Psychomotor therapy and aggression regulation: A pilot study]. *Tijdschrift Voor Vaktherapie, 2*:11–18.

Bolhuis, H., & Reynders, K. (1983). *Sensorelaxatie: Een methode tot ontspanning [Sensory relaxation: A method to relax]*. Self-Published Publication.

Bowden-Jones, O., Iqbal, M.Z., Tyrer, P., Seivewright, N., Cooper, S., Judd, A., et al. (2004). Prevalence of personality disorder in alcohol and drug services and associated comorbidity. *Addiction, 99*:1306–1314. https://doi.org/10.1111/j.1360-0443.2004.00813.x

Bräutigam, C. (2013). *Evaluatie van schemagerichte therapie: Een kwalitatief onderzoek van het patiëntenperspectief op de behandeling in een klinische setting* (Master's thesis, University of Twente).

Broek, E. van den, Keulen-de Vos, M., & Bernstein, D.P. (2011). Arts therapies and schema focused therapy: A pilot study. *The Arts in Psychotherapy, 38*(5):325–332. https://doi.org/10.1016/j.aip.2011.09.005

Brooks, C.W. (1974). *Sensory awareness*. Viking Press.

Claassen, A. M., & Pol, S. (Eds.). (2015). *Schematherapie en de Gezonde Volwassene: Positieve technieken uit de praktijk*. Springer.

Cohen, B.M., Hammer, J., & Singer, S. (1998). The diagnostic drawing series: A systematic approach to art therapy evaluation and research. *The Arts in Psychotherapy, 15*:11–21.

Coid, J., Yang, M., Tyrer, P., Roberts, A., & Ullrich, S. (2006). Prevalence and correlates of personality disorder in Great Britain. *British Journal of Psychiatry, 188*:423–431.

Dent-Brown, K. (1999). The six-part story method (6SPM) as an aid in the assessment of personality disorder. *Dramatherapy, 21*:10–14.

Dent-Brown, K., & Wang, M. (2004). Pessimism and failure in 6-part stories: Indicators of borderline personality disorder. *The Arts in Psychotherapy, 31*:321–333.

Dijk, S.D.M. van, Bouman, R., Lam, J.C.A.E., Den Held, R., Alphen, S.P.J. van, & Oude Voshaar, R.C. (2018). Outcome of day treatment for older adults with affective disorders: An observational pre-post design of two transdiagnostic approaches. *International Journal of Geriatric Psychiatry, 33*(3):510–516. https://doi.org/10.1002/gps.4791

Dijk, S.D.M. van, Veenstra, M., Bouman, R., Peekel, J., Veenstra, D., Dalen, P. van, … Old Voshaar, R. (2019). Group schema-focused therapy enriched with psychomotor therapy versus treatment as usual for older adults with cluster B and/or C personality disorders: A randomized trial. *BMC Psychiatry, 19*(1):26. https://doi.org/10.1186/s12888-018-2004-4

Dimaggio, G., Ottavi, P., Popolo, R., & Salvatore, G. (2020). *Metacognitive interpersonal therapy: Body, imagery and change*. Routledge.

DJI. (2012). *Forensic care in numbers 2007–2011*. DJI.

DJI. (2018). *DJI in numbers 2013–2017*. DJI.

Drewes, A., Nijkamp, M.N., & Roemen-van Haaren, M.W. (2019). Psychomotor interventions for personality disorders. In J. de Lange, O. Glas, J. van Busschbach, C. Emck, & T. Scheeuwe (Eds.), *Psychomotor interventions for mental health - Adults: A movement- and body-oriented approach* (pp. 221–242). Boom.

Evidence-Based Medicine Working Group. (1992). Evidence-based medicine. A new approach to teaching the practice of medicine. *JAMA, 68*:2420–2425.

Fonagy, P., Gergely, G., Jurist, E., & Target, M. (2002). *Affect regulation, mentalization, and the development of the self*. Other Press.

Fowler, J.P., & Ardon, A.M. (2002). Diagnostic drawing series and dissociative disorders: A Dutch study. *The Arts in Psychotherapy, 29*:221–230.

Franken, C.P.M., JAde, V., Westerhof, G.J., & Bohlmeijer, E. (2019). *De Mental Health Continuum Short Form (MHC-SF), een handleiding voor behandelaren in de geestelijke gezondheidszorg voor het interpreteren en bespreken van scores met patiënten*. Universiteit Twente.

Friborg, O., Martinussen, M., Kaiser, S., Overgård, K.T., & Rosenvinge, J.H. (2013). Comorbidity of personality disorders in anxiety disorders: A meta-analysis of 30 years of research. *Journal of Affective Disorders*, *145*(2):143–155. https://doi.org/10.1016/j.jad.2012.07.004

Friborg, O., Martinsen, E.W., Martinussen, M., Kaiser, S., Overgård, K.T., & Rosenvinge, J.H. (2014). Comorbidity of personality disorders in mood disorders: A meta-analytic review of 122 studies from 1988 to 2010. *Journal of Affective Disorders*, *152–154*:1–11. https://doi.org/10.1016/j.jad.2013.08.023

FVB (Federatie Vaktherapeutische Beroepen). (2017). *Strategische Onderzoeksagenda voor de Vaktherapeutische beroepen [Strategic Research Agenda for Arts Therapies Professions]*. Available online at: https://fvb.vaktherapie.nl/strategische-onderzoeksagenda (accessed January 18, 2024).

Gebhardt, S., Kunkel, M., & Georgi, R.V. (2014). Emotion modulation in psychiatric patients through music. *Music Perception: An Interdisciplinary Journal*, *31*(5):485–493.

Gold, C., Assmus, J., Hjørnevik, K., Qvale, L.G., Brown, F.K., Hansen, A.L., Waage, L., & Stige, B. (2014). Music therapy for prisoners: Pilot randomised controlled trial and implications for evaluating psychosocial interventions. *International Journal of Offender Therapy and Comparative Criminology*, *58*(12):1520–1539. https://doi.org/10.1177/0306624X13498693

Gold, C., Mössler, K., Grocke, D., Heldal, T., Tjemsland, L., Aarre, T., & Rolvsjord, R. (2013). Individual music therapy for mental health care clients with low therapy motivation: Multicentre randomised controlled trial. *Psychotherapy and Psychosomatics*, *82*(5):319–331.

Gold, C., Solli, H., Kruger, V., & Lie, S. (2009). Dose-response relationship in music therapy for people with serious mental disorders: Systematic review and meta-analysis. *Clinical Psychology Review*, *29*(3):193–207.

Green, B.L., Wehling, C., & Talsky, G.J. (1987). Group art therapy as an adjunct to treatment for chronic outpatients. *Hospital & Community Psychiatry*, *38*(9):988–991.

Guyatt, G.H., Oxman, A.D., Kunz, R., Vist, G.E., Falck-Ytter, Y., & Schunemann, H.J. (2008a). What is "quality of evidence" and why is it important to clinicians? *BMJ (clinical Research Ed)*, *336*(7651):995–998.

Guyatt, G.H., Oxman, A.D., Vist, G.E., Kunz, R., Falck-Ytter, Y., Alonso-Coello, P., et al. (2008b). GRADE: An emerging consensus on rating quality of evidence and strength of recommendations. *BMJ (Clinical Research Ed)*, *336*(7650):924–926.

Guyatt, G., Oxman, A.D., Akl, E.A., Kunz, R., Vist, G., Brozek, J., et al. (2011a). GRADE guidelines: 1. Introduction-GRADE evidence profiles and summary of findings tables. *Journal of Clinical Epidemiology*, *64*(4):383–394.

Guyatt, G.H., Oxman, A.D., Kunz, R., Atkins, D., Brozek, J., Vist, G., et al. (2011b). GRADE guidelines: 2. Framing the question and deciding on important outcomes. *Journal of Clinical Epidemiology*, *64*(4):395–400.

Guyatt, G.H., Oxman, A.D., Kunz, R., Brozek, J., Alonso-Coello, P., Rind, D., et al. (2011c). GRADE guidelines: 6. Rating the quality of evidence-imprecision. *Journal of Clinical Epidemiology*, *64*(12):1283–1293.

Guyatt, G., Oxman, A.D., Sultan, S., Brozek, J., Glasziou, P., Alonso-Coello, P., et al. (2013). GRADE guidelines: 11. Making an overall rating of confidence in effect estimates for a single outcome and for all outcomes. *Journal of Clinical Epidemiology*, *66*(2):151–157.

Gyllensten, A.L., Hansson, L., & Ekdahl, C. (2003). Outcome of basic body awareness therapy. A randomized controlled study of patients in psychiatric outpatient care. *Advances in Physiotherapy*, *5*(4):179–190.

Haeyen, S. (2018). *Effects of art therapy: The case of personality disorders cluster B/C* (Dissertation manuscript). Radboud University, March 14, 2018.

Haeyen, S. (2020). *De krachtige ervaring: Emotie- en zelfbeeldregulatie bij persoonlijkheidsstoornissen via vaktherapie* [*The powerful experience. Emotion and self-image regulation in personality disorders through arts and psychomotor therapies*]. Lectureship, Academy of Health and Vitality of the University of Arnhem and Nijmegen (HAN).

Haeyen, S., Chakhssi, F., & Hooren, S. van (2020). Benefits of art therapy in people diagnosed with personality disorders: A quantitative survey. *Frontiers in Psychology*, *11*:686.

Haeyen, S., Hooren, S. van, Veld, W.M. van der, & Hutschemaekers, G. (2018a). Efficacy of art therapy in individuals with personality disorders cluster B/C: A randomized controlled trial. *Journal of Personality Disorders*, *32*:527–542.

Haeyen, S., Hooren, S. van, Veld, W.M. van der, & Hutschemaekers, G. (2018b). Promoting mental health versus reducing mental illness in art therapy with patients with personality disorders: A quantitative study. *The Arts in Psychotherapy*, *58*:11–16. https://doi.org/10.1016/j.aip.2017.12.009

Hutchinson, D.S., Skrinar, G.S., & Cross, C. (1999). The role of improved physical fitness in rehabilitation and recovery. *Psychiatric Rehabilitation Journal*, *22*:355–359.

Hutsebaut, J., & Hessels, C.J. (2017). Clinical staging and early intervention for borderline personality disorder [Clinical staging and early intervention for borderline personality disorder]. *Journal of Psychiatry*, *59*(3):166–174.

Ingenhoven, T., Berghuis, H., Colijn, S., & Van, R. (2018). *Handboek persoonlijkheidsstoornissen* [*Handbook of personality disorders*]. De Tijdstroom.

Jacobson, E. (1929). *Progressive relaxation*. University of Chicago Press.

Karterud, S., & Pedersen, G. (2004). Short-term day hospital treatment for personality disorders: Benefits of the therapeutic components. *Therapeutic Communities*, *25*(1):43–54.

Karterud, S., & Urnes, O. (2004). Short-term day treatment programs for patients with personality disorders. What is the optimal composition? *Nordic Journal of Psychiatry*, *58*:243–249.

Kehr, T. (2020). *Report focus group 'Vaktherapie bij persoonlijkheidsstoornissen'*. HAN University of Applied Sciences. Internal document.

Keulen-de Vos, M., Broek, E.P.A. van den, Bernstein, D.P., Vallentin, R., & Arntz, A. (2017) Evoking emotional states in personality disordered offenders: An experimental pilot study of experiential drama therapy techniques. *The Arts in Psychotherapy*, *53*:80–88. https://doi.org/10.1016/j.aip.2017.01.003

Kipper, D.A., & Ritchie, T.D. (2003). The effectiveness of psychodramatic techniques: A meta-analysis. *Group Dynamics: Theory, Research, and Practice*, *7*(1):13.

Kleinlooh, S.T., Samaritter, R.A., Rijn, R.M. van, Kuipers, G., & Stubbe, J.H. (2021). Dance movement therapy for clients with a personality disorder: A systematic review and thematic synthesis. *Frontiers in Psychology, 12*:581578. https://doi.org/10.3389 /fpsyg.2021.581578

Knapen, J., Vliet, P. van de, Coppenolle, H. van, David, A., Peuskens, J., Knapen, K., & Pieters, G. (2003a). Improvements in physical fitness of nonpsychotic psychiatric patients following psychomotor therapy programs. *Journal of Sports Medicine and Physical Fitness, 43*:513–522.

Knapen, J., Vliet, P. van de, Coppenolle, H. van, David, A., Peuskens, J., Knapen, K., & Pieters, G. (2003b). The effectiveness of two psychomotor therapy programs on physical fitness and physical self-concept in nonpsychotic psychiatric patients: A randomized controlled trial. *Clinical Rehabilitation, 17*:637–647.

Koch, S., Kunz, T., Lykou, S., & Cruz, R. (2014). Effects of dance movement therapy and dance on health-related psychological outcomes: A meta-analysis. *The Arts in Psychotherapy, 41*(1):46–64.

Köck, P., & Walter, M. (2018). Personality disorder and substance use disorder—An update. *Mental Health and Prevention, 12*:82–89. https://doi.org/10.1016/j.mhp.2018 .10.003

Kuin, F.M. (2005). Op tijd stoppen: Behandeling van impulscontroleproblematiek bij cluster B-persoonlijkheidsstoornissen en dissociatieve stoornissen [Stopping in time: Treatment of impulse control problems in cluster B personality disorders and dissociative disorders]. In J. de Lange & R. Bosscher (Eds.), *Psychomotor therapy in practice* (pp. 43–63). Cure & Care Publishers.

Krietsch-Mederer, S. (1988). Die Funktionelle Entspannung - Eine Methode für die Einzeltherapie in psychiatrischer Praxis und Klinik. *Krankengymnastik, 40*:277–279.

Laurenssen, E.M.P., Luyten, P., Kikkert, M.J., Westra, D., Peen, J., Soons, M.B.J., ... Dekker, J.J.M. (2018). Day hospital mentalization-based treatment v specialist treatment as usual in patients with borderline personality disorder: Randomized controlled trial. *Psychological Medicine, 48*(15):2522–2529. https://doi.org/10.1017/ S0033291718000132

Lehembre, J. (2003). Autogene training in de praktijk [Autogenic training in practice]. *Psychopraxis, 1*:12–17.

Leirvåg, H., Pedersen, G., & Karterud, S. (2010). Long-term continuation treatment after short-term day treatment of female patients with severe personality disorders: Body awareness group therapy versus psychodynamic group therapy. *Nordic Journal of Psychiatry, 64*(2):115–122. https://doi.org/10.3109/08039480903487525

Malterud, K., Bjelland, A.K., & Elvbakken, K.T. (2016). Evidence-based medicine - An appropriate tool for evidence-based health policy? A case study from Norway. *Health Research Policy and Systems, 14*(1):15.

Manders, E. (2020). *Report focus group 'Vaktherapie bij persoonlijkheidsstoornissen'.* HAN University of Applied Sciences. Internal document.

Meekums, B. (1999). A creative model for recovery from child sexual abuse trauma. *The Arts in Psychotherapy, 26*(4):247–259. doi: 10.1016/S0197-4556(98)00076-8

Mills, A. (1989). *A statistical study of the formal aspects of the DDS of borderline personality disordered patients, and its context in contemporary art therapy.* Unpublished master's thesis. Concordia University.

Mills, A. (1994). *The DDS style guide.*

Mills, A., Cohen, B.M., & Meneses, J.Z. (1993). Reliability and validity tests of the diagnostic drawing series. *The Arts in Psychotherapy*, *20*:83–88.

Mustafa, R.A., Santesso, N., Brozek, J., Akl, E.A., Walter, S.D., Norman, G., et al. (2013). The GRADE approach is reproducible in assessing the quality of evidence of quantitative evidence syntheses. *Journal of Clinical Epidemiology*, *66*(7):736–42; quiz 42.e1–5.

Muste, E., Weertman, A., & Claassen, A.M. (2010). *Handboek klinische schematherapie*. Bohn Stafleu van Loghum.

National Steering Committee on Multidisciplinary Guideline Development in Mental Health Care. (2008). *Multidisciplinary guideline personality disorders: Guideline for the diagnosis and treatment of adult patients with a personality disorder*. Trimbos Institute.

NICE [National Institute for Health and Care Excellence]. (2021). *Personality disorders - Products*. Accessed from www.nice.org.uk/guidance/conditions-and-diseases/mental -health-and-behavioural-conditions/personality-disorders/products?Status=Published

NVVP [Dutch Association for Psychiatry]. (2021). *Personality disorders - General*. Accessed from www.nvvp.net/website/patinten-informatie/aandoeningen-/persoon lijkheidsstoornis

Parmar, A., & Kaloiya, G. (2018).Comorbidity of personality disorder among substance use disorder patients: a narrative review. *Indian Journal of Psychological Medicine*, *40*(6):517–527. https://doi.org/10.4103/IJPSYM.IJPSYM_164_18

Phagoe, S. (2018). Changes in schema modes and well-being after inpatient admission in clients with complex personality problems [Master thesis], University of Twente. Accessed from: https://essay.utwente.nl/75862/

Phagoe, S.A., Timmerman, K., Claassen, A.M., & Westerhof, G.J. (2022). Well-being and personality problems in clinical schema therapy. *Journal of Psychiatry*, *64*(2):73–79.

Popolo, R., MacBeth, A., Brunello, S., Canfora, F., Ozdemir, E., Rebecchi, D., Toselli, C., Venturelli, G., Salvatore, G., & Dimaggio, G. (2018). Metacognitive interpersonal therapy in group: A feasibility study. *Research in Psychotherapy (Milano)*, *21*(3), 338. https://doi.org/10.4081/ripppo.2018.338

Post, P. (2020). *Format richtlijntekst: Interne notitie 19 mei 2020 [Format guideline text. Internal note May 19, 2020]*. Trimbos Institute.

Punkanen, M., Saarikallio, S., & Geoff, L. (2014). Emotions in motion: Short-term group form Dance/Movement therapy in the treatment of depression: A pilot study. *Arts in Psychotherapy*, *41*:493–497. https://doi.org/10.1016/j.aip.2014.07.001

Roethof, G., & Meijden-van der Kolk, H. van der (2000). Psychomotorische therapie voor cliënten met een antisociale persoonlijkheidsstoornis, in de impulscontrole leidend tot delicten [Psychomotor therapy for clients with antisocial personality disorder, in impulse control leading to delinquency]. In M. van Hattum, & G. Hutschemaekers (Eds.), *In motion: The development of psychomotor therapy products* (pp. 151–156). Trimbos Institute.

Sanderlin, T.K. (2001). Anger management counseling with the antisocial personality. *Annals of the American Psychotherapy Association*, *4*(3):9–11.

Schaap, G.M., Chakhssi, F., & Westerhof,G.J. (2016). Inpatient schema therapy for nonresponsive patients with personality pathology: Changes in symptomatic distress, schemas, schema modes,coping styles, experienced parenting styles, and mental well-being. *Psychotherapy (Chicago, Ill.), 53*(4):402–412. https://doi.org/10.1037/pst0000056

Schmidt, H.U. (2002). Musiktherapie bei Patienten mit Borderline-Persönlichkeitsstörung. *PTT: Persönlichkeitsstörungen Theorie und Therapie, 6*:65–74.

Soler, J., Elices, M., Pascual, J.C., et al. (2016). Effects of mindfulness training on different components of impulsivity in borderline personality disorder: Results from a pilot randomized study. *Borderline Personality Disorder and Emotion Dysregulation, 3*(1):1–10.   https://bpded.biomedcentral.com/   https://doi.org/10.1186/s40479-015-0035-8

Solli, H.P., Rolvsjord, R., & Borg, M. (2013). Toward understanding music therapy as a recovery-oriented practice within mental health care: A meta-synthesis of service users' experiences. *Journal of Music Therapy, 50*(4):244–273. https://doi.org/10.1093/jmt/50.4.244

Straus, S.E., Glasziou, P., Richardson, W.S., & Haynes, R.B. (2011). *Evidence-based medicine: How to practice and teach it*, 4th ed. Churchill Livingstone, Elsevier.

Styla, R. (2014). Differences in effectiveness of intensive treatment programs for neurotic and personality disorders. Is it worth monitoring the effectiveness of a therapeutic team? *Psychiatria Polska, 48*(1):157–171.

Thunnissen, M.M., & Muste, E.H. (2002). Schematherapie in de klinisch-psychotherapeutische behandeling van persoonlijkheidsstoornissen [Schema therapy in the clinical-psychotherapeutic treatment of personality disorders]. *Tijdschrift voor Psychotherapie, 28*(5):385–401. https://doi.org/10.1007/BF03061969

Torgersen, S., Kringlen, E., & Cramer, V. (2001). The prevalence of personality disorders in a community sample. *Archives of General Psychiatry, 58*(6):590–596. https://doi.org/10.1001/archpsyc.58.6.590

Torgersen, S. (2014). Prevalence, sociodemographics and functional impairment. In J. Oldham, A. Skodol, & D. Bender (Eds.), *Textbook of personality disorders*, 2nd ed., pp. 109–129. American Psychiatric Publishing.

Trull, T.J., Jahng, S., Tomko, R.L., Wood, P.K., & Sher, K.J. (2010). Revised NESARC personality disorder diagnoses: Gender, prevalence, and comorbidity with substance dependence disorders. *Journal of Personality Disorders, 24*(4):412–426. https://doi.org/10.1521/pedi.2010.24.4.412

Wilberg, T., Katerud, S., Umer, O., Peterson, G., & Friis, P. (1998). Outcomes of poorly functioning patients with personality disorder in a day treatment program. *Psychiatric Services, 49*(11):1462–1467.

De Witte, M. (2014). Muziektherapie en emotieregulatie: Een pilotstudie bij forensische patiënten met een licht verstandelijke beperking [Music therapy and emotion regulation: A pilot study for forensic patients with mild intellectual disability]. *Tijdschrift voor Vaktherapie, 10*(3), 13–21.

Working Group on Revision of MDR Personality Disorders. (2022). *Revised Multidisciplinary Guideline Personality Disorders. Authorization version 2021.* Dutch Society for Psychiatry (NVvP).

Zimmerman, M., Chelminski, I., & Young, D. (2008). The frequency of personality disorders in psychiatric patients. *Psychiatric Clinics of North America, 31*(3):405–420, vi. https://doi.org/10.1016/j.psc.2008.03.015

Zwets, A., Hornsveld, R., Muris, P., Kanters, T., Langstraat, E., & Marle, H. (2016). Psychomotor therapy as an additive intervention for violent forensic psychiatric inpatients: A pilot study. *International Journal of Forensic Mental Health, 15*(3):222–234. https://doi.org/10.1080/14999013.2016.1152613

About the editor and authors

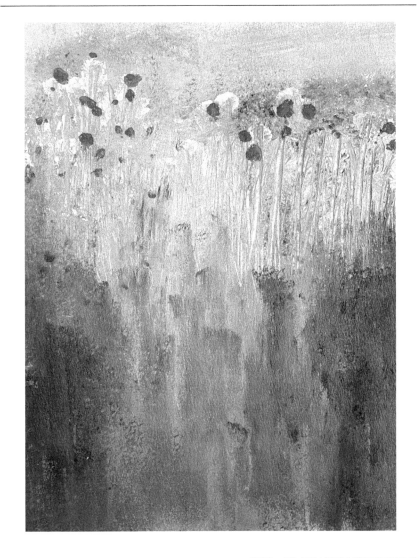

DOI: 10.4324/9781003456988-8

Editor

S.W. Suzanne Haeyen, Professor, Research Group Arts and Psychomotor Therapies in Health Care, Coordinator of Content Master Arts & Psychomotor Therapies, HAN University of Applied Sciences, Arnhem and Nijmegen (HAN), Academy Health & Vitality, Nijmegen.

Art Therapist, Senior researcher, and Chair of the Arts & Psychomotor Therapies Staff, GGNet, Center for Mental Health Care, Scelta Apeldoorn and Nijmegen, The Netherlands.

Authors

Italic text denotes each author's contribution to the chapters and sections listed.

K. Katrin Bange, Drama Therapist, Senior Schema Therapist, Private practice for Arts therapies and Coaching, Nijmegen.

- *Chapter 4: 4.17 Tableau Vivant—memory in pictures (also via Michiel de Gier); 4.31 Stand up! This is my chair; 4.32 I know a silly walk; 4.33 The Healthy Adult in Interaction; 4.34 Echo of the Happy Child.*

M.T. Thieme van Beek, Art Therapist, GGzIngeest, Poli Persoonlijkheidsstoornis & Trauma, Amstelveen/Amsterdam.

- *Chapter 2: 2.1 Modi setup in pictures; 2.32 Schema boat with crew.*

S.J.J. Stijn van Boven, Neurological Music Therapist, ZorgSpectrum, Department of Music therapy, Nieuwegein.

- *Chapter 5: 5.2 The energy of anger; 5.4 Recognize your schema; 5.11 Together alone; 5.12 Who's singing? 5.13 Self-care.*

P. Pauline Briguet, Dance Therapist MA, Fivoor Parnassia Group, Center Intensive Treatment (CIB)/Top Reference Trauma Center (TRTC), The Hague.

- *Chapter 3: 3.7 Inter-personal dialogue between Healthy Adult and Vulnerable Child; 3.8 Internal dialogue between Healthy Adult and Vulnerable Child; 3.14 Guessing game; 3.15 Being empathetic and moving along; 3.16 Warm-up embodying modes.*

E.P.A. Elsa van den Broek, Drama Therapist, lecturer Drama Therapy, Kairos Pompestichting, HAN University of Applied Sciences Arnhem and Nijmegen, Academy Health & Vitality, Nijmegen.

- *Chapter 4: 4.20 The magic shop (also via Ties Wesseling); 4.21 The 10 worst ways to ... 4.22 Angel Devil; 4.25 Late-night talk show; 4.26 Wimp.*

A.M.T.S. Anne-Marie Claassen, Psychotherapist/Program Manager, Mediant, De Boerhaven, Specialist Center for Personality Disorders, Hengelo.

- *Prologue and Introduction: co-authored (with Greta Günther and Suzanne Haeyen).*

J.I.H. Jeanne Cousijn, Art Therapist, Forensic Psychiatric Center De Rooyse Wissel, Therapeutic Service/FPC, Oostrum.
- *Chapter 2: 2.12 Edward Hopper; 2.25 Land grabbing; 2.41 Fulfilling missed basic needs; 2.44 Clay throwing contest.*

I.R. Rianne van Dalen, Psychomotor therapist/ Health psychologist, pmtActief, Deventer.
- *Chapter 6: 6.2 Ball Shower; 6.4 Creator; 6.17 Fussbudget; 6.18 Sparring Together; 6.19 Tower of Hanoi.*

J. Janneke Dogger, Art Therapist, Mediant GGZ, CoNNectum department, Center for social and neuropsychiatry adults and 60-plus, Enschede.
- *Chapter 2: 2.23 Exploration in Clay; 2.30 Window work; 2.33 Expressive glossy paper; 2.36 Drawing threads.*

I. Imelle Dohle, Music Therapist, GGz Praktijk, Arnhem.
- *Chapter 5: 5.14 Happy Child music; 5.15 Passing the beat; 5.16 Musical modes dialogue; 5.17 Drum-battle; 5.18 From blues to swing.*

E.J.C. Liesbeth Doomen, Lecturer Drama Therapy and (Psycho)Drama Therapist, HAN and Stichting 1inP, HAN University of Applied Sciences Arnhem and Nijmegen, Academy Health & Vitality, Nijmegen.
- *Chapter 4: 4.23 Visualizing internal atoms in modes; 4.24 yes-no strength exercise; 4.27 Rescripting in psychodrama; 4.28 Role-playing with modes; 4.29 Theater characters as subpersonalities.*

L.E.M. Loes van Ekeren, Music Therapist, GGNet, Center for Mental Health Care, Apeldoorn Ambulant Adults, Apeldoorn Ambulant Elderly, Apeldoorn.
- *Chapter 5: 5.8 The playlist; 5.22 The sound portrait; 5.29 Voice it!; 5.30 Djembé; 5.31 Feeling nothing (all work forms together with Irene van Sprang).*

J. Julia Engelbrecht, Music Therapist, Psychodrama Therapist, Private Practice for Arts Therapies Breda, Breda.
- *Chapter 5: 5.1 Base and release—connection and autonomy; 5.3 A song of my mode; 5.5 Body-based improvisation from basic needs; 5.6 Nurture song; 5.10 Turn up the volume; 5.23 Listen with your body (all work forms together with Greta Günther).*

M. Michiel de Gier, Drama and System Therapist, Reinier van Arkel, CAP department, Den Bosch.
- *Chapter 4: 4.17 Tableau Vivant—memory in pictures (also via Katrin Bange); 4.18 Market merchant; 4.19 Portray your coping modes.*

E.J.G.M. Emilia de Gruijter, Drama Therapist, (learning) supervisor, lecturer, University of Applied Sciences Arnhem and Nijmegen (HAN), Academy Health & Vitality, Nijmegen.

- *Chapter 4: 4.1 Somebody at the Door; 4.2 Doing What Mother Does; 4.3 Cluedo; 4.5 The Invisible Leader; 4.9 Starring Role; 4.11 Killer (also via Jack Verburgt); 4.12 Red-Green Game; 4.14 Comfort Chair; 4.30 Hints.*

G. Greta Günther, Art Therapist, Body-oriented therapist (Pesso), Schema Therapist, De Viersprong, Department KST-V, Halsteren.

- *Prologue and Introduction: co-authored (with Annemarie Claassen and Suzanne Haeyen). Chapter 2: 2.7 Circles of power (with Fransje Nolet); 2.18 The same piece of work; 2.20 Ideal parent; 2.22 Children's photographs; 2.26 Examining Materials; 2.27 My Healthy Self-Soother; 2.28 Body-oriented name drawing; 2.29 Parental home; 2.43 Walk through modes. Chapter 5: 5.1 Base and release - connection and autonomy; 5.3 A song of my mode; 5.5 Body-Based Improvisation from basic needs; 5.6 Nurture song; 5.10 Turn up the volume; 5.23 Listen with your body (from 5.1 together with Julia Engelbrecht). Chapter 6: 6.1 Letting an elastic band be shot (with Jaap Verreijen).*

M.W. Minne (Roemen-) van Haaren, Psychomotor Therapist and Drama Therapist, lecturer Therapeutic Skills, GGNet, Center for Mental Health Care, Scelta Nijmegen, Windesheim, Scelta, Master Psychomotor Therapy, Nijmegen/ Zwolle.

- *Chapter 4: 4.4 The Basic Needs Store. Chapter 6: 6.6 The Lighthouse; 6.9 Obliging people can bear much; 6.14 My Healthy Adult Attitude.*

S.W. Suzanne Haeyen, Professor, Research Group Arts and Psychomotor Therapies in Health Care, Coordinator of Content Master Arts & Psychomotor Therapies, HAN University of Applied Sciences Arnhem and Nijmegen, Academy Health & Vitality, Nijmegen. Art Therapist, Senior researcher, and Chair of the Arts & Psychomotor Therapies Staff, GGNet, Center for Mental Health Care, Scelta Apeldoorn and Nijmegen.

- *Prologue and Introduction: co-author (together with Annemarie Claassen and Greta Günther); Chapter 2: 2.2 Future view Healthy Adult; 2.5 Inside & outside; 2.6 Happy Child assignment for someone else; 2.8 Control versus letting go; 2.16 No rules; 2.35 Objections to Critical Parent; 2.38 Safety for Vulnerable Child; 2.39 Who is your Healthy Adult? (also via Joyce van Wijk); 2.40 Exploring the Happy Child; 2.42 Taking care of the basic needs of the other person's Vulnerable Child (also via Joyce van Wijk). Chapter 7: Author.*

M.C. Michiel Koenen, Psychomotor Therapist, GGNet, Scelta, Apeldoorn.

- *Chapter 6: 6.22 Changing trees; 6.23 Live bowling; 6.24 Ping pong plop; 6.25 Rolling is also fooling; 6.26 Counting ten in the jungle.*

K.J.M. Kattelijne Kraak, Psychomotor Therapist, GGNet, Center for Mental Health Care, Scelta Apeldoorn.

- *Chapter 6: 6.3 Body chart with modes; 6.5 The Healthy Adult anchored; 6.7 This makes me happy; 6.11 Children's party; 6.16 Modes with material.*

E.O. Eric van der Meijden, Psychomotor Therapist, Private Practice Belloods, Epe.
- *Chapter 6: 6.10 Yes and no; 6.12 Hitting bat with restriction; 6.13 Walking across inverted bench; 6.15 Exploring my space; 6.20 Varying circle size.*

A. Anke Michiels, Dance Movement Therapist, ETZ Department of Psychiatry, Tilburg Dance Teacher, Nieuwe Veste, Breda.
- *Chapter 3: 3.1 Blind Free Child dance; 3.2 Healthy Self-soother in dance; 3.3 Part of the whole; 3.4 Setting the pace together; 3.5 Mirroring; 3.6 Dance improvisation with materials.*

M. Maria Munain Moral, Body Oriented and Movement Therapist, Senior Schema Therapist, Ipsy-PsyQ (Parnassia Group), Amsterdam.
- *Chapter 3: 3.9 Battle of Protectors; 3.10 Happy Child plays freely; 3.11 Anger is allowed; 3.12 Emotion circles; 3.13 Discard critical pebbles.*

F. Fransje Nolet, Art Therapist GGzBreburg, Private Practice Beeld-lokaal, Tilburg.
- *Chapter 2: 2.7 Circles of Power (with Greta Günther).*

L. Linda Winters-van Oosterom, Psychomotor Therapist, De Viersprong, Department of Schema Therapy, Halsteren.
- *Chapter 6: 6.21 Wobble course.*

I. Inerajka van Renesse, Music Therapist, GGNet, Center for Mental Health Care, Scelta Apeldoorn.
- *Chapter 5: 5.24 Each to their own experience; 5.25 Explore boundaries with djembés and eggs; 5.26 Invitation to spontaneity and playfulness; 5.27 Sound of connection; 5.28 Let us hear what you feel!*

I. Irene van Sprang, Music therapist, experience expert, GGNet, Center for Mental Health Care, Scelta Apeldoorn and Apeldoorn Ambulant.
- *Chapter 5: 5.8 The playlist; 5.22 The sound portrait; 5.29 Voice it!; 5.30 Djembé; 5.31 Feeling nothing (all work forms together with Loes van Ekeren).*

N. Nicole Strijbos, Internal staff supervisor (until March 2021 Art Therapist), FPC de Rooyse Wissel, HRM department, Oostrum.
- *Chapter 2: 2.9 Crisis drawing; 2.15 Error fun; 2.19 Homage to yourself; 2.21 You and the causer of your schema; 2.37 Resilience assignment.*

K. Karin Timmerman, Art Therapist and Scientific Researcher, Mediant, De Boerhaven, Expertise Center for Personality Disorders, Hengelo.
- *Chapter 2: 2.3 Two colors: positive and negative; 2.10 Schema triptych past-present-future; 2.11 Ecoline wet and dry; 2.17 Group disruption assignment; 2.24 Scratch exercise; 2.34 Mirror assignment.*

G.D. Gerdi Tuender, Lecturer Drama Therapy and Psychodrama Therapist, HAN University of Applied Sciences Arnhem and Nijmegen, Academy Health & Vitality, Nijmegen, Private Practice, Nijmegen.

- *Chapter 4: 4.6 A place of one's own; 4.10 Favorite role; 4.13 Fairy tales; 4.15 Writing stories; 4.16 Wishful thinking.*

J.D.J.M. Jack Verburgt, Music Therapist, Private Practice.

- *Chapter 4: 4.11 Killer (also via Emilia de Gruijter). H5: 5.19 The musical family sculpture; 5.20 Musical Modes sculpture; 5.21 Beautiful and ugly.*

J. Jaap Verreijen, Psychomotor therapist, De Viersprong, clinical schema therapy department, Halsteren.

- *Chapter 6: 6.1 Letting an elastic band be shot (with Greta Günther); 6.21 Wobble course (with Linda van Oosterom).*

M. Marjon Voskamp, Psychomotor Therapist, GGNet, Center for Mental Health Care, Department Amarum, Zutphen.

- *Chapter 6: 6.27 Seeing the Healthy Adult; 6.28 The floor is lava; 6.29 Overcoming Parenting Mode with the Healthy Adult; 6.30 Parenting Modes pilloried.*

T. Ties Wesseling, Music Therapy lecturer, HAN University of Applied Sciences Arnhem and Nijmegen, Academy Health & Vitality, Nijmegen.

- *Chapter 4: 4.20 The magic shop (also via Elsa van den Broek). Chapter 5: 5.7 Multiple-chair music; 5.9 Rescripting.*

J.F. Joyce van Wijk, Art Therapist, Antes, Expertise Team Personality Disorders, Department of Schema Therapy, Spijkenisse.

- *Chapter 2: 2.4 Acrylic pouring; 2.13 Island assignment; 2.14 Nice place for the Vulnerable Child; 2.31 Life-size self-portrait; 2.39 Who is your Healthy Adult? (also via Suzanne Haeyen); 2.42 Taking care of the basic needs of the other person's vulnerable child (also via Suzanne Haeyen); 2.46 Circle exercise.*

English translation

- Alison Edwards
- Elske Klijnsma

Photo credits

Several photos in this book were taken by Eva Broekema. Other photos were provided by the different authors of the relevant chapters.

The illustrations on the cover and at the start of each chapter were taken by Eugene Arts.

Index

Milton Keynes UK
Ingram Content Group UK Ltd.
UKHW022048141024
449569UK00023B/845

9 781032 599571